THE
CONSUMER'S
LEGAL GUIDE
TO TODAY'S
HEALTH CARE

THE
CONSUMER'S
LEGAL GUIDE
TO TODAY'S
HEALTH CARE

Your Medical Rights
And How to Assert Them

Stephen L. Isaacs, J.D.
Ava C. Swartz, M.P.H.

HOUGHTON MIFFLIN COMPANY
Boston • New York • London
1992

To Ariel and Ilan

For information about permission to reproduce
selections from this book, write to
Permissions, Houghton Mifflin Company,
215 Park Avenue South, New York, New York 10003

Library of Congress Cataloging-in-Publication Data
Isaacs, Stephen L.
The consumer's legal guide to today's health care : your medical
rights and how to assert them / Stephen L. Isaacs and Ava C. Swartz.
p.   cm.
Includes index.
ISBN 0-395-57438-2. — ISBN 0-395-63277-3 (pbk.)
1. Medical laws and legislation — United States — Popular works.
2. Medical care — Law and legislation — United States — Popular works.
I. Swartz, Ava C.   II. Title.
KF3821.Z9I83   1992
344.73'041 — dc20   92-4208
[347.30441]   CIP

Printed in the United States of America

MP 10 9 8 7 6 5 4 3 2 1

ACKNOWLEDGMENTS

Many legal and health professionals gave generously of their time in reviewing the manuscript and offering suggestions for its improvement. We wish to thank Lori Andrews, J.D., research associate, American Bar Association; Diane Archer, J.D., executive director, Medicare Beneficiaries Defense Fund; Mark Barnes, J.D., former director of policy, AIDS Institute of New York State; Ronald Bayer, Ph.D., professor of public health, Columbia University; Ruth Bennett, Ph.D., professor of public health, Columbia University; Joan Bertin, J.D., associate director, Women's Rights project, American Civil Liberties Union; Margaret Brooks, J.D., director, Legal Action Center; Rebecca Cook, J.D., M.P.A., professor of law and medicine, University of Toronto; Bernard Dickens, Ph.D., LL.D., professor of law and medicine, University of Toronto; Harold Edgar, J.D., professor of law, Columbia University; Ilise Feitshans, J.D., M.P.H., research associate in the legislative drafting program, Columbia University; Harold E. Fox, M.D., vice-chairman, Obstetrics and Gynecology Department, Columbia-Presbyterian Medical Center; Lynn Freedman, J.D., M.P.H., professor of public health, Columbia University; M. Rose Gasner, J.D., former general counsel, Choice in Dying; Eric Gertner, M.S, WSO, professor of industrial engineering, Empire State College; Frank Grad, J.D., professor of law, Columbia University; Robert L. Herbst, J.D., attorney-at-law; Lynne S. Katzmann, J.D., president, Juniper Associates; David Levidow, J.D., attorney-at-law; Abraham Monk, Ph.D., professor of social work, Columbia University; David M. Namerow, M.D., pediatrician; Stephen Nassau, J.D., attorney-at-law; Sharon Rennert, J.D., associate director, American Bar Association Commission on Mental and Physical Disability Law; Stephen N. Rosenberg, M.D., professor of public health, Columbia University; Allan Rosenfield, M.D., dean, Columbia University School of Public Health; Bradford H. Sewell, J.D., M.P.H.; Granville H. Sewell, Ph.D., professor of public health, Columbia University; and Gail Shearer, director of policy analysis, Consumers Union.

The staff of the Columbia Law School library, headed by James Hoover, was an invaluable resource. Reference librarian Philip Oxley guided us to the appropriate materials and greatly eased the task of gathering information.

In writing this book, we interviewed many people who opened their hearts to us. While we have protected their wish for anonymity, we deeply appreciate their candor in sharing sometimes painful stories with us. Others whom we interviewed helped us clarify points of law or medical practice. We are grateful for their time and professional expertise.

Our literary agent, Mitchell Rose, worked closely with us in developing the idea for this book. He is a person of uncommon foresight and skill.

Our editor at Houghton Mifflin, Ruth Hapgood, deserves special thanks for her guidance, gentle prodding, and belief in the book. Her assistant, Susanna Tecce, was always enthusiastic and efficient. Our manuscript editor, Gerry Morse, accomplished her assignment with care and thoroughness.

Aundres Brenyah worked tirelessly typing the manuscript. She spent long hours at the computer and was always cheerful and supportive. We also appreciate the time she and Fernanda Berman spent fact checking.

We extend special thanks to Olivia Ward of the *Toronto Star* for her wit, perception, and advice; Victoria and Sheldon Secunda for their knowledge and wisdom; Bill Mindlin, publisher of *Photography in New York,* for always being there; Dick Stolley for his support and interest; Romana Kryzanowska for teaching the value of a strong mind and body; and David Isaacs for his keen interest and insights.

CONTENTS

1

FINDING YOUR WAY
THROUGH THE MEDICAL MAZE

IF YOU ARE like most people, you find the health care system confusing and intimidating. Doctors in crisp white coats, officious administrators, insurance companies with forms written in what appears to be a foreign language, all seem designed to reduce you to a helpless child. To deal successfully with today's complex health system, you must learn how it works and make it work for you. This means knowing your rights.

Until something goes wrong, most of us don't think about our rights; fewer still think about how our health and the law intertwine every day. Consider the following:

- Your employer asks you to choose between an HMO, a PPO, and an indemnity health insurance plan. You have no idea what these are or where you can get a clear explanation.
- You were hospitalized and sent home before you felt well. How can you prevent this from happening in the future?
- Your elderly mother has early signs of Alzheimer's disease. How can you find out what the government covers?
- You are horrified every time you read about comatose patients in a vegetative state being kept alive by machines. How can you prevent this from happening to you?
- You are planning to move out of state. Your doctor refuses to give you a copy of your medical records. Are you legally entitled to them?
- You had cosmetic surgery to get your nose fixed. The result is grotesque. The plastic surgeon says it's not his fault and, be-

sides, nobody's perfect. Do you have a case? How do you find a good malpractice lawyer?

Without resorting to complicated Latin phrases or legalese, *The Consumer's Legal Guide to Today's Health Care* answers these and hundreds of similar questions. We tell you what your rights are, how to assert them, and what to do if you need help. Knowing your rights and standing up for yourself will enable you to protect your health and, in the bargain, get the best care for your dollar. Whether you are frustrated by the medical system, have been injured and don't know whether to sue, or simply want to be aware of your rights, *The Consumer's Legal Guide to Today's Health Care* can put *you* in control.

The book grew out of our personal experience and professional expertise. Here are our stories.

Ava Swartz

I was thirtysomething, in optimum health and pregnant. With an obstetrician I'd known for years, one who had a voice like Valium and manner like Dr. Welby, I planned on Lamaze classes, birthing rooms, and breast-feeding. But eight months later, I lay in a hospital bed, IVs in both arms, listening to the Dr. Welby look-alike tell me that my condition was "catastrophic."

It began somewhere in my sixth month. Without warning, a steak dinner sent me straight to bed with sharp, shooting abdominal pain. Indigestion, I thought, not bothering to call the doctor. But after several more days and sleepless nights of the worst pain I have ever known, I called. "Braxton Hicks contractions, perfectly normal," he replied in his most soothing voice. The pain got worse. By day it made routine tasks almost impossible. At night I lay in bed gasping for relief, afraid to take an aspirin for fear of harming the baby. I went back to the doctor. In honeyed tones he gently talked to me about the fears of first-time, older mothers. Was it all in my head? Willing to try anything, I dragged myself to a psychologist, a lovely lady who lived in a loft on a small, crooked street in Greenwich Village. Once a week I talked through the pain. I talked about my mother, my sister, my family, and my fear of having a baby. Still the pain continued. I tried yoga, practiced Lamaze.

After the psychologist diagnosed "psychic pain," I marched over to my obstetrician and demanded a blood test. When it showed low platelets and elevated liver enzymes, he sent me to an internist, who suggested mononucleosis or pneumonia and insisted on taking an X ray. I wasn't crazy after all. After my platelets dropped to an alarming level, my doctor insisted I go straight to the hospital, where he called another internist — this one hypothesized lupus. A hematologist took a painful bone marrow biopsy from my hip and grinned. "Well, you don't have leukemia." An ear, nose, and throat specialist left his tennis game to treat me for an infected salivary gland. The one person the good Dr. Welby look-alike should have called but didn't was the most obvious choice: a high-risk-pregnancy specialist.

After becoming progressively weaker, unable to eat, and barely able to stand, I delivered my daughter by emergency Caesarean section under general anesthesia in the middle of the night. My doctor deferred to his partner to perform the surgery. She botched the job, severing muscles and leaving my stomach deformed and with an infected scar.

So much for birthing rooms and breast-feeding. Rushed to the intensive care unit as soon as my daughter was born, I first saw her days later through a haze of drugs. The miracle of this story is that she was born healthy, albeit underweight, and continues to be a delightful little person filled with joy.

As for my condition, it turned out I had HELLP (for hemolysis elevated low platelets) syndrome, an unusual, but not uncommon, pregnancy-related syndrome that has been recognized for about thirty years.

This did not happen at a backwater clinic, but at the renowned Mount Sinai Hospital in New York City. When I got out of the hospital, I spent hours in a medical library poring over journals that described my condition. I consulted with obstetric specialists in high-risk pregnancy. When I described my symptoms, the majority of them said, without missing a beat, "Oh yes, you had the HELLP syndrome." But when I challenged my obstetrician's partner with this and with the botched surgery, she said, "How dare you! I saved your life."

To add insult to injury, when I asked Mount Sinai Hospital for a copy of my medical records, I was told that the cost was $1 per *page*, plus a $15 "administrative fee." When you've been in the hospital for weeks, this can add up to hundreds of pages — and dollars. Under New York law, a hospital has to provide a patient's medical records on receipt of a written request, but photocopying charges are not supposed to be exorbitant. Rather than pay, I asked a doctor friend to request the records for me; the hospital sent them as a courtesy.

Even though this experience took place more than five years ago, it still haunts me. Why didn't I insist that my doctors call in a high-risk-pregnancy specialist? What more could I have done? Could I have been more assertive? Should I have asked more questions? Should I have sued the doctors? (Ultimately I decided not to and tried to put the entire episode behind me.) If this could happen to me, a relatively knowledgeable patient with a master of public health degree, what is it like for those who have even less experience with the health system?

That's why I wanted to write this book.

Stephen Isaacs

When Ava and I talked with our friends and acquaintances, we discovered that just about everybody has a story to tell about run-ins with the health care system. They range from the hair-raising — a woman who broke her hip and damaged her kidney in an on-the-job accident had to fight for five years to receive workers' compensation — to the merely difficult — a health club refused to refund money to an unhappy customer. Almost all involved the law in one way or another.

As a lawyer and a professor at Columbia University, I have seen how the law affects health care in countless cases. In my law practice, I advise clients on a wide variety of such health-related problems as denial of insurance benefits, protecting health and assets in old age, and drafting documents for people who do not want to be "kept alive" in a vegetative state by machines.

In my classes at Columbia, I teach my students how the law will affect them as doctors, nurses, and hospital administrators. They learn what the law is, what the trends are, and what can and cannot be done under the law.

Yet until now, nothing — no book, no class — gave *you* this same "insider" information. Without it, you are at the mercy of the health system. With it, you can make the system work to your advantage. *The Consumer's Legal Guide to Today's Health Care* leads you through the health system, giving you the power to take charge and avoid being victimized by a system you don't understand.

The information we present is based on the latest laws, court decisions, and administrative regulations. Throughout the book, we use actual case histories to illustrate key points. When a person's identity is a matter of public record, as in law cases and congressional testimony, or the subject is willing to be identified, we use full names. In other cases, we protect the person's identity by using only a pseudonymous first name and last initial. We include checklists of questions that you can photocopy and use in times of need — for example, when selecting a health plan and before surgery. We also give the name, address, and telephone number of many organizations that offer further help.

Laws differ from state to state. On subjects as diverse as malpractice, drug testing in the workplace, and the right-to-die, there are fifty different sets of laws. For matters governed by state law, we discuss the common issues and principles, majority and minority rules, and trends in the law.

Many important medical-legal issues are controlled by federal law — legislation passed by the Congress, decisions handed down by the Supreme Court, and regulations issued by a federal agency such as the Food and Drug Administration. Federal law is applicable in every state in the nation. In matters of federal law, we explain your rights under the national standard.

The Consumer's Legal Guide to Today's Health Care is designed to make you aware of your rights as a health consumer and advise you how to protect them. It will not make you a lawyer. We advise you to seek the counsel of an attorney when appropriate. With that note of caution, we invite you to learn more about how to take command of your health care.

2

YOUR RIGHTS AS A PATIENT: SEVEN PATHS TO PATIENT POWER

CONTENTS

Not long ago, a doctor's word was law. Patients were taught to follow orders, not to ask questions. If something went wrong, a patient would no more sue a physician than take a beloved relative to court. Today, high-tech specialists have replaced the fabled family doctor who did everything from delivering babies to setting broken legs.

Superficially, the health care system appears to be tilting away from physician omnipotence and toward patient power. Notices of patients' rights hang on hospital walls. Women demand a greater role in gynecological and obstetrical care. Medical textbooks laud the health benefits of active rather than passive patients. Leaders in the health field publicly extol the importance of serving patients. "I would like to see hospitals become true advocates for the interests of hospital patients," said Dick Davidson, president of the American Hospital Association, in *Hospital* magazine.

Still, most people are intimidated by the health care system. Scared and often in pain, patients enter the land of the sick. Stripped of their clothing and identities, they are pricked, prodded, and told what to do. Even the definition of patient as "bearing pain without complaint" reinforces an image of passivity.

But it is when you are sick and vulnerable that you need to be most aware of your rights. In this chapter, we give you seven paths to patient power to put you on a more equal footing with the medical profession. They are:

- Informed consent
- Your right to medical treatment
- Refusal of medical treatment
- Keeping your records confidential and conversations with your doctor private
- Your right to see your own medical records
- Selecting a health professional
- How to complain

Informed Consent

Knowledge Is Power

Before undergoing any surgical or medical procedure, you are legally entitled to an explanation in plain language you understand of what is going to happen to you so that you can give what is called informed consent. Informed consent is such a fundamental principle in American law that a doctor who does not obtain your permission prior to operating or performing other medical procedures could be found guilty either of battery (unauthorized touching) or negligence. Almost seventy-five years ago, Benjamin Cardozo, one of America's most respected judges, wrote, "Every human being of adult years and sound mind has a right to determine what shall be done with his own body." (Obviously you can't give your consent when you are unconscious or bleeding profusely. In these and similar types of emergencies, such consent is implied.)

Crucial Elements of Informed Consent

Before you can give informed consent, your physician must tell you the nature of the treatment, its benefits and risks, alternatives to the treatment, and the probability of success.

The Diagnosis

The physician must tell you what's wrong with you. If you do not understand, ask for a further explanation. It's your body and your right.

The Nature of the Treatment

You have a right to a detailed explanation of the procedure or treatment. Surgery raises particular concerns. Remember that you are authorizing an operation to correct a specific problem, not a general search-and-destroy mission. In one venerable case, Belinda Chambers went to her doctor suffering from abdominal cramps. He said the cause was a cyst on her left ovary. The young Maryland woman authorized an operation to remove her left ovary and left fallopian tube. But while she was under anesthesia, the doctor also removed her right ovary, right tube, and uterus. As she told the jury during her 1979 lawsuit, "He woke me up, asked how I felt, and then told me he had given me a complete hysterectomy. I thought I was having a nightmare." The jury awarded her $1.2 million.

If the surgeon discovers an unanticipated problem during the course of an operation, it can be corrected, although there must be reasonable limits.

The Benefits and Risks

Most people are nervous before an operation or medical treatment. Knowing the potential risks and anticipated benefits can help calm your fears — or give you reason to walk away.

Learning about the benefits is rarely a problem. Doctors gladly tell you why the treatment is good for you. But risks and side effects are another story. No area of informed consent arouses such passion or incites more lawsuits. There is no simple mathematical formula to govern how much you should know about the risks of an operation or treatment. A lot depends on the seriousness of the risk and the likelihood of its occurring. A 1 percent chance of death or paralysis is serious. A 3 percent chance of a mild stomachache isn't.

Courts have ruled that physicians don't have to tell you about remote risks, although what this means in practical terms varies from state to state. In one influential case, decided in 1972, nineteen-year-old Jerry Canterbury, a clerk-typist for the FBI in Washington, D.C., saw Dr. William Spence, a neurosurgeon, about his agonizing back pain. After performing a series of tests, Dr. Spence recommended surgery for a probable slipped disc. Not wanting to alarm his patient, Dr. Spence failed to warn Canterbury about the 1 percent chance of paralysis and told Canterbury's mother that the risk was no more serious "than with any operation." Then the worst happened: Canterbury became paralyzed. In the resulting lawsuit, the court said that a doctor must tell his patient about all serious side effects — even those with a minimal risk.

As this example tragically illustrates, doctors are not omnipotent fortunetellers. No matter how well you think you know and trust your physician, the rule is to *ask* about any procedure. If your doctor brushes you off or doesn't have time for your questions, go elsewhere. Even if there is only a 1 percent risk of serious damage, you don't want to be that statistic.

On the other hand, many physicians argue that telling patients about risks that rarely occur might alarm them and scare them away. "Trust me, don't ask me," they say. The decision not to disclose certain risks is known as therapeutic privilege. This use of medical discretion — or medical paternalism — was the norm and still is in some states. Current legal thinking limits its use. A doctor is neither legally nor ethically justified in withholding information because he feels the patient might refuse treatment. Remember: knowledge is power.

Treatment Alternatives

Since one condition can be treated several ways, doctors may disagree about which is best. Cancers can be treated by chemotherapy, radiation, or surgery. Anesthesia can be local, spinal, or general. More than a dozen methods of birth control are available. Every option has advantages and disadvantages, and it is your right to be informed about each of them, including their risks and benefits. Ask about alternatives to recommended treatment, including the alternative of doing nothing.

Eleven-year-old Maria Marino and her parents learned this the hard way. While on vacation in 1980, Maria fell off a snowmobile and broke her arm. As the court records attest, her parents took her to a nearby hospital, where Roberto Ballestas, an orthopedic surgeon, told them he had to operate immediately. When Maria's parents said they wanted to go home to see their family doctor, Dr. Ballestas told them that any delay might cause permanent nerve damage. At no time did he tell them of a medically accepted alternative to surgery — putting the child's arm in a splint and letting time heal the break. Maria was left with a metal plate and two screws in her arm (later removed by her family surgeon), ugly scars, and the trauma of an unnecessary operation. Her parents sued, and the court ruled that the surgeon had failed in his duty to tell them about the alternative treatment.

The Probability of Success

This can be tricky. You should know about your doctor's success rates as well as your overall chances for a successful result. Although it takes some nerve, ask your surgeon how many times he or she has performed an operation and with what success. If the doctor tells you that an operation is "100 percent effective," beware. It ain't so. Even male sterilization (vasectomy), which is almost foolproof, runs a small risk of failure. In one old case, a cosmetic surgeon who promised to make his female patient a "model of harmonious perfection" was held liable for breach of contract when his reconstructive surgery resulted in a repellent mess.

What to Do with What You've Got
Say you know the surgeon's success rate, the risks, benefits, and alternatives. You're not a doctor. How do you evaluate the information or know what is the best choice for you? One way is to get a second medical opinion. Many insurance companies now demand — and pay for — a second opinion before surgery and may help you locate a doctor who can give it. The Department of Health and Human Services runs a toll-free second surgical opinion hotline: (800) 638-6833.

When Informed Consent Is Not Valid
Informed consent is null if it is given under pressure or if the patient is hysterical, drunk, or on drugs. In an emergency, consent is assumed. In most nonemergency situations, there is time to think about the options, to consult family and friends, and to seek a second opinion. Take advantage of it.

Informed consent is void if the patient is not legally capable of understanding the nature of the procedure and its risks and consequences. Adults are presumed to have this capacity. (The unique problems of informed consent for children are discussed in Chapter 10.) Mentally incapacitated people may or may not be able to consent to treatment, depending on the nature and severity of their condition. As a practical matter, but one that has been accepted as law, close family members are often asked to authorize decisions to treat — or increasingly, not to treat — an incapacitated relative. Only rarely is it necessary to get a court order to appoint a relative as a guardian or conservator with the power to make treatment decisions.

Consent Forms: Read Before You Sign

Take time to read the consent form before you sign it. If there is ever a dispute, your signature can be used as proof that you knew what was going to happen. But you can still protest. "The signature on a consent form is not *conclusive* evidence of informed consent, particularly if no real information was given to the patient," says Professor Frank Grad of Columbia Law School.

The consent form should be specific and reflect your discussions with the doctor. If there is anything in the form that you have doubts about or that you don't agree with, cross it out or change it. It's your right. Just be sure to initial any changes you make.

Many hospitals insist that you sign a general consent form when you enter, which is supposed to protect them against future legal action and give them the right to treat you as they believe necessary. In reality, these forms are vague and, unlike the detailed forms for specific procedures, have limited legal clout. Even if you signed and something goes wrong, you can still go to court. Judges have found that patients did not have any choice and are, in effect, coerced into signing.

Although general consent and admissions forms may indicate your willingness to have your temperature and blood pressure taken, they are not binding when questions arise about your consent to specific procedures, such as exploratory surgery. Consent does not always have to be written. It can be oral or implied by behavior. For example, a man who went to an immunization clinic, rolled up his sleeve, and said, "Go ahead," could not argue later that he did not know what was happening, even though nothing was in writing. In practice, for procedures other than minor ones in which the risks are obvious or well known (for example, taking a blood sample), doctors and hospitals require a written consent form. If you are in a hospital and have questions about the consent form, ask to see the patient representative, an employee whose job is to deal with patients' questions. Most hospitals now have one on staff. Or simply ask for more time to consider it.

Avoid Cost Shock

One question that is not normally considered part of informed consent but should be is "How much will it cost?" It is not unusual for a person to go into a state of shock when the bills come. And they do come — from the hospital, doctors, anesthesiologists, pharmacy, and others you never even heard of. Only rarely does insurance cover all treatment. To avoid cost shock, find out beforehand approximately how much the total bill will come to.

If there is a disagreement about your medical or hospital bill, first ask for an explanation. "When a hospital is involved, make sure to get an itemized bill and go over it with the administrator or patient representative. Under the American Hospital Association's [AHA] Patients' Bill of Rights, this is your right," advises Ila Rothschild, an attorney with the AHA. If the disagreement cannot be settled amicably, report the matter to your county medical board. You can find the number in the white pages of your telephone directory. If it's not listed, call the American Medical Association, (202) 789-7400. If the local medical board cannot solve the problem, your next step is to seek the advice of an attorney. (See Chapter 14 for guidance on finding a lawyer.)

Before agreeing to surgery or treatment other than simple and relatively harmless procedures, discuss the following questions with your doctor:

CHECKLIST: BEFORE AGREEING TO SURGERY OR MEDICAL TREATMENT

- What is wrong with me? What is my illness or condition?
- What will happen during my surgery or treatment? What is the name and nature of the treatment?
- What is likely to happen if I decide not to be treated?
- What are the benefits of the treatment?
- What are the risks and side effects? What is the probability of their occurring?
- What is the name of the doctor who will treat me or perform the surgery? How many times has he or she done it? What is his or her success rate?
- What is the probability that the treatment will succeed?
- What alternative treatments are available? What are the risks and benefits of each of them?
- How much will it cost?

• Finally, ask yourself, Have I had enough time to decide in an unpressured environment?

Consent for Medical Research and Experiments
"The history of medical progress is to a large extent the history of medical experimentation," writes George Annas, professor of health law at Boston University. Without research on people, there would be no polio vaccine, kidney dialysis, or birth control pill. Yet mention human experimentation and some see repeats of Dr. Josef Mengele's experiments at Auschwitz or the Tuskegee, Alabama, study. In that infamous project, begun in 1932, four hundred black sharecroppers with syphilis were followed for forty years, but were never treated or told they had the disease.

As a result of public outrage, the federal government passed regulations governing the rights of human experimentation subjects. The states mandated additional protections. The most important safeguard was the creation of institutional review boards whose job it is to review medical research proposals, judge the risks and benefits, examine the methodology, and make sure that the rights of participants are protected.

If you are asked to be a subject of medical research, follow the rules of informed consent described above. In addition, be sure that

• the research has been approved by an institutional review board.
• you understand the purpose of the experiment.
• your name will be kept confidential unless you authorize its use.
• you know where to turn for assistance in case of side effects or unanticipated problems.
• it is clear who pays the cost of treating side effects (it is often free).

By law, you cannot be penalized for refusing to take part in medical research. Don't be afraid to say no if you do not want to participate.

Your Right to Treatment

In an Emergency Room

Under federal law and the law of nearly every state, if you show up at an emergency room, the hospital staff must examine you. If it's an emergency, or if you're a woman in active labor, the hospital must treat you and keep you there until your condition has stabilized, to quote federal law. Although the definition of "stabilized" is not wholly clear, at the very least, emergency room personnel cannot legally turn you away because your Blue Cross card is at home or you don't have health insurance. An emergency room physician or hospital that refuses to treat a person in need of immediate care risks fines from the government, loss of accreditation, and lawsuits.

The first major lawsuit brought under this law designed to prevent patient "dumping" involved Dr. Michael Burditt, a Texas obstetrician/gynecologist. According to court documents, Dr. Burditt, head of obstetrics and gynecology at the DeTar Hospital in Victoria, Texas, refused to admit Rosa Rivera, an indigent woman in labor with her sixth child, who had come to the hospital's emergency room. When Ms. Rivera arrived, her blood pressure was dangerously high. Dr. Burditt ordered her transferred by ambulance to a hospital 170 miles away, saying, "Until DeTar Hospital pays my malpractice insurance, I will pick and choose those patients that I want to treat." En route, Ms. Rivera gave birth to a healthy baby.

The U.S. Department of Health and Human Services (HHS) charged Dr. Burditt with violating the patient-dumping law. In his defense, Dr. Burditt argued that Ms. Rivera's blood pressure was so high that she could not be treated properly at DeTar Hospital. HHS fined him $20,000, and Dr. Burditt went to court to appeal the fine. In 1991, five years after the incident had taken place, a federal court of appeals upheld the fine.

If you have a medical emergency and someone tries to deny you entry because you can't prove you're insured, insist on seeing a doctor or the hospital's patient representative if there is one. But once safely inside, don't think that a doctor will see you immediately. Emergency rooms are chaotic, jammed with people who have been shot, stabbed, mangled in car accidents, or have over-dosed on crack. They have also become the primary source of health care for many poor people. Doctors take the most serious cases first and let others wait their turn, a system called triage. Sometimes the beds are filled, and there is no place to put new patients. The wait can drag on for many hours.

Outside an Emergency Room
Outside an emergency room, a doctor does not have to take you as a new patient nor must a hospital admit you. A doctor can refuse to accept you as a new patient no matter how arbitrary the reason, as long as federal, state, or local antidiscrimination laws are not violated. A physician could refuse to see you because of your blue eyes but not because of your skin color. Once you have established a doctor-patient relationship, a physician cannot arbitrarily drop you. This would be "abandonment," which is both illegal and unethical. He or she must give you sufficient time to find another doctor.

When a Hospital Wants to Discharge You
Before You've Recovered
To cut health costs, insurance companies, hospitals, and health maintenance organizations contract with private, often profit-making utilization review companies whose job is to determine whether hospitalization is necessary, and if it is, for how long. Typically, before you enter a hospital or during your stay there, your doctor's request for hospitalization is examined by a utilization review firm. If the company determines that hospitalization is not necessary or that it should be for a shorter period than the doctor recommends, your insurance or HMO will not cover the part of the stay deemed unnecessary.

The bottom line is that patients are being denied admission to hospitals or are being released "quicker and sicker," and you could be the loser.

What can you do if a hospital wants to send you home before you feel fully recovered? In many states, patients and doctors have the right to appeal a premature discharge to the utilization review firm. (If Medicare is paying, you can appeal to a peer review organization. See Chapter 11.) The guidelines of the Utilization Review Accreditation Commission, a Washington, D.C., group that is attempting to set standards for the industry, authorize doctors to lodge an appeal, on which a utilization review committee must rule within two working days. If you believe you are being discharged early, complain immediately to your doctor and the hospital's patient representative, if there is one. They can tell you how to lodge a protest.

If you are released prematurely and are injured because of it, you may have a lawsuit against the doctor, the hospital, the insurance company, and the utilization review company. Whether you have grounds for a suit depends on state law and the facts of the case. Consider the two leading cases, both heard in California.

In the first, decided in 1986, Lois Wickline was admitted to the Van Nuys Community Hospital for complicated surgery on her back and leg. Her doctor requested that Ms. Wickline remain in the hospital for observation an additional eight days because of the possibility of an infection or a blood clot. Medi-Cal, the California Medicaid agency that approves the length of hospital stays, rejected the request and granted only a four-day extension. The doctor did not protest and released Ms. Wickline when the four days were up. After she was sent home, her right leg became infected and she was rushed to the hospital, where it was amputated. Ms. Wickline sued Medi-Cal for negligence in not approving her doctor's request for the eight-day extension. She lost because her doctor did not object to Medi-Cal's ruling as he was entitled to do by law. The decision makes clear that Ms. Wickline had a strong case against her doctor *and* the hospital if she chose to sue them (which she didn't).

In the second case, twenty-five-year-old Howard Wilson, a patient in College Hospital in Los Angeles, was suffering from depression, drug dependency, and anorexia. His physician, Dr. Warren Taff, determined that Mr. Wilson needed to spend an additional three or four weeks in the hospital. Blue Cross sent the request to its utilization review firm, Western Medical Review, which determined that further hospitalization was "not justified or approved." Based on this decision, Blue Cross of Southern California refused to pay for further hospital care. Dr. Taff broke the news to his patient, who left the hospital crying — and three weeks later committed suicide.

Wilson's father brought a lawsuit against the utilization review company, among others allegedly responsible for his son's death. In 1991, the same California court that had decided Lois Wickline's case five years earlier said that Wilson's father could sue the utilization review company for the premature discharge of his son. The court said that it was up to a jury to determine whether the utilization review company's decision "was a substantial factor in causing Mr. Wilson's death."

Refusal of Treatment

You have the right to refuse medical treatment, even if it's good for you. It may not always be healthy, but it's part of the autonomy that you enjoy as a patient. You cannot be forced to have an operation, take medicine, or stay in a hospital against your will. Contrary to what you see on television, you can walk out of a hospital at any time. "We have an obligation to warn our patients about the risks they run if they leave against our advice and to urge them to stay," says Fred Landes, an emergency-medicine physician. "But if they are competent, we can't force them to stay. It's their choice." If you decide to leave over the objections of your doctor, the hospital will ask you to sign a form agreeing not to sue them or the doctor should your condition deteriorate.

You are free to leave even if it puts your life in jeopardy. Dr. Landes tells the story of Jack R., a fast-track investment banker rushed to a hospital with a heart attack. "The cardiologist treated him with a new medication to break up the clots," Dr. Landes said. "This succeeded, but put him at risk of bleeding elsewhere because of thinned blood." When his physician wanted to monitor Mr. R.'s condition in the hospital, Mr. R. told him, "Doc, I feel great. I'm out of here." The physician responded, "You don't understand," and explained the risk of internal bleeding. "No, *you* don't understand," Mr. R. said. "I've been working on a big merger for the past three years. Tomorrow's the big day. I've got to be there." And he left. That's the last Dr. Landes heard from him.

Since it is a serious step to leave a hospital against your doctor's orders, think very hard before taking it. If you decide to leave, make sure to find out about follow-up treatment and what to do if you need further medical care.

Some people refuse treatment because of their religious convictions. Newspapers frequently report stories about Jehovah's Witnesses who refuse blood transfusions. When a hospital asks a court to approve a transfusion over a patient's objection, judges almost always rule in favor of the patient, except when children are involved. If a child needs a lifesaving transfusion, judges usually authorize it over the parents' objections. This is discussed in Chapter 10, "Parents and Children."

The right to refuse treatment is the justification for withholding lifesaving or life-prolonging treatment for terminally ill patients. As part of a growing movement to allow people to die with dignity, almost all states and the District of Columbia have enacted laws that recognize living wills, durable powers of attorney, or health proxies. See the discussion in Chapter 13, "The Right to Die."

Confidentiality

Your medical records and your conversations with your doctor are confidential. They cannot be made available to your employer, your insurance company, or anybody else without your permission. The Hippocratic oath established the sanctity of the physician-patient relationship, and state laws today prohibit doctor-patient conversations and records from being disclosed without the patient's consent, except in limited circumstances, which vary from state to state. These circumstances are:

- If you sue your doctor, you waive the protection of confidentiality and your records can be used as evidence.
- Contagious diseases like typhoid fever must be reported, as must cases of gunshot and knife wounds and suspected cases of child abuse.
- In the interest of protecting the public's health, the names of people carrying sexually transmitted diseases such as gonor-

rhea and syphilis must be reported to the health department. In some states, the names of those with AIDS or those who are infected with the AIDS virus must be reported to the health department. Many states authorize doctors to instruct patients carrying the AIDS virus to tell their partners. If the patient refuses, the physician can legally warn the partners directly. When names are reported, health departments must protect the identity of the diseased person. To date, their record is excellent.

• If a patient poses a threat to somebody's life, a doctor probably must warn the intended victim. In one case, a student told his psychotherapist that he planned to kill his former girlfriend. The therapist did not warn the girlfriend. Shortly after this threat, the patient murdered the young woman. When the victim's parents sued, the judge ruled that the therapist had a duty to warn the young woman.

In practice, medical records are common knowledge to dozens of people. The American College of Hospital Administrators estimates that seventy-five people have access to any patient record. You waive your right to keep your records confidential all the time; you have no choice. Every time you file a medical claim, you sign a statement authorizing the release of your records to an insurance company. The data goes into a giant computer operated by the Medical Insurance Bureau (MIB), a company maintained by a consortium of eight hundred insurance companies. With so many people having access to medical records and the many exceptions to the rule on confidentiality, it is not surprising that leaks to unauthorized people occur all too frequently.

What can you do if you are the victim of a computer glitch? Say you are turned down for an insurance policy for inexplicable reasons — perhaps a mistake in your medical records. Once you're in the computer, you need a healthy capacity for perseverance to deal with bureaucratic doublespeak. Don't be lulled into thinking you can correct a computer error easily. It's very hard, but not impossible. This is what to do:

First, call the insurance company and ask why your application was rejected. Someone will probably tell you it was because of information in your medical records, or something equally vague. Try to track down the source. More likely than not, this will lead you to the MIB. When an insurance company wants to learn the health history of an applicant, it taps into the MIB computer for the person's medical records.

Call or write the MIB — P.O. Box 105, Essex Station, Boston, MA 02112, (617) 426-3660. The MIB will send you a form to fill out and forward a copy of the requested file to your doctor within thirty days of receiving the form back from you. (Note that the bureau releases information only to physicians, not to individuals.) After reviewing the records with your doctor, you may be able to figure out why your application was rejected. If you were turned down because of an error in the file, have your doctor write the insurance company to set the record straight. All correspondence should be sent by certified mail, return receipt requested.

Access to Medical Records

In the past, patients had almost no right to see or copy their medical records, which were considered doctors' property. But times change, and that concept is considered outmoded. At least twenty-seven states have laws granting patients access to their medical records. To find out about your state's laws, contact the medical society in your state. You can get its address and telephone number from the American Medical Association's Washington, D.C., office, (202) 789-7400.

State laws place conditions on the availability of records. In New York, physicians and hospitals must provide a copy of medical records upon receipt of a written request. In Maryland, hospitals must give patients a copy of their medical records, but doctors don't have to. In many states, a doctor who believes — and can demonstrate — that the information would harm a patient's health doesn't have to release the records. This applies particularly to mental health records.

Although patients are legally entitled to their records in most states, the medical profession doesn't make it easy. As noted in Chapter 1, some hospitals charge a dollar a page, plus an "administrative fee." For a hefty medical file, this can add up to a lot of money. It might be easier to ask a friendly physician to request your records, since they are provided free of charge to doctors as a professional courtesy.

Despite the variations among states, certain steps should be followed just about everywhere. First ask your doctor or hospital what procedure to follow to obtain a copy of your records. If you meet resistance, send a written request — by certified mail, return receipt requested. If that doesn't get results, write the agency or group that oversees access to medical records. The New York State Department of Health, for example, has set up an office just to handle complaints from people who can't get their medical records. But not all states have such an organization. To find out if there is one near you, call the state branch of the American Health Information Management Association. You can get the number by calling its headquarters, (312) 787-2672.

Finding the Right Health Professional

Breaking the Code of Silence
If you are one of the many people who are perfectly content with their doctor — who have found the combination of knowledge, experience, warmth, and availability that we all crave — skip this section. But if you are frustrated because your doctor is too busy to answer your questions, angry because you sit fuming for hours in the waiting room after taking a taxi to be on time, or plagued by doubts about your doctor's competence, read on. Or perhaps you are moving to a new community and have to find health professionals to meet your family's needs.

In this section, we advise you how to find a doctor and other health professionals — for example, a pediatrician for your children, a family practitioner for your overall health needs, a dentist, an allergist for your chronic asthma, or a chiropractor. Although we talk specifically about finding a doctor, the same guidelines can be modified to locate any health professional.

If you've ever tried to conduct a thorough, rational search for a health professional, you probably already know that the deck is stacked against you. "Obtaining access to complete, up-to-date, and verified information about physicians is all but impossible," wrote Dr. Julia Reade and Dr. Richard Ratzan in the *New England Journal of Medicine.* You cannot, for example, get such basic information about doctors' competence as whether they have been disciplined for incompetence, lost their license, or been successfully sued for malpractice.

Doctors do not like to say bad things about one another. When they do, or are forced to, the medical profession rises as a body to throw a thick blanket over the release of negative information to the public. Take the National Practitioner Data Bank, for example. Ordered by Congress in 1986, this computerized data bank is supposed to store information about doctors who have lost their license for incompetence or been censured, disciplined, or sued for malpractice. Hospitals must check with the bank before offering staff privileges to a physician. But is the information in the National Practitioner Data Bank available to you and me? Absolutely not. In fact, a leak to an unauthorized person is punishable by a fine of up to $10,000.

This code of medical silence might be justifiable if the systems designed to protect patients from inept doctors and other health professionals worked, but they don't. "State medical boards are our first line of defense against bad medical care, and the evidence shows that there are too many leaks in these defenses," said Oregon Congressman Ron Wyden as he opened congressional subcommittee hearings on physician discipline in 1990. "They are plagued by understaffing, case backlogs, insufficient resources, and limited access to information. As a result, too many incompetent physicians can slip through the disciplinary net and continue to inflict bad medical care on patients for an extended period of time." Similarly, medical associations — professional organizations made up of doctors — state and federal governments, and insurance companies, do not adequately protect the public against inept doctors.

Now that we've told you how hard it is to crack the code that medical students probably learn along with Anatomy 1, how do you go about finding the right doctor or health professional? If you are letting your fingers do the walking toward the *Yellow Pages* right now, we can advise you in one word: Don't. As a source of information about doctors, the *Yellow Pages* get very low marks, according to Dr. Reade and Dr. Ratzan.

To increase your chances of finding a qualified and competent health professional, follow the nine steps outlined below. Whether you need a primary care physician for routine care or a high-tech specialist for a rare disease, this list can be a reliable guide to separating the cream from the milk.

CHECKLIST: FINDING A HEALTH PROFESSIONAL

• **Get recommendations from a number of sources:**
Family and friends. There is no stronger recommendation than a satisfied customer. Just remember that your needs are probably different from those of your Uncle Louie. He may be thrilled with his cardiologist, but if you are worried about an enlarged mole on your back, you probably need someone else. But the cardiologist can probably give you some names. Get at least three.
Your current doctor. Through contacts at professional associations, continuing medical education courses, medical publications, and the old-boy network, your current doctor may be able to suggest a physician if you are moving to a new community or to recommend a specialist if you need one. Nurses are often a great resource. "They tend to have the inside story," says Ellen Sanders, first vice-president of the American Nurses Association. "They have sound practical knowledge and know who's good."
Public education/advocacy groups. If you need an infertility specialist, turn to RESOLVE. If asthma is the problem, call the Asthma and Allergy Foundation. For just about any illness or condition, an organization exists that can refer you to doctors, educational materials, and others with the same problem. Two booklets that provide names, addresses, and phone numbers are *The Directory of National Helplines* (Consumers Index, Pieran Press, Ann Arbor, MI 48106, [800] 678-2435), and *The Self-Help Sourcebook* (St. Clares–Riverside Medical Center, Denville, NJ 07834, [201] 625-7101). There is a small charge for the booklets.
City and county health departments. These should be able to give you the names of nearby doctors practicing the

specialty you require. Consult your telephone directory or call your state health department (addresses and phone numbers are listed at the end of this chapter).

City and county medical societies. These are professional associations of physicians, which can usually supply the names of members.

Hospitals. Say you need a pediatrician. One way to start your search is to call the head of the pediatrics department at a nearby hospital or medical center and ask for recommendations. Many hospitals have begun to advertise their own physician referral services. When you call a published number, you will be given the names of doctors affiliated with a particular hospital. But keep in mind that a reference from a hospital department or physician referral service tells you nothing about qualifications. It guarantees only that the doctor is affiliated with the hospital. You may be getting the names of those physicians who are most in need of the business, not those who are most highly reputed. Some referral services even charge doctors a fee to be listed.

- **Check out the doctor's educational background.** You want to know where a doctor went to school and served a residency. If the doctor graduated from a prestigious medical school like Johns Hopkins or Harvard, you know only that he or she was academically qualified to be admitted to a very selective institution. While this is likely to be a plus, it does not follow that the person has good doctor skills. Two books, available in most libraries, supply information about doctors' credentials: the American Board of Medical Specialties' *Compendium of Certified Medical Specialists* and Marquis's *Directory of Medical Specialists*.

- **Look for a board-certified or board-eligible physician.** The books in which you look up doctors' educational credentials can also tell you whether they are board certified. *Board certified* indicates that a doctor has completed a number of years of residency — usually two to four — involving intensive study of a specialty, and passed a rigorous examination in the discipline. The exams are given by so-called specialty boards in different areas of medicine, for example, ophthalmology and pediatrics. It is one of the ways the medical profession attempts to maintain high standards.

But beware. Not all medical boards are alike. Any group of physicians can set up a specialty board. Some may have high standards, others almost none. Of the approximately 150 different medical boards in existence, the American Board of Medical Specialties (ABMS) has certified only twenty-three as meeting its standards. Call its hotline — (800) 776-2378 — to find out whether a physician is certified by a board the ABMS recognizes. If the doctor is not so recognized, it does not necessarily mean that you have to look elsewhere. You should, however, inquire carefully into the doctor's qualifications.

If you cannot locate a board-certified physician, look for one who is *board eligible* — a doctor who has taken a residency in a specialty but has not yet passed the certification examination.

• **Find out whether the doctor you are considering has been disciplined.** Every year the Public Citizen Health Research Group ferrets out a list of doctors, dentists, chiropractors, and podiatrists who have been formally disciplined by federal or state agencies and lists them in a publication called *Questionable Doctors*, which may be in your local library. If it isn't, you can order a copy of the list for your state by sending $12 to the Health Research Group, 2000 P Street, NW, Washington, DC 20036.

• **Find out where the doctor has staff privileges.** Doctors are not allowed to practice in just any hospital. Rather, they are limited to those hospitals where a committee of doctors has reviewed their credentials and found them competent to practice their specialty. Only then are they awarded staff privileges in the hospital.

If your potential doctor has privileges in a highly reputed hospital, so much the better. If he or she has privileges in a hospital whose reputation doesn't meet your standards, it should give you pause. And if you simply *must* go to a specific hospital — perhaps because it is known for its excellent work with cancer patients — make sure you choose a doctor who has privileges there.

- **Interview potential candidates.** Don't be intimidated by the thought of interviewing a physician. It is an important and accepted part of medical practice. You will probably have to pay for the doctor's time, but the expense is certainly worthwhile in time saved and anxiety relieved. Here are suggested questions to help you evaluate potential physicians:

Where did you go to school and serve your residency? You probably know this from the credentials check, but it is useful to have the information in narrative form.

What is your specialty or particular area of interest? Medicine is filled with subspecialties and sub-subspecialties. An internist may be particularly knowledgeable about heart or liver problems, an oncologist about breast cancer.

Are you or another doctor available twenty-four hours a day in case of emergency? Medical crises do not always occur during office hours. Find out who is the back-up support.

How long does it take to get an appointment? If a doctor is so busy that he or she can't see you for months, think what will happen if you require immediate care.

What is your policy toward telephone conversations? You want a doctor who returns nonemergency phone calls within a reasonable time — preferably the same day. Some doctors, notably pediatricians, set aside an early morning hour for patients' calls.

Do you handle routine matters yourself or do you rely on nurse practitioners or other nonphysicians to take care of them? Depending on your individual taste, a doctor's delegation of routine work to others may be a plus or a minus.

What is your philosophy about medical care? You should know whether a physician has an aggressive or conservative approach to treatment decisions.

What is your diagnosis of my condition and how do you propose to treat it? If you are visiting a doctor for a specific problem, this is obviously a critical question that will illustrate the doctor's philosophy about medical care and whether you both think along the same lines.

Have you had experience in treating cases like mine, and what has your success rate been?

Will you give me a copy of the results of my medical tests?
Although it is still not standard medical practice, an increasing number of doctors give their patients a copy of test results.
What is your attitude toward terminating life-support systems? Make sure your doctor will carry out your wishes. If you have prepared a living will, health proxy, or durable power of attorney, give a copy to the doctor you select.

• **Ask about fees, payment terms, and insurance.** Many people are hesitant to discuss money with a doctor — with some justification. We recently heard about a young woman who consulted a plastic surgeon at Columbia Presbyterian Hospital about removing a scar. After he described a very detailed operation, the young woman asked how much the procedure would cost. Pulling himself to his full five-foot-six height behind his massive desk, the surgeon looked her in the eye and said huffily, "I am a professor at Columbia University. I never discuss money." The young woman pulled herself out of her chair and left.

   Since you are the one who has to pay — at least a part — do not be bashful about asking about fees. It is your right to know how much the medical services will cost, when the doctor expects to be paid, and whether he or she will take assignment, that is, agree to be paid directly by the insurance company.

• **Describe your situation fully and honestly.** When you talk with prospective physicians, be sure to give them a full description of your symptoms, your condition, and your needs. Don't forget to mention your allergies to certain medication. Good physician-patient relations are built on trust, whose foundation is an honest sharing of information. Since doctors tend to make decisions quickly, provide the important information early.

• **Follow your instincts.** Even with all the information at your disposal, it is hard knowing how to choose. Everybody's needs and priorities are different. Some people prefer an older, experienced doctor, others a younger person recently out of medical school. Many women insist on a female gynecologist. It is perfectly all right to make your decision based on "feeling" or "gut reaction" as long as you have done your best to assure that the doctor you select has the qualifications and skills to provide the care you need.

Telephone Diagnosis and Outpatient Clinics

Two fairly new medical phenomena are designed to speed diagnosis and treatment. The first is consultation via a 900 telephone number. For $3.00 a minute, or whatever the current price, you can confer with a doctor by phone. It may be okay for simple ailments, but for any serious complaint, you should see a doctor in person, as your telephone consultant will be the first to tell you. Think about whether you want to spend $180 an hour for medical advice from a person you don't know and who knows nothing about you.

The other service is outpatient clinics, a booming alternative to hospitals and emergency rooms. Some of these are walk-in clinics, known as doc-in-the-box centers, that provide immediate care for simple medical problems. More sophisticated outpatient clinics specialize in specific types of care. One clinic may be devoted only to surgery, another to diagnostic imaging such as MRI (magnetic resonance imaging), a third to chemotherapy.

For convenience and cost, outpatient clinics are hard to beat. That's probably why nearly half of all surgical and diagnostic procedures are now performed out of hospitals. This number is expected to grow to two thirds by 1995. Far better to have a bleeding hand taped up in minutes than spend hours waiting in a hospital emergency room. *How* the hand is bandaged is another story. Quality of care in outpatient clinics is a crapshoot. Although ambulatory surgical centers, home health care agencies, and freestanding substance abuse treatment centers may be licensed, the majority of outpatient facilities are unregulated, according to a 1990 report of the U.S. General Accounting Office. They are neither licensed nor monitored by state governments, nor are they accredited by professional societies that set and oversee standards.

"Millions of procedures are performed each year in unlicensed or underregulated facilities," said Congressman Ron Wyden in 1991. "There is little or no quality review of the doctor's expertise. The training of the assisting personnel may be suspect. There is no check on whether adequate lifesaving equipment is on hand."

Since so many freestanding clinics operate without anybody checking on them, it is particularly important that you investigate:

• whether the clinic is licensed by the state government.
• whether it is accredited by a recognized body such as the Joint Commission on Accreditation of Health Care Organizations or the American Association for Ambulatory Health Care.
• whether the clinic has emergency lifesaving equipment on hand and, if not, how it would handle a life-threatening situation.
• the credentials of the doctor who will see you.
• whether the doctor who referred you to the clinic has a financial interest in it. Although it may be legal for doctors to refer patients to clinics in which they have a financial interest (the law is in flux at the moment), there may be a conflict of interest. At the very least, you should know about it.

How to Complain

If an experience with your medical care has ever made you sick, learning how to complain creatively can get dramatic results. While increasing numbers of dissatisfied patients realize that they don't have to take it anymore, few know where to go, whom to talk to, or how to navigate through the medical labyrinth.

A word of caution: Don't get mad as hell. Angry confrontations do little good in getting your problems solved.

Start with the source. It may be a doctor, nurse, or dentist. Or a hospital, in which case you would ask to speak with the patient representative or administrator. Be polite, clear, and firm in explaining the problem and how you would like it to be resolved. If you get no satisfaction, write out your complaint and mail it.

If conversations and letters don't work, get on the telephone or start corresponding with the following people or organizations:

- The local or state medical (or nursing, dental, or other professional) society. These professional associations often have mechanisms to resolve disagreements between health professionals and patients.
- The state licensing authority. Health professionals must be licensed in the state in which they practice. Flagrant violations can lead to suspension or revocation of a license. Short of that, many state licensing boards are equipped to try to settle disputes. Contact the state department of health (see the list below for the address and phone number).
- Your elected representatives. Part of any legislator's job is helping constituents solve problems. That's what they are paid to do, and, besides, it's good politics. Contact your senator, congressman, or state representatives.
- Radio, television, and newspapers. Never underestimate the power of a juicy story splashed over the six o'clock news. Some radio and television stations have special hotlines or segments of news programs that offer aid to unhappy consumers.
- Lawyers. You'd be surprised at how quickly a letter on an attorney's letterhead gets results. Moreover, if you believe that you were the victim of malpractice, see a lawyer. In Chapter 14 we offer advice on finding an attorney.

STATE DEPARTMENTS OF HEALTH

Note: Addresses and telephone numbers sometimes change. If you have difficulty locating the department in your state, check with the Association of State and Territorial Health Officials, 415 Second Street, NE, Washington, DC 20002, (202) 546-5400.

Alabama
Department of Public Health
434 Monroe Street
Montgomery, AL 36130-1701
(205) 242-5095

Alaska
Division of Public Health
P.O. Box H
Juneau, AK 99811-0601
(907) 465-3030

Arizona
Department of Health Services
1740 W. Adams Street
Phoenix, AZ 85007
(602) 542-1000

Arkansas
Department of Health
4815 W. Markham Street
Little Rock, AR 72205
(501) 661-2111

California
Department of Health Services
714 P Street
Sacramento, CA 94234-7320
(916) 445-4171

Colorado
Department of Health
4210 E. 11th Avenue
Denver, CO 80220
(303) 320-8333

Connecticut
Department of Health Services
150 Washington Street
Hartford, CT 06106
(203) 566-4800

Delaware
Division of Public Health
P.O. Box 637
Federal Street
Dover, DE 19901
(302) 739-4726

District of Columbia
Department of Public Health
1660 L Street, NW
Washington, DC 20036
(202) 673-7700

Florida
Department of Health and
   Rehabilitative Services
1317 Winewood Boulevard
Tallahassee, FL 32399-0700
(904) 488-6294

Georgia
Division of Public Health
Department of Human Resources
878 Peachtree Street, NE
Atlanta, GA 30309
(404) 894-7505

Hawaii
Department of Health
P.O. Box 3378
Honolulu, HI 96813
(808) 586-4400

Idaho
Department of Health and Welfare
450 W. State Street
Boise, ID 83720-5450
(208) 334-5500

Illinois
Department of Public Health
535 W. Jefferson Street
Springfield, IL 62761
(217) 782-4977

Indiana
State Board of Health
1330 W. Michigan Street
P.O. Box 1964
Indianapolis, IN 46206-1964
(317) 633-0100

Iowa
Department of Public Health
Lucas State Office Building
East 12th and Walnut Streets
Des Moines, IA 50319-0075
(515) 281-5787

Kansas
Department of Health and
  Environment
Landon State Office Building
Topeka, KS 66612-1290
(913) 296-1500

Kentucky
Department of Health Services
Cabinet for Human Resources
275 E. Main Street
Frankfort, KY 40621-0001
(502) 564-7736

Louisiana
Office of Public Health
P.O. Box 60630
New Orleans, LA 70160-0629
(504) 568-5050

Maine
Bureau of Health
State House, Station 11
Augusta, ME 04333
(207) 289-3201

Maryland
Department of Health and Mental
  Hygiene
201 W. Preston Street
Baltimore, MD 21201
(301) 225-6860

Massachusetts
Department of Public Health
150 Tremont Street
Boston, MA 02111
(617) 727-0201

Michigan
Department of Public Health
P.O. Box 30195
Lansing, MI 48909
(517) 335-8000

Minnesota
Department of Health
717 Delaware Street, S.E.
Minneapolis, MN 55440
(612) 623-5000

Mississippi
State Health Department
2423 N. State Street
P.O. Box 1700
Jackson, MS 39215-1700
(601) 960-7400

Missouri
Department of Health
P.O. Box 570
Jefferson City, MO 65102
(314) 751-6400

Montana
Department of Health and
  Environmental Services
Cogswell Building
Helena, MT 59620
(406) 444-2544

Nebraska
Department of Health
301 Centennial Mall, South
P.O. Box 95007
Lincoln, NE 68509
(402) 471-2133

Nevada
Department of Health
505 E. King Street
Carson City, NV 89710
(702) 687-4740

New Hampshire
Department of Health and Human
  Services
6 Hazen Drive
Concord, NH 03301
(603) 271-4685

New Jersey
Department of Health
CN 360
Trenton, NJ 08625-0360
(609) 292-7837

New Mexico
Department of Health
1190 St. Francis Drive
P.O. Box 26110
Santa Fe, NM 87502-6110
(505) 827-0020

New York
New York State Health
   Department
Corning Tower II
Empire State Plaza
Albany, NY 12237-0001
(518) 474-2121

North Carolina
Division of Health Services
Department of Environmental
   Health and Natural
   Resources
1330 St. Mary Street
Raleigh, NC 27605
(919) 733-7081

North Dakota
Department of Health
State Capitol
600 E. Boulevard Avenue
Bismarck, ND 58505-0200
(701) 224-2370

Ohio
Department of Health
246 N. High Street
P.O. Box 118
Columbus, OH 43266-0118
(614) 466-3543

Oklahoma
Department of Health
1000 N.E. 10th Street
P.O. Box 53551
Oklahoma City, OK 73152
(405) 271-4200

Oregon
Health Division
Department of Human Resources
1400 Southwest Fifth Avenue
P.O. Box 231
Portland, OR 97201
(503) 378-3033

Pennsylvania
Department of Health
Health and Welfare Building
P.O. Box 90
Harrisburg, PA 17108
(717) 787-5901

Rhode Island
Department of Health
3 Capitol Hill
Providence, RI 02908-5097
(401) 277-2231

South Carolina
Department of Health and
   Environmental Control
2600 Bull Street
Columbia, SC 29201
(803) 734-4880

South Dakota
Department of Health
445 East Capitol Avenue
Pierre, SD 57501-3185
(605) 773-3361

Tennessee
Department of Public Health
344 Cordell Hull Building
Nashville, TN 37247-0101
(615) 741-3111

Texas
Texas Department of Health
1100 W. 49th Street
Austin, TX 78756-3199
(512) 458-7111

Utah
Department of Health
288 North 1460 West
Salt Lake City, UT 84116
(801) 538-6101

Vermont
State Health Department
60 Main Street
Burlington, VT 05401
(802) 863-7200

Virginia
State Health Department
Main Street Station
1500 East Main Street
Richmond, VA 23219
(804) 786-3561

Washington
Department of Health
MS ET-21
Olympia, WA 98504
(206) 586-5846

West Virginia
Department of Health
1800 Washington Street
Charleston, WV 25305
(304) 348-0045

Wisconsin
Division of Health Services
P.O. Box 7850
Madison, WI 53707
(608) 266-3681

Wyoming
Department of Health and Human
   Services
117 Hathaway Building
Cheyenne, WY 82002-0710
(307) 777-7656

3

HEALTH INSURANCE: HOW TO PROTECT YOURSELF AND YOUR FAMILY

CONTENTS

Unraveling the Mysteries of Health Insurance

What does a trillion and a half dollars look like? That's what the United States is expected to spend on health care by the year 2000. Skyrocketing medical costs place health care in danger of becoming a luxury. Insurance companies are charging more and tightening eligibility requirements. Businesses are slashing health benefits for their employees and herding them into plans that save money but restrict their freedom to choose their own doctor. Health planners are coming up with alphabets of alternative medical plans and ideas about "rationing" health care. Overhauling the health care system is high on the national political agenda. States such as Hawaii and Oregon have taken the lead in dramatically reorganizing the way that health services are delivered and paid for.

In these confusing times, when cost consciousness threatens to erode health benefits, it's hard to find your way through the maze of plans and options. To protect yourself and your family, you must become an educated health care shopper. Whether you are self-employed or work for a large corporation, you must know what to look for when choosing a health plan and learn a whole new vocabulary of words like "HMO," "PPO," "deductible," and "coinsurance." You must know what to do if an insurance company turns down your application or hassles you about a claim you have filed. You must learn your rights under federal and state law.

In this chapter we guide you through the ins and outs of health insurance. Cutting through the gobbledygook of insurance company brochures, we tell you what to look for when choosing a health plan, what to do if an insurance company turns you down, ways to get coverage even if you're hard to insure, and how to keep your insurance if you lose your job, get divorced, or your spouse dies. Finally, we tell you how to minimize the hassle of filing claims and what to do if an insurance company refuses to pay you the money to which you are entitled.

The High Cost of Health Care

"If I'm *really* sick, I'll go to the Plaza Hotel and order room service," Florence R., a sixty-year-old New York painter in astonishingly good health, is in the habit of telling her friends. The reality is that Ms. R., who has taught portrait painting for thirty years and regularly shows her work, cannot afford health insurance premiums.

She is like the estimated 35 million Americans who have no health coverage at all and another 60 million who have such inadequate coverage that a major catastrophe would mean financial — as well as physical — ruin. More than two-thirds of these people are employed. They may be the aerobics instructor at your health club, the part-time computer teacher at your local college, the graphic designer, the real estate broker, or, like Florence, the portrait painter. In fact, anyone. Indeed, the need for health coverage has become a rallying cry for workers. Pick up any newspaper report of a strike. What are they fighting — or negotiating — about? You guessed it. Health coverage.

Unless you are covered, and covered well, by health insurance, you cannot afford to get sick in our society. Pediatricians routinely charge $50 and more for a fifteen-minute visit. Radiologists get $10 to $15 a minute to read an X ray. If you need the latest high-tech medicine, the cost is astronomical. Perhaps the most stunning example is that of Cindy Martin, an executive secretary from a small Pennsylvania town. In 1989 she received a new heart, liver, and kidney in the same operation. The bill came to $1.25 million. She died in the intensive care unit of the hospital four months after the operation.

As a nation, we have the most expensive health care system in the world. We pay more than $700 billion a year for health care, up from about $50 billion in 1965. The percentage of our gross national product that we spend on health care has nearly doubled in twenty-five years to a whopping 12 percent and is expected to reach 15 percent by the year 2000. No wonder that lawmakers talk about the "crisis" in health care. But more important than the global picture is the impact on you as businesses, insurance companies, and government try to stem the tide of rising health costs. You are faced with the following:

Higher Premiums

Insurance companies pass the rising cost of health care directly to you by raising premiums. Small businesses are particularly hit hard. It is no longer unusual for insurance companies to jack up rates for these enterprises by 30 to 50 percent each year. Many people find it difficult to find insurance coverage at a price they can afford — if they can get a policy at all. "Forget about finding cheap health insurance if you have to buy on your own," wrote *Newsweek*'s Jane Bryant Quinn. "Good low-priced policies don't exist."

Fewer Benefits

As insurance companies raise their rates, many businesses try to recoup by reducing the benefits they offer their employees. Health benefits have become the greatest source of friction between labor and management, says Stephanie Poe of the Employee Benefits Research Institute.

Increased Cost

Employers make their employees pay for a larger share of their health care. "The company's policy used to pick up everything. I didn't have to pay a cent," says Fred D., a thirty-six-year-old computer programmer. "Now I pay a deductible and 20 percent of the doctors' bills. With two young children and a mortgage on a new house, I have to worry every time we even sneeze." The number of businesses that pay the full amount of health insurance premiums dropped by one-third between 1980 and 1988.

Difficulty Getting Insurance

Insurance companies prefer to insure healthy people who aren't going to file claims. The industry does not want to cover people with cancer, kidney failure, or other long-term illnesses. Individuals with medical problems have trouble getting insurance. Either they are rejected outright or the "pre-existing" condition is excluded from coverage — sometimes for a specific length of time, sometimes forever. More and more people stay in unsatisfactory jobs because they are afraid of losing their health coverage.

Managed Care

New forms of health organizations are supposed to offer health care at lower rates and curb unnecessary medical procedures. Health maintenance organizations (HMOs) are the best known, but they have competitors in the form of preferred provider organizations (PPOs), exclusive provider organizations (EPOs), and other, even newer kinds of health care entities. To cut health costs, some large companies, like Allied Signal Corporation with 85,000 employees, offer such great financial inducements to join an HMO or a PPO that their employees are really left with no choice. Traditional health plans now require insurance company approval or second opinions before surgery and have utilization review committees to determine how long you can stay in a hospital. This active intervention in deciding what kind and how much health care patients get — with an eye to the bottom line — is called managed care.

Health Insurance Made Easy

The Players

In 1929, Dr. Justin Ford Kimball, administrator of the Baylor University Hospital in Dallas, Texas, conceived the nation's first health plan. For the sum of fifty cents a week, Dallas schoolteachers received up to twenty-one days of free hospital care. The idea quickly caught on in other communities and led eventually to the creation of Blue Cross and Blue Shield, the health insurance giant that covers nearly one out of every three Americans.

Largely because of the tax benefits given to employer-sponsored health plans, more than four out of five insured people are enrolled through their jobs. Their coverage is provided by Blue Cross–Blue Shield, a commercial insurance company, or the company itself. In addition, federal and state governments pay for the health care of millions of Americans.

Blue Cross–Blue Shield

Blue Cross pays hospital room, board, and other costs. Blue Shield pays doctors' bills. The seventy-four state and local Blue Cross–Blue Shield plans cover approximately 73 million people. Originally, Blue Cross–Blue Shields were set up as nonprofit corporations to provide benefits to healthy *and* sick people at affordable rates. To a large extent, this still holds true. Many Blue Cross–Blue Shields still insure high-risk people for comparatively low rates. However, forced to compete with private insurance companies, some Blues are now excluding unhealthy people or fending them off by charging high rates.

Commercial Insurance Companies

Unlike the nonprofit Blue Cross plans, commercial insurance companies such as the Travelers and Prudential, to name only two, are out to make a profit on the sale of health insurance policies. By selling to relatively healthy people who make few claims, commercial insurance companies can often undercut Blue Cross, which in some states must offer insurance at subsidized rates to high-risk people. Ninety-four million Americans are covered by commercial insurers.

Self-insurance by Business

About half of all large and medium-size companies insure their own workers. Instead of buying protection from an insurance company, they invest the money they would have to spend on premiums and use it to pay their employees' claims directly. Companies that insure their own employees are governed by the federal Employee Retirement Income Security Act (ERISA), not by state insurance laws. This allows them to avoid state laws requiring insurance companies to cover specific medical services, such as in vitro fertilization, mental health, or chiropractors. About 55 million people are covered by companies that self-insure.

Government

The U.S. government sponsors two large programs, Medicare and Medicaid, which, though frequently confused, are quite different. *Medicare* covers medical costs for about 33 million elderly and disabled people, rich or poor (see Chapter 11). *Medicaid,* funded and administered by both the federal and state governments, covers about 25 million poor people of all ages, including many senior citizens who go broke paying for nursing home care (see Chapter 12). The U.S. government also makes payments to disabled people under Social Security Disability Insurance (see Chapter 4), funds a variety of health programs, and provides health care for members of the armed forces, their dependents, and veterans. The states furnish health care, primarily for people of limited means, out of their own budgets.

The Choices

If you got sick in the Ozzie-and-Harriet era, you went to a doctor who diagnosed your condition, recommended a treatment, and billed you. You paid the bill, submitted it to Blue Shield or another insurance company, and were reimbursed for all or part of the charges. If you were hospitalized, Blue Cross or another insurer picked up the hospital charges directly.

This is traditional fee-for-service insurance. Many analysts feel that this system is largely to blame for the current crisis in health care. Stanford University economist Alain Enthoven contends that doctors who are paid for whatever they recommend are prone to prescribe expensive treatment and order many tests. And if their insurance pays for most health care, patients have no incentive to demand lower costs and every reason to demand the latest technology. The traditional system rewards hospitalization, high technology, and extensive testing at the expense of prevention, "well-body" care, and less costly treatments.

The traditional system may be on its way out, replaced by health maintenance organizations, preferred provider organizations, and other forms of managed care. In 1984, the health needs of 96 percent of insured Americans were covered by the traditional fee-for-service system. That dropped to 28 percent in 1991, and some experts predict that it will be only 20 percent within the next ten years.

As a result of all these changes in the health care system, many employers are asking their employees to choose among a bewildering assortment of health plans. Here is what they mean to you.

Traditional Fee-for-Service Plans

These usually have three parts. The first two, hospital charges and doctors' bills, are often called the base plan.

- *Hospital charges.* The insurance company or Blue Cross often pays these bills directly to the hospital, either fully or up to a set dollar or percentage limit or number of days. You are usually covered for a semiprivate room, routine nursing care, laboratory tests, and other hospital expenses.
- *Doctors' bills.* Most commonly, the patient pays his or her physicians' bills directly, and then submits a claim to the insurance company or Blue Shield. The company reimburses the patient according to its schedule of "usual, customary, or reasonable" fees.
- *Major Medical.* The third part fills in the gaps, covering longer illnesses, visits to doctors' offices, and some other charges not included in the base plan. The plans have a lifetime limit, say $500,000 or $1,000,000.

In almost all policies, reimbursement begins only after a *deductible* has been paid, that is, after the client has paid the first $200, $500, or other specified amount. After that, an insurance company usually reimburses a percentage (commonly 80 percent) of the medical costs and you have to pick up the remaining 20 percent (called *coinsurance*) from your own pocket. Some doctors accept *assignment*, that is, they agree to accept the amount paid by insurance as the total fee. Insurance companies pay them directly. It is to your advantage to find such a doctor. You will save money, spare yourself the paperwork of filing claims, and eliminate the wait for your expenses to be reimbursed.

While traditional insurance policies protect against the financial costs of illness, preventive health care such as regular physical checkups, well-baby care, breast examination, and birth control are rarely covered.

Health Maintenance Organizations

Enter the world of one-stop shopping. Unlike traditional fee-for-service, a health maintenance organization provides a comprehensive range of medical care in return for a fixed monthly fee. Instead of paying, say, $75 each time you visit a doctor, plus extra charges for X rays and lab tests, you pay a fixed amount, say, $150 a month, at an HMO. This covers all visits to doctors except for a $3 to $5 per visit charge that some HMOs levy, tests and treatment that the doctors order, and any necessary hospitalization. The monthly fee includes preventive care as well.

Under the original HMO models, such as the Kaiser-Permanente plan in California, patients received their health care under one roof. Today, newer models of HMOs, called independent practice associations, let you visit doctors in their own offices, waiting with the fee-paying patients.

In whatever type of HMO you select, you choose a primary physician — who could be an internist, family physician, or pediatrician — whom you consult for normal health matters. You have to give up your own family physician unless he or she participates in the HMO you join. The primary physician (also known as a gatekeeper) refers you to a specialist if he or she believes you need to see one. If the gatekeeper refuses to refer you to a specialist or order tests for you, the HMO won't pay. Except in an emergency, if you see a doctor not associated with the HMO, you have to pay out of your own pocket.

Federal law requires employers with twenty-five or more employees to offer an option to join an HMO if one is available. According to the Group Health Association of America, the trade association for HMOs, 37 million Americans are enrolled in approximately six hundred HMOs.

Preferred Provider Organizations

In the alphabet soup of health plans, preferred provider organizations are the hottest. In 1991, more than 26 million Americans belonged to them, an increase of over 600 percent since 1986. Preferred provider organizations come in many forms. The key is that an insurance company, a large business, or a union contracts with a group of doctors (the PPO) to provide services to its members at discounted prices. You aren't forced to use the PPO doctors, but it is certainly to your financial advantage to do so. Since PPOs are a recent invention and contain elements of both traditional plans and HMOs, they have fallen through regulatory cracks in some states and are not as carefully monitored as other health plans.

Choosing a Plan That's Right for You

"Can you believe it," one of my Columbia University colleagues, Jason G., groused one morning. "Now, they're giving us six different options to choose from. As nearly as I can figure out, I have to choose between a traditional plan with three different options, two health maintenance organizations, and one other — I can't understand what it is — maybe a PPO. How do I know what to do? Maybe I'll just stick with what I've got."

This is not a surprising reaction to health planning these days. We are bombarded with a dizzying array of choices and not given the tools to make decisions. If Mr. G., a professor of public health, couldn't understand the options, what hope is there for people less savvy than he about health care?

Once you cut through the jargon, however, the reasons to decide on one health plan over another become comparatively clear. As a general rule, traditional fee-for-service plans give you complete freedom to choose your doctor but cost more than HMOs and PPOs. Their focus on hospitalization and curing sickness is not to everybody's liking. Critics say that the traditional system leads to unnecessary surgery and tests. In contrast, HMOs and PPOs may restrict your choice of doctor, but they cost less than the traditional plans. Almost all HMOs and some PPOs cover preventive as well as curative care.

Whether HMOs and PPOs offer the same quality of care as traditional fee-for-service plans is still hotly debated. According to New York University law professor Sylvia Law, "Incentives for economy can also be incentives for no care or inferior care." Others argue that HMOs and PPOs eliminate *unnecessary* surgical operations and that the quality of their care is every bit as good as that of the traditional system. A twelve-year study by the RAND Corporation concluded that people who got their health care through HMOs were no less healthy than those who did not.

Choosing a health plan is very much an individual decision. If you adore your family doctor who belongs to neither an HMO nor a PPO, you have only one option — traditional fee-for-service insurance. Similarly, if you need a lot of care from specialists and do not want the potential obstacle of a gatekeeper approving referrals,

TABLE 1

Comparing Traditional Insurance, HMOs, and PPOs

Traditional Plans	HMOs	PPOs
Patient Choice		
Patient has complete choice of doctor. There may be restrictions, e.g., pre-approval of surgery, required second opinions, and length of hospitalization approved by a review committee.	Patient chooses primary physician from a panel of HMO-approved doctors. Primary physician refers patient to specialists when necessary.	Strong financial incentives limit choice of doctors to those associated with the PPO.
Cost		
Generally, more expensive than HMOs and PPOs. Patient pays doctor and is reimbursed by the insurance company. Patient is responsible for payment of deductible and coinsurance up to a certain dollar limit. There is also the hassle of dealing with insurance forms.	Monthly fee covers all care. Sometimes there is a nominal charge (say, $5.00) for visits to doctor's office. No insurance forms to fill out.	Patient pays for visits to the doctor as in a traditional plan. But only PPO-affiliated doctors offer the advantage of discounted prices.
Coverage		
Covers sickness-related care: hospitals, doctors. Catastrophes and visits to doctors' offices may be covered by major medical. Excludes preventive care such as well-baby checkups, vaccinations, routine physicals, birth control.	Monthly payment includes all covered medical and hospital care, including preventive care. HMOs often encourage antismoking, stress reduction, weight loss, and other health improvement programs.	Coverage depends on the specific plan. Some PPOs offer broad coverage similar to that of HMOs.
Quality of Care		
Incentives are to care for sick people — to hospitalize them — and to order more extensive and costly tests. Saving money doesn't count to the same extent it does in HMOs and PPOs. Critics cite the hazards of unnecessary surgery.	Incentives to keep people out of hospitals and to stress disease prevention and health promotion. Critics contend that incentives for doctors to keep costs down might lead them to skimp on care.	Some critics have asked whether cut-rate prices mean cut-rate service.

traditional insurance is likely to be your choice. If, on the other hand, you have young children who need frequent checkups and vaccinations, you might opt for an HMO.

Table 1 summarizes the key elements and pros and cons of the three major kinds of health plans available. Before deciding, examine your needs carefully. Then look at the comparisons in the table and the checklists that follow. They will help you make the right choice of the best health plan for you and your family.

CHECKLIST: CHOOSING
TRADITIONAL HEALTH INSURANCE

- **Are hospital charges completely covered?** A good policy offers complete coverage of a semiprivate room, food, nursing care, lab tests, and other hospital charges. You should have to pay only for miscellaneous items such as the telephone and television. If your plan pays for a certain number of days in a hospital, it should be at least 120 days and be backed up by a major medical policy.

  Beware of a specified dollar maximum per year, which you could easily exhaust, or, even worse, a specified dollar amount per "spell of illness" (meaning insurance won't cover you again until you've been out of the hospital for a period of time, perhaps up to six months).

- **How much is the deductible?** Once you are enrolled in a plan, insurance companies require you to pay your medical bills each year up to a certain amount before your coverage starts — the deductible. The amount you have to pay is usually $100 to $200 per person, with a family cap, although we know of deductibles that go up to $2,000. The higher the deductible the lower the premium you pay. As a general rule, choose the highest deductible you can afford to keep premium charges down.

- **How much of the doctors' fees are covered?** Most policies pay 80 percent of a doctor's "usual, customary, or reasonable" charges based on a formula intelligible only to the insurance company. After you have paid the annual deductible, you are responsible for the remaining 20 percent — the coinsurance — of the doctor's bill. You may have to pay more if the amount the doctor charges is more than the insurance company considers reasonable.

• **What is and is not covered?** Most policies cover only sick care. They do not pay for such preventive care as routine physicals, vaccinations, screening (for example, for breast cancer and glaucoma), and birth control. Check to see whether your policy covers the following:

> Prescription drugs — an important and increasingly common benefit. You often have to pay the first $3.00 or $5.00, but your insurance covers the rest.
>
> Nursing care — *remember that health insurance policies do not cover custodial care in a nursing home.*
>
> Home health care
>
> Hospice care
>
> Mental health care, both inpatient and outpatient
>
> Vision care
>
> Dental work
>
> Ambulance
>
> Durable medical equipment, such as wheelchairs and oxygen tents
>
> Drug- and alcohol-abuse treatment
>
> Outpatient surgery, care, and treatment
>
> Intensive and coronary care units at their full rate
>
> Chiropractors, acupuncturists, and other nonphysicians
>
> Maternity benefits

Check the "Exclusions" section of your policy carefully to find out what is *not* covered. If items such as dental care and eyeglasses are excluded, don't worry. Few companies pay for them.

• **What is the limit on my out-of-pocket costs?** After you have paid your deductible and a specified amount of coinsurance, your insurance should cover 100 percent of all medical costs. This is a *stop-loss* clause in insurance company jargon. If a stop-loss is not written into your policy, you could be liable for unlimited medical expenses.

• **What is the maximum lifetime coverage?** A serious illness can wipe you out financially. Make sure your lifetime coverage is at least $500,000; a million is even better.

- **When does coverage begin?** Some policies specify a thirty- or sixty-day waiting period. Others are in effect when you sign. Make sure to ask about this. Find out when coverage for pregnancy begins if that is a consideration.
- **What is the company's policy about pre-existing conditions?** Insurance companies don't like to insure sick people. If you had a recent illness or have a chronic condition, you may be turned down altogether or have to wait until you can be covered for your condition.
- **How long are children covered?** Coverage of children usually ends on their nineteenth birthday. If your children are in college, check to see whether they are covered.
- **What are the restrictions on hospitalization and surgery?** You want to know whether nonemergency stays in a hospital must be approved in advance, whether second opinions prior to surgery are required, and whether the length of your stay in the hospital is determined by a review committee.
- **How much does the policy cost?** Knowing the premium for one year gives only temporary peace of mind. Although insurance premiums are often regulated by state governments, they are frequently raised by astronomical amounts. After Phillip M., a freelance photographer, left his job in 1982, he bought a health insurance policy for which he paid $400 a year. By 1988 his premiums had risen to $1,600 a year. Then he had a back operation. When his premiums jumped to $4,600 annually, he changed to Blue Cross–Blue Shield during an open enrollment period. His new rates were $2,400 a year. But a year later, the premiums rose to $2,800 a year. "They are now threatening to raise them to $4,400 a year," he says, which will put him right back to the postoperation rates. "You just don't win." Yet he is relieved that he is insured. Without open enrollment, he isn't sure he could be. "Nobody wants to insure a person with a back problem," he says.
- **Do you have the right to renew?** Few companies guarantee renewal of your coverage. Most policies are "conditionally

renewable," which means that the company can refuse to renew your policy only if it cancels all other similar policies in the state. That at least provides some protection because the company can't single you out. It doesn't, however, protect you against increased premiums.

- **Is the insurance company financially sound?** With some insurance companies having gone the way of S&Ls, it's vital to check the financial health of a potential insurer. There are companies that rate insurers. The major ones are A. M. Best, (900) 420-0400 (the charge is $2.50 per minute); Standard and Poor's, (212) 208-1527; Moody's Investors Service, (212) 553-0377; and Duff & Phelps, (312) 368-5500. A newcomer is Weiss Research, (800) 289-9222 (the charge is $15 per report). The same information is also available at some public libraries. Buy only from a company given a top rating by two of these firms.

CHECKLIST: DOS AND DON'TS FOR BUYING TRADITIONAL HEALTH INSURANCE

If you decide to go with a traditional insurance policy, paying attention to a number of "dos and don'ts" can help protect you and save you money.

- *Do* **buy a group policy if possible.** It saves money over an individual policy.
- *Do* **take advantage of the "free look" provision when you receive a policy.** Most companies let you examine the document for at least ten days and refund your premium if the policy is not for you.
- *Don't* **replace a policy just because you think it is out of date.** Switching may subject you to new exclusions and waiting periods. Be aware that agents get a hefty commission for new enrollees. If you do switch, don't cancel your old policy until your new one has become effective.
- *Don't,* **on the other hand, keep policies merely because you've had them a long time.** You get no credit for being a loyal customer.
- *Don't* **try to profit by carrying overlapping policies.** If you

have two policies — which is expensive and wasteful — the companies will combine their benefits and limit your reimbursement to a maximum of 100 percent. It's known as *coordination of benefits.*

- *Do* **purchase major medical along with your basic hospital/ medical policy.** The Health Insurance Association of America says that the most important feature of a policy is to protect you in case of catastrophic illness, which is what a good major medical does.
- *Don't* **purchase dread-disease policies, such as cancer insurance.** The National Insurance Consumers Organization says they are an expensive rip-off with limited benefits. Your primary policy should cover catastrophic illness.
- *Don't* **hide an illness or condition that could lead to your application being denied.** If the insurer discovers your "mistake" within two years — the usual length of an "incontestable clause" — it can fight your claims and perhaps cancel the policy.
- *Don't* **pay cash.** Always pay your insurance premiums with a check, a money order, or a bank draft. Make the check payable to the insurance company, not the agent.
- *Do* **ask questions beforehand.** If you aren't sure about what's covered, ask. It's better to know that maternity benefits or pre-existing conditions are not included before you sign than be zonked by a huge bill later.
- *Do* **put everything in writing.** A telephone answer to your question is not worth the paper it's (not) written on.

CHECKLIST: CHOOSING AN HMO OR A PPO

Not all health maintenance or preferred provider organizations are the same. Before you sign up, visit the facility or the office of the primary physician. Talk to patients. Get a feel for the place. Then use the following questions to help you decide if it's right for you.

- **Is my primary physician board certified or board eligible? What about the specialists I am most likely to use?** Board certification or eligibility is no guarantee of quality medical care, but it is considered an objective indicator of a doctor's qualifications (see Chapter 2).

It's a good idea to call a specialist or two to make sure they really are available to subscribers. When the daughter of one of my students tore her shoulder, she went to her HMO in New York City. Her primary physician, a gynecologist, gave her a list of orthopedic surgeons supposedly affiliated with the HMO. My student, who is a nurse, carefully checked the credentials of all eight physicians on the list and narrowed the choice to the top three orthopedists. She then discovered that all three no longer operate on any HMO patients. Her daughter was forced to go to one of the other listed surgeons, whom her mother considered second rate.

- **Is the HMO or PPO affiliated with a good hospital?** It's not scientific or objective, but word of mouth tells a lot about a hospital's reputation. Hospitals affiliated with university medical centers are generally a good bet. At the very least, you want the hospital to be certified by the Joint Commission on Accreditation of Healthcare Organizations.
- **Is the organization accredited by a recognized professional organization or considered "qualified" by the U.S. government?** Two private organizations set standards for HMOs and accredit those that maintain their standards: the National Committee for Quality Assurance and the American Association for Ambulatory Health Care. The American Accreditation Programs, Inc., accredits PPOs. Accreditation by one of these groups is akin to receiving a *Good Housekeeping* seal of approval. It indicates that the HMO or PPO has met the qualifications for patient care, management capability, and financial stability. Accreditation is not a guarantee of quality, but it is probably the best indicator available.

About three-quarters of all HMOs are "federally qualified," that is, they comply with the quality-control standards of the federal government. The standards of the federal government are not as rigorous as those of the accrediting agencies. Nonetheless, it is an additional way to measure quality. If the HMO you are considering is not federally qualified, ask why.

- **How strong are the organization and management?** This is hard to discover, but important to know, particularly in the case of PPOs, which often are loosely regulated by state governments. "You want to know that there's really an organization out there, not just a bunch of guys operating out of a back room," says Douglas Elden, a Chicago attorney specializing in PPOs. He suggests that you ask, "How many doctors are affiliated with the organization? How many other employees are there? What is the turnover rate? How long has the organization been in business? What other HMOs or PPOs does the company administer?"

- **Is the HMO or PPO in good financial health?** Don't assume that size or popularity indicates a solid financial base. "Ask the state insurance department how sound an HMO or PPO is," suggests Margaret O'Kane, executive director of the National Committee for Quality Assurance. And request a copy of the company's latest annual report. If you're not an expert at deciphering data, ask a knowledgeable friend to interpret.

- **Can I choose my own doctor?** Remember that you have to give up your family doctor unless he or she is part of the HMO or PPO. Once you sign up, most of your contact will be with the primary physician who will be in charge of your basic health needs. It's vital that you like and trust him or her.

- **Is routine care given by the doctor or delegated to nurse practitioners or physician's assistants?** HMOs and PPOs are characterized by doctors' heavy reliance on nurse practitioners, physician's assistants, and other health aides for routine matters. Depending on your personal preferences, this could be a blessing or a curse.

- **Are there incentives that would lead doctors to skimp on care?** Remember that HMOs (and some PPOs) make money by cutting back on unnecessary surgery and excessive tests. You want to be sure, however, that you get *necessary* surgery and tests and that financial considerations do not influence your doctor's medical judgment. It may be hard to get a straight answer, but ask whether doctors are rewarded for keeping their patients out of the hospital and not ordering tests.

- **How long does it take to get an appointment?** Long delays for routine care and elective surgery are one of the big complaints about HMOs. Ask patients about their experiences.
- **Does the HMO or PPO offer a full range of such preventive health services as nutrition and stress-reduction programs?** You should know exactly what preventive services are available.
- **What services are not covered?** Check to see whether dental, vision, psychological, drug- and alcohol-abuse, and contraceptive services are excluded.
- **Am I covered immediately for pre-existing conditions and pregnancy?** If you were ill or incapacitated shortly before joining an HMO or PPO, you may have to wait before your condition is covered. Similarly, prenatal and maternity care may not be covered immediately. Find out about the length of the waiting period.
- **How much does it cost?** In addition to the monthly fee, many HMOs charge a small amount for routine doctors' visits and prescriptions.
- **What happens if I need a doctor outside the HMO's or PPO's geographic area?** What if you get an upset stomach while on vacation in Florida? Or sprain your wrist on a slot machine in Las Vegas? Most HMOs and PPOs cover *emergency* treatment at a nonaffiliated facility either within or outside their geographic area. Some HMOs and PPOs allow you to see outside doctors if you first call for approval. Learning the policy beforehand can save you needless aggravation later.
- **In case of a disagreement, what is the grievance procedure?** How do you appeal a decision? Many HMOs and PPOs require you to settle differences through binding arbitration.

The COBRA's Bite: Retaining Coverage

What happens to your health insurance if you lose your job? Or your spouse through divorce or death? Not long ago, you had to join the ranks of the uninsured. But in 1986, Congress passed the COBRA (Consolidated Omnibus Budget Reconciliation Act), which gives some protection to those who are divorced, widowed, or recently unemployed and their dependent children. It applies to all employers (except religious groups) with twenty or more employees that provide group health insurance for their employees.

If you leave your job (unless you are fired for gross misconduct) or have your hours cut back so that you are no longer eligible for insurance, you have the right to keep your benefits in your company's group health plan for up to eighteen months. If you become disabled and can't work anymore, you have the same right for up to twenty-nine months. If you divorce, are legally separated, or your insured spouse dies, you have the right to continue participating in the company plan for up to thirty-six months. Children who lose their dependent status under the health plan — for example, by reaching the age of twenty — also have the right to thirty-six additional months of insurance coverage.

While COBRA benefits should give you peace of mind, the security of knowing you won't have to face medical catastrophes without insurance isn't free. If you decide to continue the insurance, *you must pay the full premiums, plus a 2 percent administration charge, yourself.* Although a company's group rate is cheaper than buying an individual policy, it may still be pricey.

If you are eligible for COBRA benefits, inform the "plan administrator" immediately. Don't delay. You have only a limited time to apply. Sometimes it is hard to find out who administers the plan. It may be the insurance company that manages the health plan or your company itself. If your company has one, check with its benefits officer. If there is any doubt in your mind, contact both your employer and the insurance company. Send all correspondence by certified mail, return receipt requested, and keep a copy for your records.

If you need information or run into problems claiming COBRA benefits, write or call the Older Women's League, 730 Eleventh

Street, NW, Suite 300, Washington, DC 20001, (202) 783-6686. The organization also assists younger women and men.

Many states have their own laws requiring employers to continue health insurance coverage. While they are similar to federal benefits for the most part, some extend broader coverage or are more generous than others. For example, Minnesota lets a divorced spouse continue coverage under the ex's group plan until he or she becomes covered under another plan.

COBRA benefits are a stop-gap measure. At most, they give you a three-year grace period while you shop for longer-term protection. Many companies give their employees the right to convert to an *individual* policy when they are no longer eligible to be members of the group. While an individual policy is more expensive and may offer fewer benefits than a group policy, it may be the best you can get, particularly if you have a condition that makes you a high risk. Ask the plan administrator about your right to convert to an individual policy — in writing.

If You Have Trouble Getting Health Insurance

A former dancer, Sari Pace is a personal trainer at a posh New York gym. Raised in South America, she can converse with her clients — who include well-known actors, models, stockbrokers, lawyers, and dancers — in three languages. A divorced mother of a teenaged girl, Ms. Pace frequents art galleries, museums, the ballet, and the opera. She is devoted to her daughter, who shows great promise as a ballerina and is enrolled at the School of American Ballet. Both Ms. Pace and her daughter are the sort of people who make New York such a mecca for people in the arts. And, like many others, neither Ms. Pace nor her daughter has any health insurance. Except for a brief period a few years ago, they have had no health coverage for the past decade.

"I always wanted it, but after my divorce I couldn't afford it," says Ms. Pace. "I had to choose between health insurance and enrolling my daughter in ballet class and private school. After all, she's not going to be this age forever. I couldn't do it all." What Ms. Pace did do was qualify for a real estate license a few years ago. "If the real estate market hadn't crashed, I would've had something extra. And because of the economy, the schools want everything up front. I had no room to breathe."

Ms. Pace is one of the 35 million people without health insurance. Most are employed by small companies that do not offer those benefits. A U.S. government survey found that almost half of uninsured workers were employed by firms with fewer than twenty-five employees. Small companies simply can no longer afford to pay the premiums. If somebody on the payroll gets sick, the next year's premiums shoot up, or the policy is canceled. Many workers for small businesses are not able to find or afford a health insurance policy.

Healthy people can usually find a company willing to sell them a health insurance policy. The premiums may be staggeringly high and go up every year, but if you can afford it, insurance is available. If you have been sick or are disabled, you may not be able to buy insurance at all. Virtually no private company and only a dozen or so Blue Cross groups sell policies to a person who has had heart disease, most forms of cancer, diabetes, stroke, adrenal disorder, or epilepsy — among other disqualifying conditions.

Still, a few options are available. As a start, you may be able to join a group in which membership entitles you to health benefits — for example, your school's alumni association or a professional association. This is not a panacea, however, as thousands of people discovered when New York's Blue Cross announced in 1991 that it was ending coverage of private associations throughout the state.

If group membership doesn't work, find out whether there are any insurance companies in the state with *open enrollment* periods. At such times the companies insure anyone, even those who have a pre-existing condition. You may have to wait before treatment of the pre-existing condition is covered, but it's better than nothing. Currently, Blue Cross–Blue Shield plans in twelve states — Alabama, Maryland, Massachusetts, Michigan, New Hampshire, New Jersey, New York, North Carolina, Pennsylvania, Rhode Island, Vermont, and Virginia — and the District of Columbia have open enrollment at some time during the year. Contact your state insurance department (see the last pages of this chapter for phone numbers) or the Blue Cross and Blue Shield Association, (312) 440-6000, for information about open enrollment.

As a last resort, you may be eligible to join a risk-sharing pool, now set up in twenty-five states. (As of early 1992, California, Colorado, Connecticut, Florida, Georgia, Illinois, Indiana, Iowa, Louisiana, Maine, Minnesota, Missouri, Montana, Nebraska, New Mexico, North Dakota, Oregon, Rhode Island, South Carolina, Tennessee, Texas, Utah, Washington, Wisconsin, and Wyoming had risk-sharing pools.) These pools enable otherwise uninsurable people to purchase health insurance. Although the requirements in each state are different, typically you must be a resident of the state and have been turned down for insurance by at least one company. If you are eligible for the pool, you are allowed to buy insurance for yourself and your family at a premium 25 to 50 percent higher than normal. It won't be cheap, but at least it's coverage. For information about a risk-sharing pool in your state, call or write your state insurance department.

Promises, Promises: Insurance after Retirement

For many years, companies used the lure of continued health benefits after retirement to attract high-quality employees and induce managers to accept early retirement. All that has changed. The high cost of health insurance, the large numbers of retirees, and new accounting regulations have led many companies to try to cut back on those golden handshakes.

Some early retirees find that they are stuck with higher deductibles or coinsurance payments than they had bargained for. Others, who counted on their retirement coverage as a generous supplement to Medicare, are disappointed to find that their benefits have been trimmed.

Big money is involved in retirees' benefits. The federal government's General Accounting Office estimates that private companies had committed themselves to pay retirement health benefits valued at more than $400 *billion*. No wonder that 60 percent of the companies surveyed by Hewitt Associates, an Illinois benefits consulting firm, were seriously considering raising the insurance premium contributions of retirees and one in twenty were thinking about eliminating health insurance for retirees altogether.

If you believe that your health benefits are about to be modified or terminated, take the following steps to protect yourself:

- Get a copy of your company's retirement plan. Scour the benefits section for clauses reserving the right of the company to modify or amend the medical plan. If there are none, the promise to provide health benefits may be legally binding.
- Look at past years' benefits handbooks for indications that the company had unequivocally committed itself to providing health benefits in retirement.
- As a last resort, contact a lawyer who has expertise in benefits or, at the least, labor relations.

If you are already retired and your ex-employer has scaled back promised health benefits, consider going to court to protect your interests. Many people have done so, including eighty-four thousand retirees who sued General Motors when the company tried to reduce their benefits. The outcome of a lawsuit is likely to depend on how the judge interprets the language of the contract or collective bargaining agreement.

Claiming Insurance Benefits

There's no getting away from it. Filing insurance claims is a royal pain — tedious, time-consuming, and if you get snowed under by an avalanche of bills, overwhelming. Some people hire others to do it for them. Kathleen Hogue, president of Mediform, a Cleveland, Ohio, company that fills out people's insurance forms for them, tells of clients coming to her in tears because they are so frustrated by the huge piles of bills — many of them from people they'd never heard of — covering the dining room table. Someone we know became so aggravated that she didn't file a claim for three years, even though *she* was owed money. More commonly, people file as best they can; many do not bother to read the insurance company's replies. This is a sure way to lose money.

CHECKLIST: FILING CLAIMS

• **Get an itemized statement of services from your doctor.** It should include at least the physician's name, the date, the diagnosis, and the nature of the services rendered. Make sure that the bill specifies the services it covers; something vague, like "consultation," is sure to be rejected.

• **File your claim quickly.** If you let too many bills pile up, you will eventually lose or forget some. The longer you wait to submit the claim, the longer the insurance company holds on to money that rightfully belongs to you.

• **Fill out the form accurately.** When you submit the claim:
   — Give only the information requested. In standard insurance forms, you have to fill out the top part of the page.
   — Sign and date the form in the place that says, "Patient's or authorized signature."
   — Do *not* sign the part that authorizes payment directly to the doctor unless he or she has agreed to accept assignment and you have not already paid the bill.
   — Staple or tape the doctor's bill to the form.

• **Make copies of the completed insurance form and medical bills before mailing them.** File your copies in a manila folder or something similar, and keep it where you can get your hands on it quickly.

• **Examine the insurance company's response** (usually a form called Explanation of Benefits or EOB for short). This is not always so easy to do. EOBs are often unintelligible or written in a language that only insurance people can understand. If the company requests more information, send it to them along with a copy of the Explanation of Benefits form.

• **If you don't understand something, call the insurance company.** If the company has an 800 number, use it (why should you have to pay to hold for a customer service representative — at daytime rates yet?). Call on a Tuesday, Wednesday, or Thursday to avoid the rush. Write down the name of the person you talk to.

• **Remember to submit the claim for major medical if it is separate from your base plan.** Most plans pay basic benefits

and major medical simultaneously. A few still require a separate submission for major medical.
- **If two insurance companies are involved, submit the claim to both.** Submit the claim first to the insurance company that has primary responsibility for it, normally your employer's or group's insurance carrier. When that company has disposed of the claim, send it to the second one.

Trouble with a Claim?

If a company turns down a claim that you believe is legitimate or pays you less than you are entitled to and a simple phone call doesn't solve the problem, take the following steps:

- Send a letter to the insurance company explaining your position and asking them to set forth theirs — in writing.
- This will probably set in motion a series of letters back and forth. Make sure to send all letters by certified mail, return receipt requested, to protect yourself against the claim that your letter never arrived. Keep a copy of all correspondence. *Never send your original policy or any original policy materials. Send copies.* If you talk to somebody on the phone or in person, note the person's name, the date, and the substance of the conversation. Keep everything in a file.
- If the matter cannot be resolved following the company's normal procedures for handling complaints, the next step is to contact your state insurance department. Ask for the section that assists consumers. Going to the insurance department does not guarantee that you will win, but it will at least put pressure on the company to respond to your complaint. When you write to the insurance department, enclose copies of all correspondence between you and the company. State the name of the company and your policy number at the top of your letter.
- If you still get no satisfaction, consult a lawyer who is knowledgeable in insurance matters. He or she should be able to let you know whether your case will stand up in court or before

an arbitration panel. See Chapter 14 for advice on finding a lawyer.

• If the situation is truly outrageous, contact your state representative and the local newspapers, radio, and television news. The media love a juicy story.

• Contact the National Insurance Consumers Organization (NICO), 121 North Payne Street, Alexandria, VA 22314, (703) 549-8050. Although NICO has too small a staff to represent individuals, the organization may be able to offer assistance or refer you to someone who can help.

STATE INSURANCE DEPARTMENTS

Note: If the address or phone number of your state insurance department has changed or you have difficulty locating it, contact the National Association of Insurance Commissioners, 120 West 12th Street, Kansas City, MO 64105, (816) 842-3600, for the current listing.

Alabama
Insurance Commissioner
135 South Union Street
Montgomery, AL 36104
(205) 269-3550

Alaska
Director of Insurance
P.O. Box D
Juneau, AK 99811
(907) 465-2515

Arizona
Director of Insurance
3030 North Third Street
Phoenix, AZ 85012
(602) 255-5400

Arkansas
Insurance Commissioner
400 University Tower Building
Little Rock, AR 72204
(501) 686-2900

California
Commissioner of Insurance
100 Van Ness Avenue
San Francisco, CA 94102
(415) 557-1126

3450 Wilshire Boulevard
Los Angeles, CA 90010
(213) 736-2572

One City Centre Building
770 L Street
Sacramento, CA 95814
(916) 445-5544

45 Fremont Street
San Francisco, CA 94105
(415) 904-5410

Colorado
Commissioner of Insurance
1560 Broadway
Denver, CO 80204
(303) 866-6274

Connecticut
Insurance Commissioner
P.O. Box 816
Hartford, CT 06142
(203) 297-3802

Delaware
Insurance Commissioner
841 Silver Lake Boulevard
Dover, DE 19901
(302) 739-4251

District of Columbia
Superintendent of Insurance
613 G Street, NW
Washington, DC 20001
(202) 727-7424

Florida
Insurance Commissioner
Plaza Level Eleven — The Capitol
Tallahassee, FL 32399-0300
(904) 922-3110
toll free in state:
(800) 342-2762

Georgia
Insurance Commissioner
2 Martin L. King, Jr., Drive
Atlanta, GA 30334
(404) 656-2056

Hawaii
Insurance Commissioner
1010 Richards Street
Honolulu, HI 96811
(808) 586-2790

Idaho
Director of Insurance
500 South 10th Street
Boise, ID 83610
(208) 334-2250

Illinois
Director of Insurance
320 West Washington Street
Springfield, IL 62767
(217) 782-4515

100 W. Randolph Street
Chicago, IL 60601
(312) 814-2420

Indiana
Commissioner of Insurance
311 West Washington Street
Indianapolis, IN 46204-2787
(317) 232-2385
toll free in state:
(800) 622-4461

Iowa
Insurance Commissioner
Lucas State Office Building
Des Moines, IA 50319
(515) 281-5705

Kansas
Commissioner of Insurance
420 S.W. 9th Street
Topeka, KS 66612
(913) 296-7801
toll free in state:
(800) 432-2484

Kentucky
Insurance Commissioner
229 West Main Street
Frankfort, KY 40602
(502) 564-3630

Louisiana
Commissioner of Insurance
950 North Fifth Street
Baton Rouge, LA 70801-9214
(504) 342-5900

Maine
Superintendent of Insurance
State House Station 34
Augusta, ME 04333
(207) 582-8707

Maryland
Insurance Commissioner
501 St. Paul Place
Baltimore, MD 21202
(401) 333-2520
toll free in state:
(800) 492-6116

Massachusetts
Commissioner of Insurance
280 Friend Street
Boston, MA 02114
(617) 727-7189

Michigan
Insurance Bureau
611 West Ottawa Street
Lansing, MI 48933
(517) 373-9273

Minnesota
Commissioner of Commerce
133 East Seventh Street
St. Paul, MN 55101
(612) 296-6848

Mississippi
Commissioner of Insurance
1804 Walter Sillers Building
Jackson, MS 39205
(601) 359-3569

Missouri
Director of Insurance
301 West High Street
Jefferson City, MO 65102-0690
(314) 751-4126

Montana
Commissioner of Insurance
126 North Sanders
Mitchell Building
Helena, MT 59601
(406) 444-2040
toll free in state:
(800) 332-6148

Nebraska
Director of Insurance
941 "O" Street
Lincoln, NE 68508
(402) 471-2201

Nevada
Commissioner of Insurance
1665 Hot Springs Road
Carson City, NV 89710
(702) 687-4270
toll free in state:
(800) 992-0900

New Hampshire
Insurance Commissioner
169 Manchester Street
Concord, NH 03301
(603) 271-2261
toll free in state:
(800) 852-3416

New Jersey
Commissioner
Department of Insurance
20 West State Street
Trenton, NJ 08625
(609) 292-5363

New Mexico
Superintendent of Insurance
PERA Building
P.O. Drawer 1269
Santa Fe, NM 87504-1269
(505) 827-4500

New York
Superintendent of Insurance
160 West Broadway
New York, NY 10013
(212) 602-0434
toll free in state:
(800) 342-3736

Agency Building One
Empire State Plaza
Albany, NY 12257
(518) 474-6600

North Carolina
Commissioner of Insurance
Dobbs Building
430 North Salisbury Street
Raleigh, NC 27611
(919) 733-7349

North Dakota
Commissioner of Insurance
Capitol Building
600 East Boulevard Avenue
Bismarck, ND 58505-0320
(701) 224-2440
toll free in state:
(800) 247-0560

Ohio
Director of Insurance
2100 Stella Court
Columbus, OH 43266-0566
(614) 644-2658
toll free in state:
(800) 282-4658

(policyholder services)
toll free in state:
(800) 843-8356
(fraud division)

Oklahoma
Insurance Commissioner
1901 North Walnut
Oklahoma City, OK 73105
(405) 521-2828
toll free in state:
(800) 522-0071

Oregon
Insurance Commissioner
21 Labor and Industries Building
Salem, OR 97310
(503) 378-4271

Pennsylvania
Insurance Commissioner
Strawberry Square
Harrisburg, PA 17120
(717) 787-5173

Rhode Island
Insurance Commissioner
233 Richmond Street
Providence, RI 02903-4237
(401) 277-2223

South Carolina
Insurance Commissioner
1612 Marion Street
Columbia, SC 29201
(803) 737-6117

South Dakota
Director of Insurance
910 East Sioux Avenue
Pierre, SD 57501-3940
(605) 773-3563

Tennessee
Commissioner of Insurance
500 James Robertson Parkway
Nashville, TN 37243-0565
(615) 741-2241
toll free in state:
(800) 342-4029

Texas
Commissioner of Insurance
333 Guadalupe Street
P.O. Box 14904
Austin, TX 78714-9104
(512) 475-2005
toll free in state:
(800) 236-8517

Utah
Commissioner of Insurance
3110 State Office Building
Salt Lake City, UT 84114-1201
(801) 538-3800

Vermont
Commissioner of Insurance
120 State Street
Montpelier, VT 05602
(802) 828-3301

Virginia
Commissioner of Insurance
1220 Bank Street
Richmond, VA 23219
(804) 786-7694
toll free in state:
(800) 552-7945

Washington
Insurance Commissioner
Insurance Building AQ21
Olympia, WA 98504
(206) 753-7301
toll free in state:
(800) 562-6900

West Virginia
Insurance Commissioner
2019 Washington Street, East
Charleston, WV 25305
(304) 348-3394
toll free in state:
(800) 642-9004

Wisconsin
Commissioner of Insurance
121 East Wilson
Madison, WI 53702
(608) 266-0102
toll free in state:
(800) 236-8517

Wyoming
Commissioner of Insurance
Herschler Building
122 West 25th Street
Cheyenne, WY 82002
(307) 777-7401

4

ON THE JOB

CONTENTS

APRIL 18, 1986, is a day neither Robin Meyerson nor her husband, Dennis, will ever forget. A New Jersey schoolteacher with a master's degree in reading, Mrs. Meyerson was traveling that morning between the two schools where she taught when a triaxle dump truck slammed into her car from behind. She ended up in a hospital with multiple injuries to her neck, head, and back. She had five operations and for four and a half months wore a "halo," a device mounted on her shoulders and bolted to her head. She was thirty-five years old.

Yet Mrs. Meyerson's injuries were only the beginning of her misery. When she applied to the school district's insurance carrier to collect workers' compensation, her odyssey of suffering began. "They paid the medical expenses for the first year and then told us to go to their doctor for more tests," says Mr. Meyerson, an accountant. "Then they said they wanted to find out how bad her injuries were." But when the results came back, the insurance company refused to pay any more. "They said, 'Sue us,'" says her husband.

Despite this, Mrs. Meyerson continued to see her own neurologist for treatment. But because the insurance company cut off her benefits, the hospital refused to treat her further. "She went from having an injury to having a major injury," says her husband. "Damage to her spine became irreparable."

In New Jersey, workers' compensation hearings are held only once every three weeks. As a result, cases drag on. And on. Mr. Meyerson estimates that his wife had more than twenty-two hearings. Finally, after five years, she won her case. But she has yet to see a penny. The insurance company immediately appealed. Mr. Meyerson expects that his wife's case will be decided by the state supreme court.

Mr. Meyerson estimates that his wife's medical expenses have come to more than $350,000. "She is totally incapacitated," he says. "And this was a schoolteacher who spent her life teaching the gifted and talented."

As the Meyersons' story indicates, it is not easy to be compensated if you are injured on the job. Every state has enacted a workers' compensation law, but benefits are low and claiming them can be a tremendous hassle. In some cases, a union will go to bat for you, but this is true only part of the time; to many unions, job security is more important than job safety. The four out of five Americans who are not union members are left pretty much to their own devices and are relatively vulnerable.

Nor is it easy to have a dangerous workplace fixed. Although Congress created the Occupational Safety and Health Administration in 1970 to get companies to clean up their act, the agency's performance has been disappointing. People have been fired for complaining about working conditions. "When you agree to take a job, you give up many of your basic civil rights," says Jim Moran, executive director of the Philadelphia Project on Occupational Safety and Health.

Despite this generally discouraging panorama, you can take some measures to protect yourself and there are places you can turn to for help. In this chapter we tell you what to do:

- if you are working in an unsafe or unhealthy workplace.
- if you are injured on the job and plan to claim workers' compensation.
- if you want to protect yourself beforehand by buying disability insurance or if you become disabled.
- if your company introduces a drug-testing program, ostensibly to improve workplace safety.

Protecting Yourself

Unsafe and Unhealthy Worksites

Every year, millions of workers are hurt on the job. A survey by the U.S. Bureau of Labor Statistics revealed that 6.8 million employees suffered job-related disabilities or injuries in 1990, the highest since 1972, when the bureau began collecting statistics. "As a form of violence, job casualties are statistically at least three times more serious than street crimes," writes Ralph Nader.

The Occupational Safety and Health Administration (OSHA) distinguishes "unsafe" from "unhealthy" working conditions. "Unsafe" conditions are those which threaten life or bodily injury, such as a boiler about to explode. Few can argue about these. However, a workplace that an employee considers hazardous may appear quite safe from management's perspective.

"Unhealthy" conditions are another matter. Arguments arise about which substances, and in what dosage, are unhealthy, particularly cancer-causing chemicals whose effects might not become apparent for twenty years or more. Tens of thousands of toxic chemicals in the nation's workplace need to be regulated, yet OSHA has produced full safety standards for only a small fraction of them.

People tend to think of job-related health in terms of industrial accidents — the unguarded chain saw that chops off a man's arm, the construction worker falling from a scaffold — or exposure to harmful substances such as coal dust, which causes black lung disease, or asbestos, which causes cancer. But these are not the whole story. Repetitive motion injuries, which can affect anyone from a tennis instructor who gets tennis elbow to a supermarket cashier who develops tendinitis, account for almost half of today's job-related injuries.

The Office as a Health and Safety Hazard

Office work, too, can be dangerous to your health. Indoor air pollution trapped inside poorly ventilated office buildings can cause respiratory problems and other diseases. Doing something about "sick" buildings has become a high priority of occupational health experts.

Computers represent another potential health hazard. According to federal government statistics, 40 percent of all workplace injuries are linked to computers. Secretaries, data processors, telephone operators, and airline reservationists spend nearly their entire day sitting at one. They may develop several health problems from the work at the computer or from the stress of the job.

The first is back pain or wrist injury, the most common of which is carpal tunnel syndrome. This occurs when a nerve in the arm is compressed as it passes through the wrist bones or carpals and a ligament under the skin. The result is numbness, tingling, or pain in the fingers or hand. It is caused by sitting in the same position and repeating the same motion over long periods of time. If your hand or wrist bothers you, take it seriously. Carpal tunnel syndrome and other repetitive-motion injuries may require surgery. The problem can be alleviated by taking periodic breaks from the computer and using adjustable tables, chairs, and display screens.

The second major hazard is eyestrain from watching a computer monitor — video display terminal (VDT) — for a long time. Its symptoms are blurred or double vision and headaches. Proper lighting and equipment plus periodic breaks can relieve the symptoms, although some people have to wear special glasses when using a computer.

Concern about repetitive-motion injuries and computer-related eye problems have led to the development of a new field, ergonomics, which strives to make the work environment more user friendly to those who inhabit it. Developing ergonomically sound policies for office workers is among OSHA's highest priorities.

A third concern about computers is radiation. Studies have indicated higher rates of miscarriages in mice that have been exposed to radiation emitted by VDTs than in those that have not, but so far there is no conclusive evidence that such radiation causes miscarriages or birth defects in humans. The fact is that we simply do not know very much about the risk to human reproductive systems or the risk of cancer from VDTs.

Columbia University's Jeanne Stellman, a workplace health expert, says, "Currently, the overwhelming opinion of scientists is that VDTs do not represent a threat to reproductive well-being." Her conclusion is buttressed by a study by the National Institute for Occupational Safety and Health, a federal agency established in 1970 to conduct research on making the workplace safer. The 1991 study found no relation between VDT use by pregnant women and miscarriage. Despite this, doubts remain. Louis Slesin, editor of *VDT News*, offers some practical tips to reduce risks of radiation from VDTs. Keep the computer at arm's length. Turn it off when you're not using it. Most important, he says, stay away from the sides and backs of computers, where most radiation originates.

San Francisco and Suffolk County, New York, passed laws regulating VDT use. San Francisco required employers to provide proper lighting and adjustable chairs and tables. The city also mandated fifteen-minute rest breaks after two hours of VDT use and periodic training of office employees. The Suffolk County law went one step further by requiring employers to pay 80 percent of the cost of annual eye examinations for VDT users and eyeglasses for those who need them. Both laws were struck down by the courts on the grounds that cities and counties did not have the authority to pass this legislation.

What to Do If You Work in a Dangerous Place

Tell Your Company

If you are represented by a union, see your union representative. Since working conditions are usually part of a labor-management contract, it is the union's responsibility to fight for you. Some unions, such as the Oil, Chemical and Atomic Workers Union, go to great lengths to protect their workers. Others are more reluctant.

If you do not have a union to fight your battle, you may have to do it yourself. Advise your company of the health or safety problem. Under federal and state right-to-know laws, a company must inform its employees of hazardous chemicals in the workplace and their potential effect. Remember, however, that you may be risking your job by complaining too loudly. A complaint to OSHA, which will keep your name confidential, might be safer. Addresses and phone numbers of regional offices are provided in this chapter.

Before complaining to the company, you may be well advised to seek guidance from a Committee on Occupational Safety and Health (COSH) (see next page) or to get the opinion of an industrial hygienist, an expert in occupational hazards. Contact the American Industrial Hygiene Association, 345 White Pond Drive, Akron, OH 44311, (216) 873-2442, or the American Board of Industrial Hygiene, 4600 West Saginaw, Lansing, MI 48917, (517) 321-2638, for a referral.

Call a COSH

Let's say you work in a totally controlled new high-rise office building. It's air-conditioned in summer, heated in winter, the windows don't open, and no fresh air enters. For months you have had a nagging headache and sore throat. You suspect that bad air may be making you sick but do not know how to find out or whom to call. Then, coincidentally, you see a local television news program on sick buildings. The name and phone number of a Committee for Occupational Safety and Health flashes on the screen for a few seconds. You call and are advised what to do and referred to a doctor specializing in occupational medicine.

Calls like this actually jammed the phone lines of the New York Committee on Occupational Safety and Health (NYCOSH). According to Joel Shufro, the committee's director, more than six hundred people called NYCOSH after its phone number appeared on the screen during such a news special.

NYCOSH is one of twenty-four Committees on Occupational Safety and Health and four COSH-related groups throughout the United States. They are nonprofit organizations whose goal is to help prevent worker injury, disease, and death. COSH groups can give advice on identifying and controlling toxic substances in the workplace and recommend doctors specializing in occupational medicine and lawyers with expertise in workplace law.

A list of COSH groups follows. Jim Moran says that his group (PhilaPOSH) will provide assistance to those who cannot locate a nearby COSH.

COMMITTEES ON OCCUPATIONAL SAFETY AND HEALTH

COSH Groups

Alaska
Alaska Health Project
431 W. 7th Avenue, #101
Anchorage, AK 99501
(907) 276-2864

California
San Francisco–Bay Area COSH
Labor Occupational Health Program
School of Public Health
University of California at Berkeley
2515 Channing Way
Berkeley, CA 94720
(510) 642-5507

Los Angeles COSH (LACOSH)
2501 S. Hill Street
Los Angeles, CA 90007
(213) 383-4416

Sacramento COSH (SACOSH)
c/o Fire Fighters, Local 522
3101 Stockton Boulevard
Sacramento, CA 95820
(916) 924-8060

Santa Clara COSH (SCCOSH)
760 N. First Street
San Jose, CA 95112
(408) 998-4050

Connecticut
Connecticut COSH (ConnCOSH)
P.O. Box 31107
Hartford, CT 06103
(203) 549-1877

District of Columbia
Alice Hamilton Occupational
  Health Center
410 Seventh Street, SE
Washington, DC 20003
(202) 543-0005

Illinois
Chicago Area COSH (CACOSH)
37 South Ashland Avenue
Chicago, IL 60607
(312) 666-1611

Maine
Maine Labor Group on Health
Box V
Augusta, ME 04330
(207) 622-7823

Massachusetts
Massachusetts COSH (MassCOSH)
241 St. Botolph Street, Room 227
Boston, MA 02115
(617) 524-6686

Western MassCOSH
458 Bridge Street
Springfield, MA 01103
(413) 247-9413

Michigan
Southeast Michigan COSH
  (SEMCOSH)
2727 Second Street
Detroit, MI 48206
(313) 961-3345

New York
Alleghany COSH (ALCOSH)
100 East Second Street
Jamestown, NY 14701
(716) 488-0720

Central New York COSH
  (CNYCOSH)
615 W. Genessee Street
Syracuse, NY 13204
(315) 471-6187

Eastern New York COSH
  (ENYCOSH)
c/o Larry Rafferty
121 Erie Boulevard
Schenectady, NY 12305
(518) 393-1386

New York COSH (NYCOSH)
275 Seventh Avenue, 8th Floor
New York, NY 10001
(212) 627-3900

Rochester COSH (ROCOSH)
502 Lyell Avenue, Suite #1
Rochester, NY 14606
(716) 548-8553

Western New York COSH
  (WNYCOSH)
450 Grider Street
Buffalo, NY 14215
(716) 897-2110

North Carolina
North Carolina COSH (NCCOSH)
P.O. Box 2514
Durham, NC 27705
(919) 286-9249

Pennsylvania
Philadelphia POSH (PhilaPOSH)
3001 Walnut Street, 5th Floor
Philadelphia, PA 19104
(215) 386-7000

Rhode Island
Rhode Island COSH (RICOSH)
340 Lockwood Street
Providence, RI 02907
(401) 751-2015

Tennessee
Tennessee COSH (TNCOSH)
1515 East Magnolia, Suite 406
Knoxville, TN 37917
(615) 525-3147

Texas
Texas COSH (TexCOSH)
c/o Karyl Dunson
5735 Regina
Beaumont, TX 77706
(409) 898-1427

Wisconsin
Wisconsin COSH (WisCOSH)
1334 S. 11th Street
Milwaukee, WI 53204
(414) 643-0928

COSH-related Groups

Louisiana
Labor Studies Program
Institute of Human Relations
Loyola University
Box 12
New Orleans, LA 70118
(504) 861-5830

New Jersey
New Jersey Work Environment
    Council
452 East Third Street
Moorestown, NJ 08057
(609) 866-9405

Ohio
Greater Cincinnati Occupational
    Health Center
2450 Kipling Avenue, Suite 203
Cincinnati, OH 45239
(513) 541-0561

West Virginia
Institute of Labor Studies
710 Knapp Hall
West Virginia University
Morgantown, WV 26506
(304) 293-3323

Another source of advice is the National Safe Workplace Institute, 122 South Michigan Avenue, Suite 1450, Chicago, IL 60603, (312) 939-0690.

Complain to OSHA

OSHA is empowered to issue health and safety standards for businesses. It can inspect worksites and fine companies that violate federal standards, including a general standard that requires employers to provide a workplace free of "recognized hazards" that can cause death or serious physical injury. The Occupational Safety and Health Act permits states to pass their own occupational safety and health laws if they are as tough as the federal law. Twenty states have OSHA-approved plans covering public- and private-sector employees and two states, Connecticut and New York, have OSHA-approved plans covering public employees only.

The law authorizes OSHA to inspect a worksite if an employee has a valid complaint, but be prepared to wait. Complaints are investigated by category. First priority is assigned to life-threatening dangers, such as a leaking gas pipe, which must be investigated within twenty-four hours. Second priority goes to incidents that have led to a death or the hospitalization of at least five people. Employee complaints rank third. Spokesperson Susan Fleming says that OSHA investigates signed, written complaints that it feels have merit on the basis of their importance, the number of people affected, the agency's priorities, and the availability of inspectors. OSHA has fewer than fifteen hundred inspectors to police more than 5 million worksites, so don't hold your breath waiting for a visit.

Despite the difficulty in getting OSHA to carry out an investigation, a complaint can be worthwhile. At the very least, it should trigger a letter from OSHA ordering the company to investigate the hazard and to report back to the agency. If you decide to lodge a complaint, write to the OSHA office in your region (see the list of OSHA's regional offices below) and include the following information:

- Your company's name and address
- The nature of the problem in as much detail as you can give
- How long the situation has gone on
- What, if anything, has been done to correct the problem
- Your name. This is important. OSHA will keep your identity confidential if you ask them, but must have it to consider your complaint a "formal" one. OSHA handles anonymous com-

plaints merely by sending a letter to the company advising that the agency has been notified of a problem.

• A place where OSHA can contact you — probably your home address

The Occupational Safety and Health Act is supposed to protect people who file complaints against retaliation by their companies. In practice, companies routinely punish employees who they find have lodged such a complaint. If you fear retaliation, be sure to request that OSHA not reveal your name.

If you have been punished for complaining to OSHA, you have few options, because only OSHA can sue on your behalf. Except in some states that administer their own plans, you do not have the right to sue the company yourself. Send a letter to OSHA — certified mail, return receipt requested — setting forth what happened. The law gives you thirty days from the time you were fired or punished to lodge a complaint. OSHA will investigate and try to arrange a settlement. If that fails, it might eventually bring a lawsuit on your behalf for reinstatement and back pay.

OSHA should be the place to turn for protection against a hazardous work environment. However, "OSHA's enforcement is ineffective," says Ilise Feitshans, an expert in occupational health law at Columbia University. "OSHA has become toothless because it gets so little support from Congress and the White House budget."

Companies have little incentive to comply with the law, and the financial penalties for noncompliance are, with few exceptions, a slap on the wrist — a small cost of doing business. Joseph Kinney, director of the National Safe Workplace Institute, tells of his brother, a construction worker who fell to his death when a scaffold collapsed. The company was fined only $800 for eight violations of the Occupational Safety and Health Act.

This may change. For the first time since 1971, penalties and fines have been increased. In 1991, maximum fines for violations that might cause death or grave physical injury jumped from $1,000 to $7,000. For "willful" violations, involving an employer who knew about and did nothing to correct extremely dangerous conditions, the penalty was raised from $10,000 to $70,000. Since a company can be charged with many violations per employee, penalties can take a big bite out of the assets of an organization with a large work force.

OCCUPATIONAL SAFETY AND HEALTH ADMINISTRATION
1825 K STREET, NW
WASHINGTON, DC 20006
(212) 634-7943

Regional Offices

Note: States and territories whose names are in italics operate their own OSHA-approved job safety and health programs (Connecticut and New York plans cover public employees only). States with approved programs must have a standard that is identical to, or at least as effective as, the federal standard.

Region 1
Connecticut, Massachusetts, Maine, New Hampshire, Rhode Island, *Vermont*
133 Portland Street
Boston, MA 02114
(617) 565-7164

Region 2
New Jersey, *New York*, Puerto Rico, *Virgin Islands*
201 Varick Street
New York, NY 10014
(212) 337-2378

Region 3
District of Columbia, Delaware, *Maryland*, Pennsylvania, *Virginia*, West Virginia
Gateway Building
3535 Market Street
Philadelphia, PA 19104
(215) 596-1201

Region 4
Alabama, Florida, Georgia, *Kentucky*, Mississippi, *North Carolina, South Carolina, Tennessee*
1375 Peachtree Street, NE
Atlanta, GA 30367
(404) 347-3573

Region 5
Illinois, *Indiana, Michigan*, Ohio, Wisconsin
230 South Dearborn Street
Chicago, IL 60604
(312) 353-2220

Region 6
Arkansas, Louisiana, *New Mexico*, Oklahoma, Texas
525 Griffin Street
Dallas, TX 75202
(214) 767-4731

Region 7
Iowa, Kansas, Missouri, Nebraska
911 Walnut Street
Kansas City, MO 64106
(816) 426-5861

Region 8
Colorado, Montana, North Dakota,
  South Dakota, *Utah, Wyoming*
Federal Building
1961 Stout Street
Denver, CO 80294
(303) 844-3061

Region 9
Arizona, California, Hawaii,
  Nevada
71 Stevenson Street
San Francisco, CA 94105
(415) 995-5672

Region 10
Alaska, Idaho, *Oregon, Washington*
1111 Third Avenue
Seattle, WA 98101
(206) 442-5930

Contact Local Government Agencies

State, county, and city governments can pass laws governing the safety of the workplace. Storage of combustible substances or a blocked emergency exit may violate a local fire department ordinance; the use of toxic chemicals may violate environmental laws; an unsafe elevator may violate the building code; smoking on the job may violate health laws. Try calling the appropriate government agency. If in doubt about whom to contact, call the department of health first.

Contact the District Attorney

If an employer's willful or reckless disregard of worker safety caused death or serious injury, it may be possible to charge the management with murder or endangering lives. Since this involves a criminal charge, it can be brought only by the government, through a district attorney's office. A lawsuit won't help dead or seriously injured employees, but it might protect others.

OSHA has the authority to ask the Justice Department to prosecute company officials, but it rarely does. The Justice Department does not give OSHA cases a high priority. Only one person has been sent to jail for violating the Occupational Safety and Health Act.

Frustrated with OSHA's inability to deter companies from behavior harmful to worker safety, district attorneys in half a dozen states have charged officers and directors of companies with murder, assault, and other crimes. In Chicago, for example, three officers of the Film Recovery Company were convicted of manslaughter in 1985. Stephen Golab, an illegal immigrant from Poland, worked for more than a year stirring tanks of sodium cyanide at the company's poorly ventilated plant in Elk Grove, Illinois. His job was to extract silver from used film. One day, overcome by cyanide fumes, Golab went into convulsions, collapsed, and died. The district attorney for Cook County filed criminal charges against the company and three of its officers. The judge, finding that they had willfully deceived employees about the hazards of working with cyanide, supplied virtually no safety equipment, and provided woefully inadequate ventilators, sentenced each of them to twenty-five years in prison.

Can You Refuse to Work under Hazardous Conditions?
As a general rule, you cannot refuse to work in unsafe or unhealthy conditions. You run the risk of being fired for doing it, even though it may save your life. Under OSHA regulations, only one situation justifies refusing to work in a dangerous environment — a reasonable belief that the conditions pose an imminent danger to life or safety and cannot be remedied in time to forestall disaster. When two workers in a Whirlpool manufacturing plant refused orders to walk on a wire mesh screen 20 feet above the floor shortly after one of their fellow employees fell to his death through a weak spot in the screen, they were reprimanded for insubordination. They sued the company for unlawful discrimination, and the case went all the way to the Supreme Court. Upholding their claim in 1980, Justice Stewart wrote that OSHA's regulations do no more than "permit employees to avoid workplace conditions that they believe pose grave dangers to their own safety."

Except in the most drastic circumstances, such as exposure to life-threatening poisonous gases, you will have a hard time justifying a refusal to work. "These are tough cases to win," says Mark Lerner, an attorney with OSHA. "If you're thinking about walking off the job, make sure you're right."

Workers' Compensation: If You're Injured

When Richard Hall, a forty-year-old machine operator with the Bostich company in Rhode Island, slipped on some oil at work and severely injured his back, he claimed workers' compensation. According to Mr. Hall, the firm's insurance company paid him benefits for one month, then stopped payments without any warning or reason and fought him every step of the way for the next year. For another sixty-five weeks, Mr. Hall did not receive any compensation. His medical bills went unpaid, his house was nearly repossessed, and he saw so many doctors and appeared in so many workers' compensation hearings that he lost count. He hired a lawyer, but the attorney knew little about the intricacies of workers' compensation and did nothing for him.

Nearly destitute, Mr. Hall learned of the Injured Workers of Rhode Island. They got him a lawyer skilled in workers' compensation, helped save his house, and encouraged him to keep going. After more than a year, a workers' compensation board judge found in Mr. Hall's favor and ordered the insurance company to pay his medical costs and back pay to which he was entitled under the law. Mr. Hall, who still cannot perform physical labor, spends his time directing the National Coalition of Injured Workers, whose affiliates throughout the country try to help people avoid the situation he faced. (See the "Where to Turn for Help" section of this chapter for addresses and phone numbers.)

What Is Workers' Compensation?
There are five key points to workers' compensation:

- It is a *no-fault* system. To be compensated, you do not have to show that your employer caused your injury or was to blame in any way. The company's negligence is irrelevant. All you have to show is that you sustained an injury in your job.
- Injured workers cannot sue their employer (with few extremely limited exceptions, which we discuss later in this chapter). Even if you were hurt because of the gross negligence of your employer, you are not permitted to sue.
- Every state has its own workers' compensation law. Although there are many common features, each law is somewhat different.
- Workers' compensation pays medical bills, death benefits, and a portion of lost wages to disabled workers.
- Workers' compensation is your right.

Workers' compensation is a child of the Industrial Revolution. As workers moved from the farm to the factory, industrial accidents took an increasing toll. Workers had little chance of being compensated for their injuries. They could sue, but because the law favored employers, they were almost sure to lose. "There was blood on the workhouse floor. Tens of thousands of breadwinners were walking around wounded with no recourse, no safety net," says Maryland attorney David Blum, a workers' compensation expert. "That's the bad news. The good news is they could vote." In 1910, New York enacted the country's first workers' compensation law. Wisconsin followed one year later, and by 1949 every state had passed such a law.

The theory behind the workers' compensation system is simple — both employees and employers trade risk for certainty. Employees exchange the risk of going to court — which could result in a financial bonanza but is more likely to result in nothing — for the certainty of receiving limited compensation for injuries. Companies agree to pay job-related injury claims, whether or not it was their fault, and in return are assured that they will not be sued. The cost of workers' compensation is passed on to the consumer in the form of higher prices.

Although workers' compensation was created to simplify claims and eliminate the need for lawyers, it has evolved into a complicated, legalistic system that all too often pits an injured worker against an employer's insurance company. "Remember, workers' compensation is an adversarial system," says Joe Mays, a New Jersey truck driver who heads a group called VOCAL (Victims of Compensation Abuse of the Law). "Insurance companies are paid to stop your benefits, and they keep trying until you lose, you die, or you give up. If you plan to claim workers' compensation for anything other than the simplest injury, prepare for a long, hard, and discouraging fight."

Since you may be in for a battle if you claim workers' compensation, it is a good idea to seek the advice of a lawyer earlier rather than later. Ask friends and coworkers if they have had positive experience with attorneys in workers' compensation cases. If you have trouble locating a lawyer or need advice about a workers' compensation claim, contact a nearby COSH or Injured Workers

Association. (See lists in this chapter.) Chapter 14 contains additional advice on finding and talking to a lawyer.

Who Is Covered?

With a few exceptions, workers' compensation covers just about everybody who works. In a handful of states, the law does not cover farm workers, domestic workers, or employees of very small companies — fewer than three to five people. Federal government employees are covered by a separate law, as are longshoremen, railway workers, sailors, and coal miners.

What Is Covered?

The language of almost every state law is identical, compensating workers for "injuries by accident arising out of and in the course of employment." In simpler terms, the law compensates people for work-related injuries. To make a claim, you must show (1) that you were injured and (2) that your injury was work related.

You Were Injured

Many injuries are the result of an accident at work. These are the clearest situations. If the door to the office supply cabinet slams on your hand and breaks one of your fingers, it is obviously a work-related accident. However, many people are injured on the job even though no accident occurs. In the past, these injuries were not covered, but many now are, depending on the state and the specific circumstances.

One problem area is injuries that develop over time, as in the case of Mark Montoya, a Salt Lake City, Utah, shop foreman. Three years after he started his job, Mr. Montoya began feeling pains in his back — pains, he said in court documents, that were caused by his work designing and building cabinets. It turned out that part of his job involved lifting eighty-pound boards. The pain forced him to miss a week of work and see an orthopedist. He claimed workers' compensation for that week plus his doctors' bills. The insurance company contested and the state workers' compensation board turned down his claim because he could not pinpoint a specific time of injury. The Supreme Court of Utah reversed the board's decision, ruling that injuries which develop over a period of time should be covered.

Another problem situation is occupational illness, namely, disease caused by long exposure to toxic substances at work. Occupational claims run into difficulty because it is hard to prove that exposure to a toxic substance twenty-five years in the past caused an illness that has recently developed. Yet that's the length of the latency period for many cancers. Also, people who have been exposed to hazardous substances in several different jobs find it difficult to pinpoint the responsible party. Or their own behavior, such as smoking, may have caused or contributed to the illness.

Coverage of occupational diseases is minimal. The U.S. Department of Labor estimates that workers' compensation covers only 5 percent of the people injured by occupationally related diseases. States handle occupational illness claims in a variety of ways. Some simply list those diseases they cover (usually pretty restrictive). Others limit the time after exposure when an injured worker can file a claim. This becomes critical if, say, a worker exposed to a toxic substance develops initial, not particularly virulent symptoms of a disease just as the statute of limitations is running out.

Mental illness, another gray area, is of growing importance, as workplace stress is recognized to cause both physical and mental illness. The traditional rule that barred compensation for mental injuries unless accompanied by physical harm has been eroded in many states. Some, such as Arizona, require a worker to prove that mental illness was caused by unexpected, unusual, or extraordinary stress. In others, such as Alaska, Oregon, and Indiana, neither physical injury nor abnormal stress is a requisite. The Indiana case involved Sharon Jean Hansen, a woman with a deep fear of guns. According to court records, her supervisor, aware of her fear, would sneak up behind her and stick his finger in her ribs as if he were holding a gun, drop books that fell to the floor with a loud *bang*, and fire cap guns at her. One day he said something that caused Ms. Hansen to become hysterical. She fled from the office, unable to stand it any longer. Her doctor said she was disabled, based on his diagnosis of her condition as severe anxiety and depression. But the insurance company contested and the workers' compensation board denied her claim. The Indiana Supreme Court reversed the board's decision, finding that Ms. Hansen had indeed suffered a work-related injury, even though it was not a physical one, and was eligible for workers' compensation benefits.

The Injury Was Work-related

In addition to proving you were injured, you must prove that your injury is work related. You don't actually have to be injured at your place of work, although it helps. A worker who suffers a heart attack at his desk is more likely to collect workers' compensation benefits than one who keels over at the breakfast table.

Whether an injury is considered work related depends on the law of your state and the circumstances under which the injury occurs. Commuters beware. You are probably not covered for injuries incurred en route to and from your office, although once you reach your employer's parking lot you can breathe safely — you are considered to be at work.

Traveling sales staff are covered when they are on company business. In one case, a traveling salesman stopped his car to have a picnic lunch and picked some blackberries across the road. While crossing the highway, he fell into a ditch and hurt his ankle. An Alabama court found that the injury did not arise out of the course of his employment, since he was off on what it termed a "personal enterprise."

Many cases involve recreational activities — a company picnic or softball game. If they take place on company time or property — or the company is really involved — the injured worker is likely to be able to claim workers' compensation benefits. Richard Scott, who played shortstop for his company's softball team, suffered a broken elbow when hit by a relay from the left fielder. The workers' compensation board turned down his claim, ruling that his injury did not arise out of and in the course of his employment. He appealed and won. The court noted that the company supplied the uniforms, paid the league entrance fee, displayed a championship trophy in the lunchroom, and in general was quite involved in the team.

Benefits

Workers' compensation is like a comprehensive insurance policy with three kinds of coverage: life, medical, and disability.

Life Insurance

Workers' compensation pays benefits to dependents of workers who are killed by work-related injuries. Death benefits are paid according to a formula and subject to a maximum amount, which varies by state.

Medical Bills

Workers' compensation pays doctors' and hospital bills resulting from a work-related injury. In theory, you should not have to pay anything. In practice, if your claim is contested by an insurance company, you may not receive anything until it is settled, which, with lengthy delays and an extended appeals process, could take up to five years or more. In the meantime, doctors may hound you for payment.

Every state has different rules governing choice of doctors. In New York, you can go to any doctor you want. (Many doctors do not accept workers' compensation patients, however, because they don't like the paperwork, the aggravation with workers' compensation officials, the possibility of losing time in hearings, and the low levels of reimbursement.) In Virginia, your employer selects the doctor. In Pennsylvania, your employer must post a list of five doctors from which you pick one to treat you in the first fourteen days after your injury. After that, you can go to any doctor you want. "Avoid company doctors if you can," urges Eleanor Filoon of the Injured Workers of Pennsylvania. "They are paid to save the company money and will look for ways to send you back to work, even if you are disabled."

Disability

If a job-related injury causes you to miss work, workers' compensation reimburses part of your lost wages. The amount you receive depends on whether the injury is *partially disabling* (you can still work, although perhaps at a less strenuous job) or *totally disabling* (you can't work at all) and whether it is *temporary* or *permanent*. Four points to keep in mind:

Most states pay two thirds of your weekly wage, up to a maximum amount, which varies wildly among the states. For an injury that leaves a worker totally and permanently unable to work, the maximum ranges from $175 a week in Georgia to $700 a week in Alaska.

Workers' compensation often does not reimburse for short absences from work. In Pennsylvania, for example, no compensation is paid during the first seven days after disability begins. If a worker misses more than fourteen calendar days of work, compensation is retroactive.

Disability benefits are based on wages at the time of injury and are *not* adjusted for inflation. This can work a particular hardship on people exposed to toxic substances causing diseases that show up many years later. A worker exposed to asbestos twenty-five or thirty years back may develop mesothelioma today. Workers' compensation, if paid at all, might come to two thirds of the 1965 salary.

In addition to compensation for lost wages, most states pay a set amount to a worker who loses the use of a body part such as an eye, ear, arm, hand, or foot. Many states also pay something to seriously scarred or disfigured employees and for rehabilitation and vocational training.

Claiming Compensation

Workers' compensation is your right. It may not be easy to claim what is yours, but that compensation may be your only source for paying steep medical bills, being reimbursed for lost wages, or obtaining vocational training and rehabilitation therapy. To claim workers' compensation, you must remember to *treat, report,* and *file.*

Treat

See a doctor to have your injury treated. "Make sure to tell the doctor that your injury occurred at work and that you plan to claim workers' compensation," says David Levidow, a New York lawyer specializing in labor law. "If you don't, he or she will not fill out the necessary forms for your employer's insurance company and the workers' compensation board."

Report

Report the injury, in writing, to your employer. State that you have been injured and that the injury is work related. Most states allow you thirty days to do this, although the notification period in some states is much shorter. Colorado, for example, gives you only two days, Alabama five. Your employer should inform its insurance company about the injury. Check to make sure it has been done.

File

File a claim with the workers' compensation board. If your employer doesn't have the proper form, get one directly from the board. In many states, injured workers have up to two years to file a claim.

Until now, you are in control of arranging to get your benefits. From here on, the scenario shifts dramatically. Once you file, you may be subjected to mountains of paperwork, insensitive examinations by batteries of doctors, long delays, hearings before workers' compensation judges, harassment from insurance companies, and even retaliation from employers, although the latter is against the law. If you ask yourself if the trouble is worth the reward, remember that it's your right.

After you file your claim, most of your dealings will be with your employer's insurance company, and you will have some contact with the workers' compensation board. The insurance company may have its doctor or doctors examine you. It may send an insurance adjuster to your home or hospital to tape an interview with you. If this happens, beware. "Don't talk to an insurance adjuster," says Maryland attorney David Blum. "If you don't already have a lawyer, get one. No good can come from the interview. The insurance company is your adversary, and the purpose of the interview is to find a way to avoid paying you."

When the insurance company gets all the necessary information relating to your case — the company's report of the injury, the doctors' reports, and whatever other information it gathers — it either accepts liability or contests the claim. Unless it is a routine matter, expect the insurance company to contest. If it does, or classifies you in a lower category than you should be in — say, partially disabled instead of totally disabled — a judge employed by the workers' compensation board will hear your case. The docket is often crowded, so be prepared to wait months before the hearing is scheduled and hours in the waiting room before your case is heard. The hearing is like a trial. You present your side; the insurance company presents its side; witnesses are heard and cross-examined, and the judge makes a determination on the merits. Hearings often stretch over months or years. Both you and the insurance company have the right to appeal an adverse decision.

Sometimes an insurance company drags its feet and then challenges the claim. This is what happened to Trish Vevera, a twenty-nine-year-old dancer who injured her hip while performing in the national touring company of *Elvis*. Ms. Vevera informed the company of her injury early in August. The company, based in New York, notified its insurer immediately. Between August 15 and November 2, Ms. Vevera called the insurance company every week, but all she got was a runaround. No papers, no money, no assigned representative — nothing. Finally she hired a lawyer, who got a response from the insurance company — it contested the claim. This led to three workers' compensation hearings, visits to many company doctors, arbitrary — and possibly illegal — termination of her disability benefits. Ms. Vevera's story has a relatively happy ending. She won her case, although she remains embittered by the treatment she received. "You can have the system," she says. "It's so frustrating and unfair."

If your condition changes, so may the disability benefits. If it deteriorates, you can go back to the workers' compensation board and request that the benefits be increased. If your condition improves, the insurance company can ask the workers' compensation board to terminate or reduce disability benefits. Both will lead to another round of doctors' examinations and hearings.

Beyond Workers' Compensation: Bringing A Lawsuit

As a general rule, you cannot sue your employer for a work-related injury, even if the company's gross negligence caused it. The law says that workers' compensation is the "sole and exclusive" remedy. Like all rules, this one has some exceptions. A few states (Arizona, Kentucky, New Jersey, and Texas) allow you to opt out of the system and take your chances in court. You must follow the state law if you choose that route; for example, Texas allows you to make the decision only when you are first hired, a highly unlikely scenario for an eager new employee. If you are thinking of opting out, make sure your health insurance covers on-the-job injuries.

Some states allow an employee to sue an employer whose malicious behavior caused an injury, but these are tough cases to win. You must show that the employer *deliberately* intended to harm you, writes Arthur Larson, author of a highly respected legal treatise on workers' compensation. To have any chance in court, you must prove that your employer acted in a truly venal manner.

For example, in California, William Iverson charged that his hearing was damaged and he suffered emotional distress when a fellow worker set up a steel horseshoe target above his workstation, forced him to stay there, and repeatedly pounded the target with a large sledgehammer and that his employer, the Atlas Pacific Engineering Company, did nothing to stop this behavior. He was allowed to sue the company for assault, false imprisonment, and intentional infliction of emotional injuries. In another California case, Reba Rudkin, a lung-diseased worker in an asbestos plant of the now-bankrupt Johns-Manville Products Corporation, sued the company for concealing information in its possession for more than fifty years that long-term exposure to asbestos could cause life-threatening illnesses. The case was settled out of court.

Even if you can't sue your employer, there may be a potential lawsuit against a manufacturer of faulty equipment or toxic chemicals that harmed you (see Chapter 6) or an insurance company that maliciously or intentionally deprived you of benefits you deserve. Contact an attorney if you think you have a case.

Where to Turn for Help
An Injured Workers Association in your vicinity can provide advice on the workers' compensation system, refer you to a lawyer, and offer emotional support at a tough time. Contact one in your own or a neighboring state.

NATIONAL COALITION OF INJURED WORKERS
12 REJANE STREET
COVENTRY, RI 02816
(401) 828-6520

California
Injured Workers Outreach
2205 Hockory Way
West Sacramento, CA 95691
(916) 371-2720

Injured Workers United
760 North First Street, #2
San Jose, CA 95112
(408) 998-4054

Applicants Alliance
P.O. Box 2144
Rocklin, CA 95677
(916) 632-0363

Colorado
Work Injured Citizens' Coalition
P.O. Box 537
Morrison, CO 80465
(303) 988-5377

Illinois
Injured Workers of Illinois
37 S. Ashland Avenue
Chicago, IL 60607
(312) 666-1611

Louisiana
Injured Workers Union
P.O. Box 1029
Baton Rouge, LA 70821
(504) 344-7416

Maine
Injured Workers of Maine
P.O. Box 611
Westbrook, ME 04092
(207) 854-4579

United Injured Workers of Maine
P.O. Box 368
Woodland, ME 04694
(207) 454-8100

Injured Workers of Maine
RFD 3, Box 5130
Skowhegan, ME 04976
(207) 784-8896

Massachusetts
Injured Workers United
P.O. Box 4357
Fall River, MA 02723-0403
(508) 993-9240

Michigan
Michigan Injured Workers
20600 Eureka Road
Taylor, MI 48180
(313) 246-9077

Nevada
Nevada Association of Injured
  Workers
P.O. Box 4871
Sparks, NV 89432
(702) 322-6843

New Jersey
VOCAL
391 Trilby Avenue
Westville, NJ 08093
(609) 848-2678

New York
Victims of Compensation
62 C.E. Penny Drive
Wallkill, NY 12589
(914) 895-3396

Injured Workers of New York
68 North Street
Camillus, NY 13031
(315) 672-5814

Ohio
The Ohio Injured Workers
   Association
P.O. Box 360775
Columbia, OH 43236-0775
(614) 868-1225

Oregon
Oregon Workers Against
   Discrimination
P.O. Box 46
Sublimity, OR 97385
(503) 769-3354

Pennsylvania
Injured Workers of Pennsylvania
36 Bristol Road
Feasterville, PA 19047
(215) 355-8917

Rhode Island
Injured Workers of Rhode Island
340 Lockwood Street
Providence, RI 02907
(401) 751-4673

Utah
Injured Workers Association of
   Utah
868 S. McClelland Street
Salt Lake City, UT 84102
(801) 328-1100

United States Government
National Association of Federal
   Injured Workers
P.O. Box 73578
Puyallup, WA 98373
(206) 848-7442

If You Become Disabled:
Insurance Coverage and Government Benefits

Evelyn T. was a high-powered lobbyist for a New York charitable organization until she hailed a taxi at a busy intersection one October evening after having dinner with a friend. A car crashed into her, knocking her into the air. She landed on her head and lapsed into a coma. For more than two years she underwent intensive therapy, first at an upstate rehabilitation center and, after she had returned home, at a nearby hospital. Fortunately, disability insurance, a fringe benefit the company provided, covered a large part of the salary she was no longer able to earn. Otherwise she would have had to live on Social Security Disability benefits.

Many people think only in terms of life and health insurance, forgetting about coverage if they become disabled. Yet the chances are greater than one in three that if you are twenty-one or older, you will be disabled before you retire, according to the Health Insurance Association of America. You should know about disability insurance, government programs that provide assistance to disabled individuals, and disabled people's rights to freedom from discrimination in employment.

Advance Protection: Disability Insurance
Disability insurance gives you and your family financial protection if you are so severely injured or ill that you are unable to work. Like life and health insurance, it is sold by commercial insurance companies. Some companies offer disability insurance to their employees as a fringe benefit.

Disability insurance replaces part of the income you lose when you can't work. Insurance companies are reluctant to sell policies that cover 100 percent of lost wages. Such complete coverage, they say, discourages disabled people from going back to work. Although it varies from company to company, you can generally purchase a policy that pays up to two thirds of your lost wages. This may not be so bad as it seems at first glance, since the benefits from a policy you pay for — as contrasted with one your company furnishes — are tax deductible.

Purchasing a disability policy is similar to buying health insurance (see Chapter 3). In both cases, it is to your advantage to join a group rather than buy an individual policy. In both cases, it is difficult to obtain individual coverage if you have a chronic illness or condition that makes it likely you will file claims. Look for the following when considering a disability policy:

CHECKLIST: BUYING DISABILITY INSURANCE

- **How is disability defined?** How a policy defines "disability" is critical. It determines whether you will be able to receive benefits. Most policies define disabilities in terms of occupation. Try to find a policy that provides coverage if you are unable to work in your *own occupation* or your *usual occupation.* Under this definition, a chiropractor whose injured hands prevent him from manipulating patients would be considered disabled. Less advantageous is a policy that defines disability in terms of *inability to perform any occupation for which you are qualified by education or training.* Under this definition, our injured chiropractor who could teach or work as a consultant would not be considered disabled. Worst of all is a policy that defines disability as *inability to perform any occupation at all.* Under this definition, unless our injured chiropractor was comatose, he probably would not be considered disabled.

- **How long will benefits be paid?** You can buy policies that will protect you for life, until you are sixty-five, or for two to five years. The longer the coverage, the more expensive the policy.

- **What are the benefits?** Most companies sell policies that cover two thirds or less of lost income. There are all sorts of variations; for example, some policies pay high benefits for up to two years, then reduce them. The level of benefits you select is reflected in the premium. At the higher end, premiums become very pricey.

  Ask two specific questions about the benefits. Are they adjusted for inflation? If not, see whether you can purchase a rider that will increase them as the cost of living rises. Are Social Security Disability Insurance and workers' compensation payments deducted from disability benefits? Obviously, you are better off if they are not.

- **How is income or salary defined?** This is important to people who earn a base salary and have additional income through overtime, bonuses, or consulting. Find out whether additional income is included in the base on which benefits are calculated.

- **How long must I wait before benefits begin?** All policies require a waiting period (called an elimination period), which can range from weeks to years. Three to six months is normal. The longer the waiting periods, the lower the premiums.

  Find out whether coverage begins immediately should you sustain a serious permanent injury. Many policies pay benefits at once under a "presumptive total disability" clause. You also want to know what happens if you are disabled, recover enough to return to work, but then are forced out again by a recurrence of the disability. Let's say you hurt your back and recover sufficiently to return to work. Two weeks later, agonizing pain sends you straight to bed. If the disability recurs within six months, many policies do not require a new waiting period.

- **Does the policy cover partial disability?** Although most policies require you to be totally disabled, some provide coverage if you can work only part time or at a lower-paying job.

- **What conditions are excluded from coverage?** Insurance companies do not cover disabilities caused by a *pre-existing condition*, that is, an illness or injury that manifested itself some time before your coverage began. They may eliminate disabilities resulting from conditions that were treated as long as two years ago.

In fact, they may refuse to cover you if you have a chronic illness, anything from a back ailment to cancer. "Companies are tougher in weeding out bad risks for disability policies than they are for normal health insurance," says Greg Moxhay, a Rye, New York, insurance agent. Do not lie about your health, even if it means being turned down.

You should know that most *individually purchased* disability policies exclude coverage of pregnancy. However, companies with fifteen or more employees that provide short-term disability coverage for their employees must, under federal law, cover pregnancy as a disability. The laws of many states require similar coverage for employees of smaller companies.

- **Must you continue paying premiums if you are disabled?** Look for a "waiver of premiums" clause, which frees you from paying premiums while you are disabled.

- **Can you renew the policy at the same premium?** Ideally, you want a policy that cannot be canceled and for which the premiums are guaranteed to remain the same.

- **How much does it cost?** This is not easy to answer, because you will be faced with many options, only some of which are worth extra money. Many experts feel that the best way to keep premiums down is to extend the waiting period for benefits as long as possible. This means, of course, that you have to cover an initial loss of income out of savings, a second income, or loans.

Government Coverage of Disabilities

Social Security Disability Insurance

Some of the money that is taken out of your paycheck goes toward a program called Social Security Disability Insurance (SSDI), which is supposed to replace a portion of the income you lose should a serious disability prevent you from holding a job.

The reality is that getting money from Social Security Disability Insurance is like squeezing water from a stone. Of the approximately one million people who apply for Social Security Disability benefits every year, 70 percent are turned down initially. The eligibility requirements are extremely narrow. To be considered disabled, you must have a physical or mental impairment that prevents you from doing *any substantially gainful work*. Your disability must be either a long-term one, expected to last (or having lasted) at least twelve months, or life threatening.

If you have worked a sufficient amount of time — there is a formula based on age and work credits that the Social Security Administration can interpret — and are totally disabled, apply for SSDI benefits. Payments can begin the sixth month after the onset of your disability. The amount you are entitled to depends on the length of time you've worked and the salary you've earned.

Apply at the nearest office of the U.S. Social Security Administration. Call its toll-free number — (800) 772-1213 — to request the necessary forms. The application process is complicated and time-consuming, requiring submission of many forms, medical reports, and other information. As you go through each step, remember that you are trying to convince skeptical government bureaucrats, whose first response is to suspect your claim is fraudulent, that you really are so totally disabled that you cannot hold a job. If you are able to file your claim in person, do so, after calling ahead to make an appointment with a claims representative. Make sure that the doctors, therapists, and others who are submitting materials on your behalf understand the importance of buttressing your claim to total disability and that they should not pussyfoot about the severity of your illness or injury.

Initially, the Social Security Administration decides on your eligibility based on whether your illness appears on a list of one hundred or so disabling conditions, including loss of both arms or legs, incurable cancer, and severe brain damage. If your condition is included, you're in. If it isn't, the reviewer next looks at the medical evidence to determine whether you are too disabled to hold a job.

If you are turned down, appeal. Over 60 percent of the people who do so are successful in overturning an adverse decision. By law, you have the right to four appeals: first, a reconsideration of your case by the Social Security Administration; second, an administrative hearing; third, a hearing before the National Appeals Council; and finally, an action in a federal district court. If you don't have a lawyer to help you in your initial dealings with the Social Security Administration, get one for the appeals process. If you need help, contact a local disabilities support group or the National Organization of Social Security Claimants' Representatives, which provides referrals to member attorneys specializing in Social Security cases. The phone number is (800) 431-2804. Because any attorney can join, membership does not guarantee expertise.

Medicare
If you have been receiving Social Security Disability Insurance for twenty-four months, you are automatically entitled to Medicare. This U.S. government program covers many of the hospital, physician, and equipment needs of disabled people. It is discussed in Chapter 11.

Supplemental Security Income
Supplemental Security Income (SSI) is a program for the elderly, blind, and disabled poor people. If you have a disability that would qualify for Social Security Disability Insurance and your earnings are low enough (in 1992, a single person must have an income of less than $400 a month and assets of less than $2,000; the exact amount changes slightly every year), apply for SSI at the nearest office of the Social Security Administration. In most states, SSI

beneficiaries are also eligible for Medicaid, which can help meet health care needs.

The Rights of Disabled People to Work

Not since the civil rights legislation of the 1960s has Congress passed such a landmark law as the 1990 Americans with Disabilities Act (ADA). The law gives disabled people unprecedented protection against discrimination in the workplace, as well as in hotels, restaurants, and other places of public accommodation; trains, buses, and other means of transportation; and in access to government services and programs. The ADA's protections against employment discrimination apply to all businesses with twenty-five or more employees as of July 26, 1992, and fifteen or more employees as of July 26, 1994. If you are one of the more than 43 million Americans who are disabled or employ more than fourteen people, you should become familiar with the ADA.

Under the ADA, it is against the law for an employer to discriminate against a qualified person who has a disability. The act bans discrimination in all aspects of employment — hiring, firing, promoting, compensation, and training. The law defines "disability" as a physical or mental impairment that substantially limits one or more of the major life activities — like walking, seeing, learning, hearing, breathing, and working. Furthermore, if an employee or job applicant is regarded as disabled, whether or not the perception is accurate, he or she is protected by the law. This protects someone with epilepsy or diabetes that is under control, or who tests HIV positive, from job discrimination based on stereotypes and prejudices. Current drug abuse, compulsive gambling, and kleptomania are specifically excluded as disabilities.

According to the law, a person is "qualified" if he or she can perform the "essential functions of a job with or without reasonable accommodation." What an employer has to do to make "reasonable accommodation" for a disabled person depends on the specific circumstances involved, including the nature of the disability, the extent of the changes needed, and the size and financial strength of the company. An employer may have to restructure a

job, adopt a modified or part-time work schedule, hire an inter-
preter or reader, or make the facility physically accessible to disabled people — by installing a ramp for wheelchairs, for instance.
If a specific accommodation causes undue hardship to an employer, it does not have to be made. The Equal Employment Opportunity Commission is taking a case-by-case approach in determining what is a "reasonable accommodation," an "undue hardship,"
and an "essential function" of a job. "Most disputes between employers and disabled employees or potential employees will be
settled informally, but court intervention will be required in some
cases," says Sharon Rennert, associate staff director of the American Bar Association's Commission on Mental and Physical Disability Law.

A job interviewer can't ask about an applicant's disabilities, but
can question his or her ability to perform a job. It is often a fine
line. Suppose a one-armed man applies for a job as a card dealer in
Las Vegas. It would be natural for an interviewer to ask the applicant whether a one-armed person can do the work. And it gives
the applicant the perfect opportunity to reply, "Let me show you,"
take out a pack of cards, shuffle, and deal.

Similarly, you can't be asked to take a pre-employment physical
before receiving a job offer. Once it makes an offer, an employer
may require a physical examination as long as all entering employees must have one and the results remain confidential. If the
physical turns up a disability, the job offer can't be withdrawn
unless the disability will keep you from doing the job. One exception is drug testing. An employer can test applicants for illegal
drug use and refuse to hire those who test positive.

Employers charged with discrimination in violation of the ADA
can defend themselves in two ways. First, even though it screens
out disabled people, a company could show that it was testing
applicants for their ability to do the job, that the test was consistent with the company's business needs, and that reasonable accommodation is not feasible. Using this defense, an airline, for
example, could use tests that eliminate blind applicants seeking a
job as a pilot. Or it could show that a job applicant posed a direct
threat to the health and safety of others in the workplace.

If you believe that an employer or potential employer has discriminated against you because of a disability, contact the head-quarters of the U.S. Equal Employment Opportunity Commission or one of its district offices listed below.

EQUAL EMPLOYMENT OPPORTUNITY COMMISSION
1801 L STREET, NW
WASHINGTON, DC 20507
(202) 663-4264

District Offices

Atlanta District
(Georgia)
75 Piedmont Avenue, NE
Atlanta, GA 30335
(404) 331-6093

Baltimore District
(Maryland, Virginia)
111 Market Place
Baltimore, MD 21202
(301) 962-3932

Birmingham District
(Alabama, Mississippi)
1900 Third Avenue North
Birmingham, AL 35203
(205) 731-0083

Charlotte District
(North Carolina, South Carolina)
5500 Central Avenue
Charlotte, NC 28212
(704) 567-7100

Chicago District
(Northern Illinois)
536 South Clark Street
Chicago, IL 60605
(312) 353-2713

Cleveland District
(Ohio)
1375 Euclid Avenue
Cleveland, OH 44115
(216) 522-2001

Dallas District
(Oklahoma, Northern Texas)
8303 Elmbrook Drive
Dallas, TX 75247
(214) 767-7015

Denver District
*(Colorado, Montana, Nebraska,
North Dakota, South Dakota,
Wyoming)*
1845 Sherman Street
Denver, CO 80203
(303) 866-1300

Detroit District
(Michigan)
477 Michigan Avenue
Detroit, MI 48226
(313) 226-7636

Houston District
(Central Texas)
1919 Smith Street
Houston, TX 77002
(713) 653-3320

Indianapolis District
(Indiana, Kentucky — Louisville
Only)
46 East Ohio Street
Indianapolis, IN 46204
(317) 226-7212

Los Angeles District
(Southern California, Nevada)
3660 Wilshire Boulevard
Los Angeles, CA 90010
(213) 251-7278

Memphis District
(Kentucky — except Louisville;
Tennessee)
1407 Union Avenue
Memphis, TN 38104
(901) 722-2617

Miami District
(Florida, Panama Canal Zone)
1 N.E. First Street
Miami, FL 33132
(305) 536-4491

Milwaukee District
(Iowa, Minnesota, Wisconsin)
310 W. Wisconsin Avenue
Milwaukee, WI 53203
(414) 291-7111

New Orleans District
(Arkansas, Louisiana)
701 Loyola Avenue
New Orleans, LA 70113
(504) 589-2329

New York District
(Connecticut, Maine,
Massachusetts, New Hampshire,
New York, Puerto Rico, Rhode
Island, Vermont, Virgin Islands)
90 Church Street
New York, NY 10007
(212) 264-7161

Philadelphia District
(Delaware, New Jersey,
Pennsylvania, West Virginia)
1421 Cherry Street
Philadelphia, PA 19102
(215) 597-9350

Phoenix District
(Arizona, New Mexico, Utah)
4520 N. Central Avenue
Phoenix, AZ 85012
(602) 640-5000

St. Louis District
(Kansas, Missouri)
625 N. Euclid Street
St. Louis, MO 63108
(314) 425-6523

San Antonio District
(Southern Texas)
5410 Fredericksburg Road
San Antonio, TX 78229
(512) 229-4810

San Francisco District
(American Samoa, Northern
California, Commonwealth of
the Northern Mariana Islands,
Guam, Hawaii, Wake Island)
901 Market Street
San Francisco, CA 94103
(415) 744-6500

Seattle District
(Alaska, Idaho, Oregon,
Washington)
2815 Second Avenue
Seattle, WA 98121
(206) 553-0968

Washington Field Office
(District of Columbia)
1400 L Street, NW
Washington, DC 20005
(202) 275-6365

You may also have a case under state human rights laws or the federal Vocational Rehabilitation Act, which applies to recipients of federal aid and government contractors. Before proceeding too far, consult a disabilities advocacy group or a lawyer knowledgeable in disabilities law.

Drug Testing of Employees

Is It Legal?
Suppose you went to work one morning and instead of being greeted with a smile and a cup of coffee, you were handed a form letter stating that the company, concerned that increased use of illegal drugs could affect worker safety and the quality of the company's products, was instituting a drug-testing program for all employees. Beginning immediately. Anyone testing positive would have to enroll in a drug rehabilitation program; second offenders would be dismissed. You are given an empty bottle in which to urinate and directed to the bathroom, under the watchful eyes of your supervisor to make sure you don't cheat.

In one form or another, such scenes occur every day at American businesses. Given employer and employee fears about threats to worker safety caused by drug abuse, a strong federal antidrug policy (which requires random testing of airline, railroad, maritime, and interstate trucking workers; it is much more than "Just say no"), and an estimated cost of drug and alcohol abuse to American society of $1.3 billion a year, it is hardly surprising that more and more organizations are instituting drug-testing policies. According to the American Management Association, 62 percent of American companies tested their employees for drugs in 1990, up from 20 percent in the previous five years. Seventy percent of the nation's largest companies test job applicants for drugs.

Many people feel that forcing someone who is not suspected of using drugs to give a urine sample violates traditional American principles of privacy. This kind of intrusive behavior is turning us into "a nation of suspects," argues Leonard Glantz, a law professor at Boston University. It also may force people to reveal personal matters that are none of the company's business, for example, that an employee takes lithium for depression or uses birth control pills. Additionally, if the goal is to make the workplace safer, drug testing may not be the way to do it. Traces of marijuana smoked on a Saturday night may show up in a urine sample taken the following Wednesday, long after the effects have worn off. "A positive result on a drug test does not indicate a person is impaired," says Lewis Maltby, director of the American Civil Liberties Union's National Task Force on Civil Liberties in the Workplace. "There are much better ways to test for impairment directly."

The law regarding drug testing is evolving. Federal government workers and employees of companies heavily regulated by the government, such as railroads and nuclear power plants, can argue that drug testing of people not suspected of being users is an unconstitutional search and seizure. If you work for a private company, you cannot argue that a drug-testing program, even a patently offensive one, violates your constitutional rights. The Constitution does not apply to you. It is written to protect people against *governmental* actions, not actions of private businesses or individuals. As a result, businesses have a lot of leeway in administering drug tests.

Generally, job *applicants* have no right to object to a drug test. You can, of course, refuse to take one, but if you do, the employer has no obligation to hire you. *Employees* have more grounds to contest a company's drug-testing policy. They could argue that it violates the state constitution or laws.

Whether drug testing is legal depends on the specific circumstances involved: who is being tested; what tests are given; how testing is conducted; and what happens afterward. There is no simple yes or no answer.

What to Ask about Your Company's Drug-testing Program
Does the company use both a screening and a confirmatory test?
Although blood, saliva, and strands of hair can reveal drug use, the preferred method of drug testing is urinalysis. According to the American Medical Association, urinalysis can detect cocaine, PCP, amphetamines, barbiturates, and heroin taken within the past two to seven days. Marijuana stays in the body somewhat longer; traces can be detected up to twenty-one days after use in the case of a chronic heavy smoker.

Standard practice dictates that drug testing be done in two

stages. The first is a screening test that measures drugs or their residue in the urine, the most common being the enzyme multiplied immunoassay test (EMIT). The problem with screening tests is that they are not very accurate. They record many drug-free people as having drug traces in their body. The tests can confuse legal substances with illegal ones. For example, an herb tea with coca leaves can show up as cocaine. Houston University law professor Mark Rothstein, author of *Medical Screening and the Employee Health Cost Crisis,* says that of 100 people identified by EMIT as users of illegal drugs, up to 66 may be wrongly accused.

Because of this inaccuracy, many companies use a second, more reliable test to confirm the results of a positive first one. The most common, gas chromatography/mass spectrometry (GC/MS), is almost 100 percent accurate in weeding out those falsely branded as drug users.

A drug-testing program that identifies employees to be disciplined on the basis of a single EMIT test without confirmation may be vulnerable to legal challenge.

Does the testing method respect employee dignity? Heavy-handed, degrading testing is susceptible to challenge. Perhaps the classic story of how *not* to test workers for drugs is that of Plainfield, New Jersey, firefighters. On the night of May 26, 1986, the fire chief and director of public affairs of the Plainfield Fire Department entered the city's firehouse, locked the doors, and woke the sleeping firefighters. Each employee was required to submit a urine sample under the watchful eyes of testing agents employed by the city. This procedure was repeated on two other nights until all of the city's 103 firefighters were tested. The city did not give any advance notice of its testing plan. There was never a written department order that set forth the basis for the testing or established standards for collecting and analyzing the samples. Sixteen firefighters tested positive and were fired immediately — without pay. At no time were they told what substances had been found in their urine. Later they received written complaints charging them with commission of a criminal act. The ousted firefighters sued the city and won. The court banned Plainfield from further directionless, departmentwide testing.

What happened in Plainfield is an example of one intrusion piled on the next — a surprise raid, holding people prisoner, forcing them to urinate while inspectors watched. Assaults on people's dignity do not often combine so many elements, but obviously, the more there are and the more degrading they get, the more likely a drug-testing program is to be struck down.

Some things to look out for: Are employees watched while they urinate? (One company was ordered to stop a drug-testing program that included videotaping workers giving their samples in a stall.) Are they kept under what is, in effect, house arrest until they urinate? Are they given notice that they will be tested? Answers to questions such as these help judges and arbitrators determine whether a drug-testing program is carried out in a reasonable way.

How are employees targeted for tests? There are a number of ways in which companies carry out employee testing.

- **Testing for cause:** an employer has reasonable grounds for believing the employee uses drugs. This kind of testing conforms to traditional principles of American justice holding that a person's bodily integrity can be violated only if there is reason to suspect he or she is doing something illegal.
- **Testing without cause:** an employee is required to give a urine sample even though there is no ground for suspicion that he or she uses drugs.
  — Workers involved in serious accidents, particularly involving public transportation, are often tested for alcohol and drugs. In 1989, the U.S. Supreme Court upheld testing of railroad engineers involved in serious accidents.
  — Workers responsible for public safety or national security may be tested. In a companion case to the railroad engineers' case, the Supreme Court held that Customs officials applying for jobs that involved halting the flow of drugs or giving them access to classified information could be tested for drugs. The legality of random testing of workers involved in public safety — police officers, firefighters, narcotics agents, air traffic controllers — is not yet clear. Many state courts have upheld it; some have struck it down.
  — Drug testing of *all* employees, generally at the time of their annual physical, is usually upheld if advance notice of the test was given.

— Random testing of employees is the most controversial and open to legal challenge. Particularly vulnerable are policies giving management the power to test anyone for any reason — or no reason at all. Most courts and arbitrators have struck down this type of testing as capricious and unreasonable, with one court terming it "a gross invasion of privacy . . . almost unheard of in a free society."

Random testing by some prearranged formula such as drawing 10 percent of the employees' names out of a bowl every month may violate state constitutions or laws. Take the case of Barbara Luck, a thirty-four-year-old computer programmer who had worked for the Southern Pacific Railway in California for six years and had an exemplary record. Ms. Luck was three and a half months pregnant when the company began its random drug-testing program. She refused to provide a urine sample, and Southern Pacific fired her. Ms. Luck sued the company for wrongful discharge, and a jury awarded her $485,000. In 1990 the California Supreme Court ruled that random drug testing of current employees violates the right of privacy guaranteed by California's constitution. It let the award stand.

Is testing part of a written, comprehensive antidrug policy? A written policy can provide justification for instituting drug testing, describe how tests will be conducted and samples analyzed, and set company policy toward employees who test positive. If no written policy exists, a company may be vulnerable. In one case, an arbitrator found that even though the company had a past practice of requiring drug testing, in the absence of a written policy it could not penalize employees for refusing to take a test.

Can an employee have a sample analyzed by a laboratory of his or her choice? Laboratories are notoriously inaccurate in their interpretations of urine specimens. One U.S. government study found an error rate of up to 66 percent. As a result, many employees ask to keep part of the sample and have it analyzed by a lab of their own choosing. It can certainly be argued that your future should not hinge on an employer's choice of laboratories or the possibility of a mix-up. "On the day of the test, give a urine sample at your doctor's office and have him or her send it out for analysis," recommends Margaret Brooks, director of New York's Legal Action Center.

Does the testing program violate state law? Fifteen states — Connecticut, Florida, Hawaii, Iowa, Louisiana, Maine, Maryland, Minnesota, Mississippi, Montana, Nebraska, Rhode Island, Tennessee, Utah, and Vermont — and the city of San Francisco have passed laws regulating drug testing. Unlike the approach of the federal government, which promotes drug testing, these state and local governments, with the exception of Utah, have placed limits on employers' rights to test employees. Courts in two other states — California and New Jersey — have found that random drug testing violates the state constitution.

Although the laws of each state are different, in general they provide the following safeguards:

- Limit testing to current employees whom an employer has reasonable grounds to believe are on drugs
- Require that a second test be done to confirm an initial positive result
- Establish guidelines for laboratory analysis
- Assure that samples be given in private
- Require that results be kept confidential

To find out about the law in your state, contact the nearest branch of the American Civil Liberties Union. If it's not in your phone directory, call ACLU headquarters in New York, (212) 944-9800.

Does the testing program violate a collective bargaining agreement? After an allegedly intoxicated motorman caused a trolley collision in Boston that injured thirty-three people, the general manager of the Massachusetts Bay Transit Authority announced it would begin random testing for drugs and alcohol. "We'll see them in court," responded a representative of the motormen's union.

Although the law has not been wholly settled, a company's drug-testing policy may be a condition of employment that is subject to labor-management negotiations. If there is any doubt in your mind, contact your union representative.

Are test results kept confidential? They should be held in confidence, available only to those people who have a need to know. A company that shares test results may be open to a lawsuit for defamation or invasion of privacy.

What is the company policy toward people who refuse to submit to drug testing? There are few grounds for refusing to take a drug test ordered upon reasonable suspicion that an employee is using drugs. Even when a company institutes a random testing program that may violate the state's constitution or laws, you place yourself at risk of being fired or disciplined by refusing to take the test.

On the other hand, employees fired because they refused to submit to a random drug test may have grounds for a lawsuit. They could charge the company with wrongful discharge. Like Barbara Luck, you may end up the eventual winner, but on the other hand, you may not, and you'll find yourself out of a job. It's a risk you should weigh carefully.

What is the company policy toward those who test positive? This is, obviously, an important piece of information. The federal government requires that people who test positive be given rehabilitation. A second positive test result is grounds for dismissal. Many large companies that test employees have also adopted this policy.

5

LEISURE, SPORTS, AND TORTS

CONTENTS

THE PURSUIT OF PLEASURE is a healthy business. Every year people all over America pack their bags and embark on a search for the perfect vacation. Sports — everything from tennis and golf to skydiving and mountain climbing — attract record numbers of eager participants who fork over impressive amounts of money. As any fan who tries to get a ticket to a big game knows, spectator sports are a huge, growing business. Last year, 120 million people watched the Super Bowl on television. That's almost one out of two Americans.

Want to work off all that popcorn, pretzels, and hot dogs? Join the more than 10 million Americans who work out in about fifteen thousand health clubs and spas throughout the United States. But the rosy picture of the formerly flabby and overworked getting into shape and taking it easy has a darker side: the growing number of people who lose weight only in their wallets and end up angry, frustrated, or worse, seriously injured.

Let's say you're tired of seeing your exercise bike gathering dust. You decide to take a more active approach to lighten gravity's pull on your thighs and join a health club. A very fit, very personable manager convinces you of the wisdom of buying a three-year membership — which just happens to be on sale. Cost? $3,600. But after a few months, your spirits sag along with everything else. The promised personal attention never materializes. Traffic at the swimming pool lanes is always rush hour. The dressing rooms are a mess. You decide to quit — and try to get your money back. The very personable, very fit manager turns his megawatt smile on you and tells you to look at your contract. Surprise! It says nothing about a refund. What can you do?

Or say you and your husband love to dance. For your anniversary, you go to a nightclub. During a tango, you fall over a chair and table that were placed at the edge of the dark dance floor. Your husband twists his knee and bangs his elbow. You fall on your face and spend the rest of your anniversary in an emergency room getting three stitches in your lip. Do you have a case against the club?

Or a dream European vacation turns into a long ordeal when you slip on the gangplank of a ship off the coast of Ireland, fracturing your ankle. Instead of sailing through the Emerald Isle, you end up in a hospital where the doctor sets the bone and hands you a bill, cash only, please. When you submit the claim to your insurance company, it refuses to pay. Is there some way to be reimbursed? If not, is there a way to be covered in the future?

Incidents like these take place all the time. In this chapter, we tell you what to look for in a health club contract, what your rights are, and what to do if something should go wrong. We also tell you what your rights are if you are injured while playing or watching a sport or enjoying a leisure activity such as camping, swimming, or dancing. Last, we give you some tips on insurance coverage of illness or injuries sustained while you are out of the country.

Health Clubs: Exercise Caution

"There are a lot of shady characters out there," says Romana Kryzanowska, a charismatic former ballerina who for the past forty years has been the driving force behind Pilates, an exercise studio in New York City. "Sometimes they take your money and run. Or maybe they don't have enough money to fix things and they let the place slowly fall apart. Or they don't train the instructors properly. That's the worst part; you pay so much and if you get any attention at all, it's from trainers who don't know what they're doing. That's how injuries happen."

Ms. Kryzanowska accurately summarizes the pitfalls people face when they join a health club: insolvency, incompetence, and injuries. You must protect yourself. If you exercise caution, you can reduce the chances of being injured, financially as well as physically, at a health club.

Insolvency: Avoiding Health Clubs on the Brink
In the 1980s the booming health club market attracted many fast operators out to make a quick buck as well as honest physical fitness enthusiasts who didn't have enough capital to keep a club going through the start-up period. "Storefront operations, with a salesman sitting at a desk with only a light bulb over his head, would sell memberships for clubs that would never open. Or if they did manage to open, it wasn't for long," says Jim Johnson, a

spokesman for the Association of Physical Fitness Centers, a Washington, D.C., trade organization. "Fortunately that period is largely behind us. Customers have wised up and state legislators finally got on the case."

Whether or not that period *is* behind us is a matter of some debate. There are no good statistics available. But if you are the one whose health club has suddenly vanished, it doesn't matter if your club was one out of three or one out of a hundred that closed.

Because the physical fitness industry has been characterized by middle-of-the-night closures, "mergers," and failures to open, states are beginning to pass laws to regulate health clubs. Thirty-six states have legislation designed to protect members of health clubs, according to Helen Durkin, director of government relations of the Boston-based Association of Quality Clubs. The laws may require health clubs to post a bond (often $50,000), to give customers a three-day cooling-off period during which they can change their minds and get their money back, and to refund part of the fee if a member moves more than twenty-five miles away. Most prohibit membership contracts for longer than two or three years.

Despite these new government protections, many clients continue to have problems with health clubs. If you are one of them, contact your state department of consumer protection. Addresses and phone numbers are listed in Chapter 6. Before you sign up, get as much information about a health club as you can. Here is what to watch out for:

CHECKLIST: JOINING A HEALTH CLUB — KNOW BEFORE YOU GO

- **Determine how long the club has been in business.** There is no guarantee that a club that has been around for a long time will be there tomorrow. But it's an indication of stability.
- **Check out the club with the state consumer protection board (see Chapter 6 for telephone numbers) or the Better Business Bureau.**

- **Make sure the contract gives you three days to change your mind and get your money back.** If you change your mind, take a friend with you when you return to the club. It should stiffen your resolve when the manager starts sweet-talking you.
- **Is the club bonded and if it is, for how much?** Although this offers only limited protection if a club goes broke (if a club owing $2 million has posted a $50,000 bond, each member gets only pennies), at least it assures you of getting something back.
- **Be sure you understand the fee arrangements.** Some clubs require you to sign a loan contract for your monthly fees and charge you interest on the balance.
- **Ask what happens if you move or become sick. Will you get your money back?**
- **What's the condition of the facility?** Visit the club during a peak activity time such as the lunch hour or after work. See whether the changing rooms, exercise facilities, and pool areas are well maintained, whether members are receiving instruction, and whether it is too crowded.
- **Sign up for the shortest time you can.** Many clubs offer a three-month, or less, trial membership. Since 90 percent of health club members drop out after three months, it makes little sense to enroll initially for a period longer than that.
- **Check the Assumption of Risk or Waiver of Liability clause in the contract.** This clause says you understand that exercise can be dangerous and won't sue the club if you are injured there. Some clubs also add a clause in which you agree not to sue even if the club's negligence causes your injury. Cross off and initial this part before you sign. If the management objects, go elsewhere. Do not join a club that won't take responsibility for its negligence or that of its employees.
- **Read the contract or have a knowledgeable friend read it.** No matter what the salesman tells you, it is the wording in the contract that counts in case of a disagreement. You will be held responsible for having read and understood the contract.

Seek Competent Instructors

"You can't legislate competence," runs an old saying. While most legal reform has been directed toward protecting clients against fraud and insolvency, there are certain steps you can take to help find competent instructors.

One is to look for a certified instructor. Three private organizations — the American Council on Exercise, (800) 825-3636, the American College of Sports Medicine, (317) 637-9200, and the Aerobics and Fitness Association of America (800) 445-5950 — certify dance exercise/aerobics instructors and personal trainers. To receive certification, an instructor must pass a written test covering such topics as injury prevention, anatomy, and risk assessment and, for the last two groups, a hands-on test as well. These organizations can give you the names of certified instructors in your vicinity.

All things being equal, a certified instructor is preferable to a noncertified one. But all things are not equal, and in the freewheeling field of physical fitness, only a small percentage of trainers are certified. Whether an instructor is certified or not, find out about his or her training, education, and experience. Try to arrange for a sample lesson, even if you have to pay for it, to see how comfortable you feel with the instructor. Richard Cotton, who directs the certification program of the American Council on Exercise, suggests that you check out the condition of the physical facilities before joining a health club. "Poorly maintained equipment is a dead giveaway," he says. "It means you are likely to get poorly trained instructors. And poorly trained instructors increase the chances of your getting hurt."

Injuries: What If You Get Hurt?

For professional athletes, injuries are the downside of perfection. For the rest of us, getting hurt is not a price we want to pay for the sweaty, sometimes painful, process of getting into shape. Yet people get hurt at health clubs all the time. They pull muscles on machines, strain ankles during aerobics, or slip on wet mats. That is not to say that you should follow the advice of the wit who said, "Every time I feel like exercising, I lie down until the urge passes." Exercise, as your mother, doctor, and countless magazine articles attest, is very good for you. But if you should get hurt, your first instinct should be to stop what you are doing and take care of the injury. "No pain, no gain" should not get in the way of common sense and safety.

Many people's second instinct is to wonder whether they can sue the health club. The answer is, It depends: on the facts of the case, on the law of the state, and on whether you can convince a judge or jury that the club's negligence caused the injury. A health club has a duty to provide a reasonably safe place to work out and must take care to avoid harming its customers. If it fails to carry out its duty, it may be found liable for negligence. A health club can defend itself by arguing that a client assumed the risk of injury on joining. Or that the customer contributed to the injury. Or that it resulted from an undisclosed pre-existing condition.

Dorothea McKinley, a fifty-one-year-old secretary of Camden, New Jersey, sued the Slenderella salon, which she had joined to lose weight and improve her posture. Ms. McKinley's treatment consisted of lying on her back on a six-foot-long vibrating table. After three or four such sessions, Ms. McKinley complained of a sore back. She continued to complain to the instructor. But instead of getting her off the table, the instructor urged her to keep shaking that flab off, assuring her that it was absolutely safe and could not hurt her. Finally, Ms. McKinley wrote to the manager and asked for a refund. "There is no way in which a Slenderella treatment can injure your body," he retorted. The results of this "treatment" landed Ms. McKinley in the hospital with an acute sprain of the ligaments in her back. She had to wear a back brace. Soon after, Ms. McKinley sued the salon for negligence, and won. "Once Slenderella knew of the painful effect of its treatments upon Ms. McKinley's back, it was under a duty to use reasonable care to avoid any further risk of harm to her," the judge wrote.

What about the clause in the contract saying that you understand exercising can be dangerous, that you assume the risk of injury, and that you won't sue the club if you get hurt? Will it stand up even if the club's negligence caused your injury? Again, maybe, depending on the wording of the contract and on state law. In some states you sign away your right to sue a health club if the waiver is clear and you were not coerced into signing it. Joanne Ciofalo of Long Island sued the Vic Tanney health club for negligently maintaining its premises after she slipped near the edge of the swimming pool and injured her wrist. But since her contract specified that she gave up her right to sue, even if she was injured by the club's negligence, the judge ruled in Vic Tanney's favor. He said that the contract provision was clear and that nobody had held a gun to Ms. Ciofalo's head, forcing her to sign. In effect, the judge ruled that if she didn't like the provision, she could have gone elsewhere.

As a result of this and other similar decisions deemed unfair to members of health clubs, New York and several other states passed laws that nullified contract clauses shielding health clubs from liability owing to the negligence of the clubs and their employees.

Recreation, Sports, and Leisure-time Activities

Injuries to Spectators
You think it couldn't happen to you, but foul balls have been known to hit fans in the bleachers, hockey pucks have caromed off spectators, and race cars have crashed through fences, creating fiery infernos. What are your rights if you are the unwilling victim of a spectator sport turned into a disaster?

As a general rule, you cannot successfully sue the management if you happen to get in the way of events that may be expected to occur during a contest. When injured spectators do sue a ball club or stadium owner, courts consistently rule that they assumed the normal risks of the sport they were watching. In other words, you pay your money and you take your chances.

Lawsuits by spectators injured by foul balls at baseball games are typical. In one case, a forty-seven-year-old Philadelphia woman went with her husband to her first baseball game, a double-header between the Chicago Cubs and the hometown Phillies. Seated in the grandstand behind first base, she was enjoying the game with the rest of the fans until a foul ball hit her. She later sued the Phillies for negligence for failing to provide her with a safe seat from which to watch the game, arguing that the club should have given her a seat behind a screen. "There is nothing in the record to indicate [she] was of inferior intelligence or had led a cloistered life," wrote the judge in his ruling for the ball club. "She must be presumed to have the 'neighborhood knowledge' with which individuals living in organized society are normally equipped." This included being struck by a foul ball while watching a baseball game.

Although a spectator assumes normal risks, nobody needs to accept the risk of an unsafe facility or inadequate protection. The owner of a sports arena has a legal duty to provide a reasonably safe place to watch a sporting event. If the owner doesn't, a jury can find negligence and award damages to an injured spectator.

Fans seated behind home plate, for example, have the right to assume that the screen will protect them from foul balls. If a ball goes through a hole in the screen and hits someone on the head, the injured person could successfully sue the management for negligently maintaining and failing to inspect the screen. Similarly, fans watching football games or auto races on bleachers that collapse under their weight have successfully sued management for negligence.

It doesn't have to be an unsafe building or stadium. In Michigan, James and Ann Rockwell were watching a golf tournament at a country club in Mount Clemens from a bridge over the Clinton River when the bridge collapsed. Mrs. Rockwell fell twenty-five feet into the river, broke her back, and was permanently disabled. She sued the club for negligence and won when she was able to show that there were eighty to one hundred people on a bridge built to withstand the weight of twenty-five, that no warning signs were posted, and that no club staff were there to keep too many people from crowding onto the bridge.

Injuries to Participants: Unsportsmanlike Conduct
Ordinarily, you cannot get very far in a lawsuit for an injury caused by the nature of the game you are playing. That's like George Foreman suing Muhammed Ali for beating him up during their heavyweight championship bout. Or San Francisco Forty-niner quarterback Joe Montana suing New York Giant linebacker Laurence Taylor for tackling him too hard. They would be laughed out of court.

When you play a sport, be it pro football or a friendly game of pickup tennis, you assume the ordinary, normal risks of the game. But what about injuries caused by something out of the ordinary — the intentional elbow in the face, the cheap-shot tackle? If you can show that another person played dirty, intentionally tried to hurt you, or behaved in a manner that could only be considered reckless, you may have a case. Whether or not you win depends on how the jury or the judge sees it.

An amateur softball game in Lafayette, Louisiana, pitting Boo Boo's Lounge against Murray's Steak House was the setting for a classic situation. Adrien Duplechin, playing for Murray's, had hit a single and was on first base. The next batter hit a grounder to short. The shortstop tossed the ball to Boo Boo's second baseman, Jerome Bourque, who stepped on the bag, threw the ball to first base, and walked five feet toward the pitcher's mound to see if his team had completed a double play. But Duplechin kept running. Going full steam and well away from second base, he crashed into Bourque, knocking him over, slamming him in the chin with his elbow, and breaking his jaw. Bourque sued Duplechin and won. "Bourque may have assumed the risk of being hit by a bat or being spiked by someone sliding into second base," wrote the judge in the case. "However, he did not assume the risk of injury from fellow players acting in an unexpected or unsportsmanlike way with a reckless lack of concern for others."

Another case resulted from a soccer game between two teams of high school–aged kids in Winnetka, Illinois. Julian Nabozny, the goalie for the Hansa team, was kneeling with the ball in the rectangular penalty area in front of the goal. The rules of soccer do not allow any member of the opposing team to touch the goalie when he is holding the ball in the penalty area. David Barnhill, playing for the opposing team, Winnetka, chased the ball into the penalty area and kicked Nabozny on the left side of his head, causing permanent brain damage. When Nabozny's father sued on his son's behalf, Barnhill argued that Nabozny had assumed the risk of injury by playing in the game. Accepting Barnhill's defense, the trial court dismissed the case. But an appeals court reversed the decision. "A reckless disregard for the safety of other players cannot be excused," wrote the appeals court judge.

Unsafe Facilities
The owner or management of a facility has a legal duty to take reasonable steps to provide a safe place to have fun, whether you are swimming, hiking, canoeing, dancing, or whatever, and to

warn about reasonably foreseeable dangers. While no facility exists in a danger-free, injury-free zone, the owner or the management can be held liable if anyone other than a trespasser gets hurt as a result of negligence.

A jury — or a judge, if a jury trial is waived — determines whether the owner or management acted "reasonably," whether dangers were "reasonably foreseeable," and whether warnings were adequate. The jury also decides whether the injured person assumed the risk of getting hurt and whether his or her own negligence contributed to the injury. In some states, a person whose own negligence contributes, no matter how slightly, to the injury, loses the entire case. In most states, however, the injured person can still win, but damages are reduced in proportion to his or her own negligence.

Whether you win or lose depends on the specific circumstances and how well your case is presented by your lawyer and argued by the opposing attorney. These three lawsuits are examples:

Rita Keefe was on a two-day "cruise to nowhere" aboard the S.S. *Vera Cruz* one balmy June evening when she slipped while dancing on a wet spot on the dance floor of the ship's upper deck and fell flat on her back. Back on land, the St. Petersburg hairdresser started making the rounds of chiropractors, orthopedists, and other specialists to find relief from the increasingly painful back spasms that prevented her from holding a steady job. This went on for a year. When Ms. Keefe sued the shipping company for negligence, she presented evidence that the dance floor was slippery, that other dancers had found it treacherous, that people frequently spilled drinks on the floor, and that it had not been cleaned since the voyage began. On the basis of this evidence, the judge found that the cruise line was negligent and awarded Ms. Keefe $7,000 for lost wages and for pain and suffering.

For Richard Miller, twenty-two, his first trip to the lake at Crab Orchard National Wildlife Refuge in southern Illinois turned into a horrible tragedy. An experienced swimmer and diver, Mr. Miller walked to the end of a dock, took off his top and sandals, and then looked around. According to court testimony, he saw one sign that read "Boat Landing" but nothing indicating that swimming was not allowed or might be dangerous. He did see some people in the lake; one of them yelled that the water was fine. Because the water was murky, Mr. Miller couldn't see the bottom, which was only three feet deep. When he dove off the pier, his head crashed to the bottom. His injuries were so severe that he became a paraplegic. He sued the United States, which owned the refuge, for negligence under the Federal Tort Claims Act and was awarded one million dollars. (In the old days, you could not sue the government; now, most states and the federal government have passed tort claim acts allowing injured people to sue them.) The judge found that the government was negligent in failing to post No Swimming or No Diving signs at the entrance to the dock and that Mr. Miller was not himself negligent by diving without first seeing how deep the water was.

In another case, Burrel Rubenstein took his son and one of his son's friends camping at Yellowstone National Park. They pitched their tent at the Fishing Bridge Campground, had dinner, and turned in for the night. At about one in the morning, Mr. Rubenstein woke to feel a bear's paw on his chest. He began yelling and struggling to get the animal off him. In the ensuing tussle, the bear mangled Mr. Rubenstein's legs before the boys, who were in sleeping bags nearby, managed to drive it off. Mr. Rubenstein sued the United States government for negligence in not warning him properly of the dangers and "lulling him into a false sense of security that if he followed the rules, he would not be attacked by a bear." He lost. The judge found that the park had properly warned Mr. Rubenstein and other campers through the "bear insert" in its brochures, which warned that bears are wild animals that may appear tame, but are actually very dangerous. "A reasonable man would have realized the dangers that exist in a wildlife park," ruled the judge. "Mr. Rubenstein either knew or should have known of the risk of an unprovoked attack."

Dangerous Sporting Equipment
When Louise Hauter bought her thirteen-year-old son, Fred, the Golfing Gizmo for Christmas, she thought it would help improve his budding golf game according to court testimony. Instead, the Gizmo, a golf ball attached to an elasticized cord secured to the ground by metal pegs, left him brain damaged. Although the package clearly stated: "Completely safe — ball will not hit player," when Fred practiced his swing on the Hauters' front lawn, the ball

somehow snapped around, hitting him in the head. The family successfully sued the company. The California Supreme Court found that the manufacturer was liable for marketing a dangerously designed product and for misrepresenting the Gizmo by putting a false claim about its safety on the box.

If you are injured by dangerous sporting or recreation equipment, you can sue the manufacturer, the distributor, or sales agents on a variety of grounds. One is that the product was negligently made or that the manufacturer breached its warranty to provide a safe product. Another is "strict liability," a claim that the product was defective and you were harmed by it. (These are discussed more fully in Chapter 6.) Whatever the grounds you choose to sue under, you have to prove to the judge or jury that there was something wrong with the product or that the manufacturer failed to warn you about a danger that was not obvious. The success of your case depends on the particular circumstances, how much you knew about the sport or product beforehand, and the nature of the warning. A lot hinges on the skill of the opposing lawyers, as in the following two cases involving trampolines, tragedies, and teenagers.

Lauren Pell was a sixteen-year-old Chicago high school student whose bad landing on a minitrampoline after doing a somersault left her permanently paralyzed with a broken back. She sued the manufacturer, AMF, Inc., for marketing an unsafe product and for failing to warn adequately about its dangers. AMF argued that the warning, which read, "Caution: Misuse and abuse of this trampoline is dangerous and can cause serious injury," was adequate and that users of a trampoline assume the risk of injury. The case went to a jury, which found that AMF had not given sufficient warning — in fact, when the injury occurred, the warnings were obscured — and awarded $5 million to Ms. Pell.

The second case concerned the Aqua Diver, a small circular trampoline that could be used instead of a diving board. A diver climbs a ladder to the top of the platform and jumps two feet onto a sixteen-inch trampoline that catapults him or her into the water. Southlake Beach, Indiana, purchased one and installed it on a platform at the beach. Thirteen-year-old Bruno Garzolini climbed to the top and jumped, but instead of landing on two feet on the trampoline and catapulting into the water, he caught his left leg in the elastic cables that supported the trampoline. When his body fell forward, he broke his leg. Complications set in and the youth's leg had to be amputated. A lawsuit against the manufacturer followed. During the trial, it emerged that the manufacturer, the Nissen Trampoline Company, provided no instructions for use and no warnings about the trampoline's potential danger. Despite this, the jury found for the manufacturer. The verdict was upheld on appeal.

Waivers: Can You Sign Away Your Right to Sue?

If you've ever entered a ten-kilometer race, gone skiing, or participated in a dangerous sport, you must have wondered about those waivers you sign, the ones saying you recognize that the sport is dangerous and that you assume all risk of injury and agree not to sue the sponsors. Are they legally binding? Can you voluntarily abdicate your right to sue as a condition of participating in a sporting event? The answer is perhaps. It depends on the particular circumstances and the law of the state where the contract was signed. Take two examples:

Daniel Williams was a law student at the University of Chicago when he entered the 10,000-meter Peachtree Road Race in Atlanta, Georgia. The application form contained this statement: "I am in proper physical condition to participate in this event, one of the most difficult 10,000-meter races in America. Heat and humidity, in addition to the hills, make this a grueling race. I waive any and all claims against officials or sponsors of the race for injuries or illness which may directly or indirectly result from my participation." During the Fourth of July race, Mr. Williams collapsed from heat prostration, which, he said in court, led to brain damage and permanent loss of motor functions. He sued the sponsors of the race, arguing that his only choice had been to sign the waiver or not race. The judges tossed out his claim, saying that as an experienced runner, a Phi Beta Kappa college student, and an Atlanta resident familiar with the summer heat, Mr. Williams knew what he was getting into.

In the second case, James Rosen was a thirty-five-year-old real estate agent when he bought a season pass at the Steamboat

Springs, Colorado, ski resort. The pass contained a waiver stating, "I understand skiing is a hazardous sport and that hazardous obstructions exist in any ski area. I accept the existence of such dangers and that injuries may result from the numerous falls and collisions which are common in the sport of skiing." During one run, Mr. Rosen lost control, hit another skier, and slammed into a metal pole set in concrete in an open area, breaking his leg. He sued the resort for negligently placing the hazardous pole in an open area of the ski trail and won, even though he had signed the waiver. The judge ruled that the waiver was so one-sided that it probably was not signed voluntarily and that, in any case, the language was too ambiguous to be meaningful.

As these cases illustrate, judges look at the language of the waiver and the conditions under which it was signed. Whether you will win depends on factors such as the following:

- If you are an experienced participant in a sport or if the waiver is for a dangerous sport such as auto racing, sky diving, or mountain climbing, a waiver is more likely to be upheld. The rationale is that you knew the dangers before you participated.
- If, as in the case of Joanne Ciofalo who slipped by the pool at Vic Tanney's, the waiver is in large print, clearly written, and you have the choice of taking your business elsewhere, it has a better chance of being upheld. This is part of a freedom of contract, say the courts.
- If, on the other hand, the waiver is written in small print, is not clear, is not signed (for example, a waiver on the back of a ticket), or the customer is in a take-it-or-leave-it position, a judge is more likely to void it.
- Waivers signed by children are almost certain to be voided. Minors cannot legally sign a contract.

In some states, liability waivers for amusement parks and sports facilities are unenforceable. Even in states without a specific law, judges do not like waivers of liability and look for reasons to invalidate them.

If you are asked to sign an agreement in which you give up your right to sue if injured by the negligence of the facility, our advice is to go elsewhere. If that is not practical, cross out the clause and put your initials above it. As a last resort, add a handwritten note, "Signed under protest."

Travel Abroad

If you travel abroad, check your health insurance policy before you go. It is hard enough being sick in foreign climes. You don't need the aggravation of wondering about quality of care and whether you will be taken to the cleaners as well as to the hospital.

If your health plan does not cover injuries or illness abroad, you can always buy a short-term policy that will. Such travel assistance policies offer toll-free, twenty-four-hour hotlines that refer you to an English-speaking doctor, provide medical evacuation if necessary, and pay your medical bills directly. Medical travel assistance policies are sold by Access America, a subsidiary of Blue Cross–Blue Shield, about a dozen commercial insurance companies, and are included in the coverage offered by some gold credit cards.

6

DANGEROUS PRODUCTS AND HAZARDOUS SUBSTANCES

CONTENTS

125

IN AN AGE of computer chips, Concordes, and electronic mail, we are bombarded with information overload. Yet when it comes to what we put in and on our bodies, we remain surprisingly ignorant. We pop prescription pills without knowing their side effects, eat foods that can poison us, have risky devices put into us, and use products that can harm us and our children. And when we dutifully try to eat healthy and buy wisely, advertising confuses us even more. Who understands what "low in sodium" really means? Or whether minoxidil actually sprouts hair on bald men? Or whether antiwrinkle cream protects you against the signs of aging? Or whether shellfish is safe? Even the commissioner of the Food and Drug Administration (FDA), Dr. David Kessler, said, shortly after taking office, that he couldn't figure out the nutritional labeling on a box of cereal.

If the commissioner of the FDA has a problem, we're all in trouble, although the situation is considerably brighter than it was in the bad old days of Franz Anton Mesmer, as in mesmerize, meaning "to hypnotize, to fascinate." Mesmer captivated Paris in the eighteenth century with his claim that "animal magnetism" was the source of all health and that a miracle cure lay in recharging the body with iron rods connected to specially magnetized jars of water, which he sold — natch. Mesmer created such a stir that a blue-ribbon commission, which included Benjamin Franklin, was formed to investigate his claims. Not surprisingly, it found Mesmer's magnets to be totally ineffective.

Nowadays, the following government organizations monitor the safety and effectiveness of products in an attempt to protect consumers from claims that have little or no basis in fact:

- The Food and Drug Administration regulates drugs, medical devices, foods, and cosmetics. Its duties include approving medicines and many devices before they are marketed, monitoring the labeling of all drugs (prescription, over-the-counter, and foods that make health claims), and overseeing the advertising of prescription drugs.

- The Federal Trade Commission oversees the *advertising* of food, cosmetics, and over-the-counter drugs.
- The Department of Agriculture is charged with assuring the safety of meat, poultry, and eggs.
- The Environmental Protection Agency is responsible for enforcing laws passed to protect us from environmental hazards such as pollution and toxic substances.
- The National Highway Traffic Safety Administration is responsible for overseeing automobile safety, including children's car seats.
- The Consumer Product Safety Commission is charged with enforcing laws that protect consumers against harmful products other than the ones mentioned above.

States and some large cities have similar consumer protection agencies to enforce state laws. Nonprofit organizations, such as the Public Citizen Health Research Group, the Center for Science in the Public Interest, and the Natural Resources Defense Council, ride herd on government regulators.

If none of these organizations can help you and you are injured by a harmful product, consider legal action. We offer this advice in light of relatively recent legal developments. Just a few years ago, the predominant philosophy was "Buyer beware." Your only chance of winning a lawsuit was to prove that the manufacturer was negligent — an almost impossible task. The onus was on the consumer. If you got hurt, too bad. Now the legal climate has warmed toward the consumer, and you have a better chance of winning in court if you were harmed by a defective product.

Despite these advances, the frustration of not knowing how to evaluate the health and safety claims of competing products, where and how to complain if there is a problem, and what to do in case of an injury can turn the most self-assured adult into a screaming two-year-old. There are, however, many resources at your disposal. In this chapter, we lead you to them, telling how best to protect yourself against unsafe and unhealthy products, where to turn for information and help, and what to do if you are injured.

Protecting Yourself from Unsafe Products

Prescription Drugs

Is Your Medicine Safe and Effective?

When FDA founder Harvey Wiley wanted to test the dangers of certain chemical food additives, he rounded up a group of government employees to volunteer for his poison squad. For a shot of whiskey before and a cigar afterward, they ate a meal laced with such chemicals as copper sulfate and sulfurous acid. If any of the volunteers got sick, the chemical was considered a hazard. How times have changed! Today, food additives and drugs must be tested extensively for harmful side effects and performance.

Before a drug reaches your medicine cabinet, it is first tested on animals for toxicity, then on small groups of fifty to one hundred volunteers, then on thousands of people. The testing can take ten years and cost upward of $50 million. The FDA will give its approval only after concluding that a drug is safe and effective for the condition it is intended to treat. Through this extensive testing, the FDA tries to prevent people from being injured or taken in by wild claims about drugs that don't work or cause tragic consequences. Although the FDA allows some unproven drugs on the market to treat people dying of AIDS or cancer, current testing procedures make it unlikely that a major medical disaster could occur today. That's the good news.

The bad news is, in the words of the Public Citizen Health Research Group, that "even at their very best, government safety standards are designed to establish a minimum level of protection for the public. The FDA does not have, nor will it ever have, the resources, authority, ability, or commitment to be the only line of defense shielding consumers." Every year, more than three hundred thousand people are hospitalized from severe reactions to medication, and eighteen thousand patients who are given drugs in a hospital die from their side effects.

Whether at home or in a hospital, most patients are kept in the dark about their medication. Neither doctors nor pharmacists dispense information with medications, and patients are too uninformed — or too intimidated — to ask. Nearly one third of all patients are told little or nothing about their medication, according to the FDA. When was the last time a doctor or pharmacist told you what side effects to watch for, what foods or other drugs you should avoid, and when to take your medicine?

Why is it so important to know what's in the drugs doctors prescribe? Shouldn't they know what's best for you? Why take the trouble to bother your doctor or pharmacist? Here's why. First, under the best of circumstances, no medicine is completely safe. By law, the FDA weighs the dangers against the benefits of a drug's use. When the FDA certifies a drug as "safe," it really means that, based on tests, the drug's benefits far outweigh its risks. Moreover, harmful side effects may not show up for many years after a drug is marketed. For instance, daughters of women who took DES during pregnancy developed cancer many years later.

Second, testing is done by the drug manufacturers, not the FDA. Many people mistakenly believe that the FDA conducts tests for new drugs. Wrong! The FDA relies on drug manufacturers to provide the information upon which it bases its approval. It is illegal to mislead the FDA, but the temptation is sometimes too great. Witness the furor over silicone-gel breast implants when the leading manufacturer, the Dow Corning Corporation, was accused of misleading the FDA about their safety. Early in 1992, an FDA advisory panel recommended that the use of silicone-gel breast implants be severely curtailed. A year earlier, but with less publicity, the FDA took action against the Hoechst pharmaceutical company for failing to notify it that the company's antidepressant drug, Merital, had caused the deaths of two women in Europe. Hoechst and one of its directors pleaded guilty to charges of violating the Food, Drug and Cosmetic Act and were fined over $200,000.

Also, the FDA is a relatively weak agency. A blue-ribbon panel reported in 1991 that the agency could not carry out its duty to protect the nation's health. It described the agency as "overextended, underfunded, and, shackled by bureaucratic restraints" and warned that "nonenforcement invites violations from unscrupulous firms."

Even if the FDA has approved a medication for one condition, doctors may prescribe it for another. Retin-A, approved as a drug to treat acne, has routinely been prescribed to prevent wrinkles. So what's wrong with this? The problem is that you don't know what side effects there may be, since the FDA approved it for only one condition and you may be taking it for another.

Finally, drugs may enter the blood stream of elderly people and children at a rate different from that of the rest of the population. Pediatricians recognized this long ago and prescribed medicine for children according to their weight, but it is a relatively recent discovery that a normal dosage for a thirty-five-year-old male may be dangerous for his seventy-year-old father. If you are elderly or the parent of a young child, it is particularly important to know about correct dosages, potential reactions to medication, and the interaction of a new medicine with other medication.

Ask Your Doctor or Pharmacist about Prescription Drugs
Under our medical system, doctors are legally responsible for telling you about the medicine they prescribe. Doctors get their information through an army of drug company salespeople and the *Physicians' Desk Reference.* This 2,000-plus-page book of pharmaceutical company ads gives doctors a great deal of information about a drug, including who should not take it and its side effects. Except in the case of some contraceptives and estrogen products, for which a manufacturer must prepare a package insert directed toward the patient, a manufacturer has no duty to let you know the risks and benefits of your medication. This is your doctor's job — and legal responsibility. Pharmacists, probably the most accessible of all health care professionals, can be a valuable source of information. They receive at least five years of training in the preparation, uses, and effects of drugs, so they should be pretty knowledgeable. Do not be afraid to ask your doctor and your pharmacist questions about the medicines you will be taking. It's your body and it's your right. Here is what to ask:

- **What is the name of the drug and what is it supposed to do?** The label should contain the name of the medication, the quantity, strength, number of refills, manufacturer, date, store name and address, and your name. If any of this information is missing or unclear, ask your pharmacist. Make sure you know what the drug is supposed to do.
- **When should it be taken and in what dosage?** Get a specific answer. "Four times a day" isn't very informative if you don't know whether it means you have to get up in the middle of

the night to take it. Be sure to note whether the medicine should be taken before, with, or after meals. Some drugs should not be taken on an empty stomach. Others are effective only if you haven't eaten. Make sure you know the correct dosage. *Parents* magazine reported the case of a four-month-old who received a prescription with dosage for a four-year-old. Luckily, the mother knew the correct dosage.

- **What side effects should I watch out for?** Some medication may cause drowsiness, nausea, dizziness, rashes, or other reactions. Know in advance what to expect. Tell your doctor if you are allergic to medication. Should you develop a severe reaction or one you were not told to expect, inform your doctor. You may be able to get an alternative. One toddler we know suffered from a red, blistery diaper rash after his pediatrician prescribed Augmentin, an antibiotic, for an ear infection. The next time the child's ear flared up, the doctor prescribed another, equally effective antibiotic.

  If a drug appears to cause you a serious or unexpected reaction, consider reporting it — or asking your doctor to report it — to the Food and Drug Administration. This will help the FDA monitor the drug's safety and may lead to the FDA's alerting doctors about the reaction, requiring a change in package labeling, or even removing the drug from the market. "Reporting adverse effects of drugs to the FDA is the single most important thing that patients can do to protect their own safety and that of others," says Mary Ponder, deputy director of the National Consumers League. The addresses of FDA headquarters and regional offices are given later in this chapter.

- **Should I avoid certain foods?** For some reason, those of us who take medication are almost never given this vital piece of information. Yet foods can interact with drugs, making them work faster, slower, or even neutralizing them completely. For example, milk slows down absorption of tetracycline, a commonly prescribed antibiotic. Large amounts of leafy vegetables, which contain vitamin K, can interfere with the effectiveness of anticoagulants. Cheese, wine, and some other foods can raise blood pressure to dangerous levels if taken with certain antidepressants.

- **Can the medicine be taken with other drugs?** Some drugs taken together can harm a patient. Daily consumption of iron pills can prevent antibiotics from being absorbed into the blood. Anticoagulants taken with aspirin can lead to excessive thinning of the blood. The American Pharmaceutical Association urges patients to let their doctors know about all medication they are taking, including nonprescription drugs.
- **Should I avoid alcohol, cigarettes, or caffeine while on the medication?** The FDA advises, "If you're taking any medicines at all, don't drink alcohol without first asking your doctor. It could be dangerous." While you're on the subject, ask about smoking and coffee, too.
- **Should I take all the medicine, even if I feel better?** A full course of treatment is often necessary to eradicate a condition, sometimes not.
- **What about storage?** This may be more important than you think. Some medicines lose potency unless refrigerated. The bathroom medicine cabinet may be the worst place to store drugs, since the heat and humidity can cause many of them to deteriorate.
- **What should I do if I forget to take my medication?**

Generic versus Brand-name Drugs

Valium. By now everybody knows its name. It was championed and reviled as the star tranquilizer of the 1970s. Valium addiction was even the subject of the book *I'm Dancing as Fast as I Can* and a movie of the same name starring Jill Clayburgh. Despite its dark side, Valium was and is a very lucrative product for its manufacturer, Hoffmann–La Roche. So it came as no surprise that when Hoffmann–La Roche's patent expired, dozens of companies rushed to make their versions of diazepam.

When a pharmaceutical company patents a drug, it receives exclusive rights to market it for seventeen years. Once the seventeen years are up, other companies can apply to the FDA to market their versions under the chemical or generic name. About half of all generic drugs are made by the same companies that manufacture the brand names. The other half are manufactured by about 350 smaller firms devoted exclusively to generic drugs.

One third of all new prescriptions are filled with generic drugs. Medicare, Medicaid, and the Veterans Administration exert great pressure on patients to buy generics. The trend toward using generics is so strong that nearly half the states have laws instructing pharmacies to fill prescriptions with generics unless the doctor orders otherwise. The next time you are given a prescription, take a look at the little box at the bottom of the paper. In most states, it has language like, "This prescription should be filled generically unless the prescriber checks the 'daw' [dispense as written] box below."

The reason for all these policies and laws can be summed up in one word: cost. Generics cost about half as much as brand-name drugs. But are they as safe and effective? That's a question asked more frequently by health professionals since 1989, when several drug companies were found guilty of fraud and bribery. In 1985, Mylan Labs suspected the FDA of delaying approval of its application to market a generic drug. After Mylan discovered that an FDA chemist was accepting payoffs from companies that manufactured generic drugs, it took its evidence to a House of Representatives subcommittee and law enforcement officers. It turned out that some generic drug companies, to gain speedy approval for their products, were bribing FDA employees. Then the scandal spread.

One case involved the Vitarine Pharmaceutical Corporation's attempt to win FDA approval for a generic version of Dyazide, a best-selling diuretic and blood pressure drug. Because the active ingredient in Dyazide is hard to replicate, Vitarine tried a novel solution to gain FDA approval. Instead of testing the generic, it substituted the brand name. Approval was swift. The investigations uncovered other instances of cheating. When the dust had settled by the spring of 1990, seven companies were implicated.

Before a generic goes on the market, it must be approved by the FDA as being approximately equal to the brand-name product. While the *inactive* ingredients may differ, generic drugs must by law contain the same *active* ingredient as their brand-name counterparts. That ingredient must be absorbed into the bloodstream at the same rate as that in the brand-name drug, plus or minus 20 percent. After the scandal, the FDA conducted an intensive investigation into the quality of generics. It concluded that virtually all of the generics it tested met FDA standards. "These results should be reassuring to consumers who use generic drugs," said Health and Human Services Secretary Dr. Louis Sullivan.

Some physicians are not reassured. They question whether the quality control is as tight, whether the 20 percent leeway in the rate of absorption makes a generic different from the original, and whether the change in inactive ingredients may affect the quality of the drug. According to a 1989 report of the American Academy of Family Physicians, which represents sixty thousand family doctors, generics should *not* be considered the equivalent of brand-name drugs. The report expressed "serious concerns about generic drugs" and recommended that their use not be mandatory.

Whether to use a generic drug is your decision. Ask your doctor whether a generic equivalent exists and what are the pros and cons of using it. It is your right to know about a cheaper alternative and its advantages and disadvantages.

Unapproved Drugs

The FDA should really label prescription drugs "Before AIDS" and "After AIDS." Before AIDS, only drugs that underwent lengthy testing procedures reached the pharmacy. After AIDS, some drugs for life-threatening or serious illnesses are fast-tracked and made available before they have gone through the time-consuming clinical trials.

As a general rule, you can buy only prescription drugs that have been approved as safe and effective by the Food and Drug Administration. But since the deadly epidemic began, AIDS activists desperately argue that they should be able to use experimental drugs that have not gone through FDA-approval channels. The alternative, they say, is death, while experimental drugs might prolong — or improve — their life.

In response to intense pressure from AIDS activists, the FDA now allows people dying of AIDS, for whom no other treatment is available, to gain access to experimental therapies. One of the most dramatic examples is a new medication for AIDS, DDI (dideoxyinosine). Based on evidence from San Francisco physicians, the FDA dropped its requirements that DDI undergo lengthy tests for safety and effectiveness before being made available to people with AIDS who could not tolerate AZT (azidothymidine). In a radical departure from its usual practices, the FDA called for ongoing monitoring of results of the studies being carried out by San Francisco doctors. FDA commissioner Kessler said that the speeding of DDI's progress to the market should set an example for the approval of drugs for other serious health conditions like cancer and Alzheimer's.

The FDA also relaxed its rules to permit the import of up to a three months' supply of a nonapproved drug as long as it is for personal use and a physician agrees to oversee treatment. This applies to just about all medicines, not just those used to treat life-threatening illnesses.

Over-the-Counter Drugs

Drugs available without a prescription at supermarkets and drugstores must also be tested for safety and effectiveness. These over-the-counter drugs include remedies for everything from coughs and allergies to upset stomachs and headaches. While such medications must be found to have a low potential to harm you, no one should be lulled into thinking that just because you don't need a prescription, these medications are entirely benign. Pediatricians regularly warn parents about aspirin because children who take it run the risk of coming down with Reye's syndrome, a rare but potentially deadly disease.

As with any drug, use over the-counter medications with caution. Many medicines to treat such conditions as allergies, athlete's foot, and yeast infections have been removed from the by-prescription-only list. Unless you never watch television, it is hard to miss the barrage of drug company advertising. Just because the drugs are heavily advertised and available without prescription does not mean they don't have the potential to harm you if used incorrectly. The ingredients haven't changed — only the marketing has.

Over-the-counter drugs differ from prescription drugs in one major area — consumer information. Those long labels and complicated package inserts are not there for decoration; they are required by the government. Federal law mandates that drug manufacturers tell you what a drug is for, what active ingredients it contains, how to use it, who shouldn't take it, what other drugs to avoid while taking it, and its expiration date. The label, which must meet the standards of the Food and Drug Administration, is your best protection. Read it if you possibly can. Unfortunately, many labels are issued in such small print that they are undecipherable. If you *are* able to read them, the information is often presented in a way guaranteed to confuse even a nuclear physicist. If you have questions or problems, never hesitate to ask your doctor or pharmacist.

Where to Get More Information

How do you know if a drug is worthless or can hurt you? Initially, check with your doctor. Obviously, he or she won't intentionally prescribe something useless or dangerous. It's up to you to tell your physician about any allergies, other pills, including vitamins, you are taking, and past reactions to medication.

Your pharmacist is another terrific, underutilized resource. A good pharmacist can answer your questions about medications, interpret package inserts, and look up published information. Or you can do your own research. Many books can tell you what you need to know about drugs. You can also go to the source that doctors consult, the *Physicians' Desk Reference.* Be aware that it is written in doctorese, and you may need a medical dictionary to decipher its contents.

Medical Devices

Touted as a miracle contraceptive, the Dalkon Shield intrauterine device caused the death of at least fourteen women who used it. More than thirty children with major birth defects were born prematurely to Dalkon Shield wearers. Thousands more suffered scarred fallopian tubes, chronic pelvic inflammatory disease, ectopic pregnancies, and infertility.

But the Dalkon Shield is not the only horror story around. In 1989, the Codis Corporation agreed to pay over $5 million to victims of pacemakers the company manufactured, knowing that they could harm users. In another case, 265 people died from a defective heart valve manufactured by Shiley, Inc., a subsidiary of Pfizer, Inc. Only after the FDA pressured it in 1990 did the company agree to notify fifty-five thousand patients that their implanted heart valve might fracture.

The sale of harmful or fraudulent medical devices goes way back. In the 1700s, Elisha Perkins, a mule trader turned physician, claimed that two brass and iron rods — which only he sold — would rid the body of disease. Perkins Patent Tractors were so popular that even George Washington bought his family a set of the three-inch rods. Soon after, cries of fraud caught up with Perkins, and he and his rods disappeared. But lest we chuckle at the naiveté of our forefathers, consider such popular twentieth-century scams as copper bracelets to cure arthritis and pyramids over beds to improve sex lives.

When it comes to our bodies, we all ache for a miracle. Those desperate to cure cancer, stop pain, become more beautiful, grow hair, or lose weight are victims of a $27 billion-a-year business run by increasingly sophisticated con artists peddling impossible dreams.

Yet only in 1976, in the wake of the Dalkon Shield scandal, did Congress grant the FDA the same power to regulate medical devices it has for prescription drugs. The law requires the FDA to separate medical devices into three categories: relatively harmless ones, such as dipsticks and tongue depressors, which can be put on the market as long as they are not misbranded or adulterated; those with the potential to do more harm, such as eyeglasses and home pregnancy tests, which can be marketed as long as they conform to performance standards and other FDA guidelines; and those which can be implanted in the body or pose a serious risk to health.

Congress required that devices in the third category — the most potentially dangerous, such as pacemakers, corneal implants, artificial limbs, and intrauterine devices — be tested by the manufacturer and approved for safety and effectiveness by the FDA *before* being placed on the market. But here's the catch: under the law, medical appliances that are about the same as ("substantially equivalent to") devices that were on the market before 1976 do not require *any* testing for safety and effectiveness. Over 90 percent of the medical devices currently in use fall under this exemption.

In 1990, Congress passed the Safe Medical Devices Act. It requires hospitals and nursing homes, as well as manufacturers, to report deaths and serious injuries caused by medical apparatuses and authorizes the FDA to order a manufacturer to stop distributing harmful devices and, if necessary, recall them. Manufacturers of implantable or life-supporting devices whose safety and effectiveness were not approved by the FDA must submit this information before the end of 1995. The FDA will then decide which devices should remain on the market.

FDA regulations require manufacturers of hearing aids and intrauterine devices to supply package inserts directly to patients. Other than that, you must rely on your doctor and your pharmacist to tell you the pros and cons. If you are not satisfied with their answers or still have doubts, you can get a quick education and help protect yourself from hazardous medical devices by following these simple rules:

• **If you have questions about a device to be surgically implanted, get a second medical opinion.** It's a good idea in any case. We discuss how to go about getting a second surgical opinion in Chapter 2.

• **If you purchase a device at a drugstore, ask the pharmacist exactly how to use it and what side effects to watch out for.** If the device is sold by prescription, request a copy of the package insert and any other written information about it. If it is sold over the counter, read the instructions, particularly the section labeled "Warnings" or "Caution."

• **If you are still in doubt, call the Food and Drug Administration.** A representative should be able to give you up-to-date findings about the safety and effectiveness of devices. The telephone numbers of headquarters and regional offices are included in this chapter.

• **Make sure that the manufacturer knows where to reach you in case something goes wrong.** For most devices, this involves filling out a warranty card and leaving a forwarding address if you move. If you have had a device surgically implanted and are moving, be sure your doctor and the device manufacturer know where to find you. Under a 1990 law, manufacturers of permanently implanted and life-sustaining devices must notify you directly if a device is found to be defective, but they have to know where you are.

Cosmetics

The Food and Drug Administration has legal responsibility for regulating cosmetics. Because of its limited budget, staff cutbacks, and belief that cosmetics are less dangerous than drugs and medical devices, the FDA does not give beauty products high priority. Less than half of one percent of its budget is spent on cosmetic surveillance.

With the exception of color additives found, for example, in lipsticks and eyeshadow, and some prohibited ingredients, such as vinyl chloride and certain toxic dyes, a cosmetics manufacturer can use any material it wishes and market its products without FDA approval. The manufacturer is supposed to substantiate that the product is safe, although FDA regulations allow the manufacturer to decide how to do so. A report of the National Academy of Sciences found that of thousands of cosmetic ingredients and food additives, "only a few have been subjected to extensive toxicity testing and most have scarcely been tested at all."

For the most part, you do not know if a cosmetic will cause a reaction until you try it. People do suffer allergic or adverse reactions to soaps, deodorants, perfumes, and other cosmetics. If you are one of them, beyond taking the obvious step of not using it, notify the FDA and the manufacturer. You should also contact the National Center for Environmental Health Strategies, 1100 Rural Avenue, Voorhees, NJ 08043, (609) 429-5358, an organization set up to assist people who are sensitive to cosmetics and other chemical products.

Food
Remember the Wonder Bread ads that promised to build bodies eight — or was it nine — different ways? Sounds great, but who bought Wonder Bread for its nutritional value? Like cotton candy, it tasted good. In our health-crazed society, which demands good nutrition, disease prevention, and good taste all wrapped in one biodegradable package, the stakes have gotten higher.

Will this breakfast cereal, which contains oat bran, really reduce your chance of a heart attack? What do lite, light, or low sodium mean? Is sushi safe? Can you really lose seventy pounds through liquid diets? Are they safe? Where can a consumer turn for reliable information?

In response to confusing and sometimes wildly inaccurate claims, Congress passed the 1990 Nutrition Education and Labeling Act. "The misleading stuff is going off the label," FDA Commissioner David Kessler told the *New York Times*. "There will be confidence that when you see claims on the labels the words will have meaning." Unless companies can cite generally accepted studies, the law forbids them from touting their products' health benefits. Labels must include certain nutritional information, such as the amount of sodium and total fat. Since fat, particularly saturated fat, is a major enemy, it is given special attention. No longer can companies claim that a food is low in cholesterol or high in dietary fiber if it is oozing with fat.

Reading labels is a start, but you don't have to rely only on what a company tells you. Here are some places to turn for reliable information about food:

- The Center for Science in the Public Interest, 1875 Connecticut Avenue, NW, Washington, D.C., (202) 332-1110; Environmental Nutrition, 2112 Broadway, New York, NY 10023, (212) 362-0424; and Tufts University (800) 525-0643, publish newsletters that compare various foods.
- The U.S. Department of Agriculture has a hotline, (800) 535-4555, for information about meat and poultry. Call for dietary as well as storage guidelines.
- The U.S. Food and Drug Administration is responsible for assuring the safety of food products that do *not* contain meat or poultry. Contact either its Maryland headquarters or the regional office nearest you. Their addresses and telephone numbers are listed under "Key Government Agencies" at the end of this chapter.

Knowing what food to put into our mouths is a problem. Learning how to keep it out is big business. Obesity has reached "epidemic proportions," according to the *New England Journal of Medicine*. At any given time, more than 20 million Americans are on a diet. More than $32 million is spent every year on weight-loss products and programs. "The diet industry is built on a foundation of false promises and false hopes," says Oregon Congressman Ron Wyden. "Customers are promised physician-supervised weight-loss programs when there is no doctor in the house. Before and after photos in ads picture persons who were never on the diet.

Endorsements from major medical organizations are implied, even though the groups have specifically repudiated the use of their names."

Ninety percent of all dieters who lose twenty-five pounds in a diet program regain that weight within two years, concludes a report issued by a subcommittee of the U.S. House of Representatives. Only by making lifelong changes in your eating and exercising habits can you keep the weight off, says the American Medical Association. No one who witnessed the saga of Oprah Winfrey's dramatic weight loss and gain has to be told that. But long-term behavior modification is not nearly as glamorous as the quick fix you get from watching pounds melt as you temporarily limit yourself to sipping three very special chocolate shakes a day.

Moreover, starvation diets can be dangerous. "While there are certainly people who can benefit from medically supervised very-low-calorie diets, they are not for everyone," Nancy Wellman, president of the American Dietetic Association, testified before a congressional subcommittee. "The most significant drawback is the potential for life-threatening side effects." Among these are heart attack, anemia, light-headedness, menstrual irregularities, and, it is claimed by plaintiffs suing Nutri/System, gallbladder damage.

The FDA, which has responsibility for regulating liquid diets, proposed a ban on 111 ingredients in over-the-counter diet products in 1991. It has been unable to decide, however, whether to ban or require special warning labels on products containing PPA (phenylpropanolamine hydrochloride), a widely used and controversial appetite suppressant. The FDA is still studying data to determine whether the drug causes high blood pressure, internal bleeding, and strokes. Meanwhile, the advertising claims of liquid diets have come under the critical eye of the Federal Trade Commission (FTC). At the end of 1991, the FTC, which has the power to stop a company from making false claims, singled out several liquid diet companies. The claims the FTC said were misleading include Optifast's slogan that it's "the one that's clinically proven safe and effective," Medifast's ads that "you will not experience a rebound phenomenon [regain lost weight] after you attain your goal," and Ultrafast's boast that it is "the quickest, safest way of losing excess body weight." If you are thinking about starting an intensive weight-loss program, consult a physician, preferably one knowledgeable about nutrition who is certified by the American Board of Nutrition, or a registered dietitian. The American Dietetic Association, 216 West Jackson Boulevard, Chicago, IL 60606, (800) 877-1600, can give you the name of a registered dietitian in your area. And ask these questions, advises the Federal Trade Commission:

- **What does the diet program require you to do?** Do you have to stick to a certain number of calories or buy special foods from the company sponsoring the program?
- **How much does the program cost and how do you pay for it?** Make sure to add up all the costs, including fees, foods, supplements, and counseling, and find out how payment is required. Some programs charge high fees up front, which you may not get back if you drop out.
- **What health risks are associated with the program?** The FTC cautions that only significantly overweight people should consider enrolling in a very-low-calorie diet program.
- **What type of professional supervision is provided?** Ask for the credentials of anybody identified as an "expert" in dieting.
- **What kind of maintenance program is provided and what does it cost?** Is the maintenance program part of the overall package or is it extra?

Consumer Products

Just about every manufactured product, from toy fire engines and children's pajamas to paint thinners and chain saws, falls under the jurisdiction of the Consumer Product Safety Commission (CPSC). Established in 1972 to "protect the public against unreasonable risks of injury and to assist consumers in evaluating the safety of consumer products," the CPSC is responsible for enforcing five federal consumer protection laws: the Consumer Products Safety Act, the Flammable Fabrics Act, the Hazardous Substances Act, the Poison Prevention Packaging Act, and the Refrigerator Safety Act.

During the cut-'em-off-at-the-knees fervor of the 1980s, the CPSC suffered along with other federal agencies charged with protecting the public's health and safety. In one year alone, it lost over

25 percent of its budget and staff. The number of regional offices dropped from fourteen to three. Rather than issue national standards to assure the safety of consumer products, the CPSC let trade associations write their own standards and police their own members. As expected, some industries have been good cops, establishing strong standards and enforcing them effectively, while others have turned their backs on the whole idea.

Children's products comprise one area in which the CPSC has some teeth. Many federal laws are specifically aimed at protecting the lives of the vulnerable young. By law, children's sleepwear must be flame retardant, cribs must have slats spaced close enough that a baby's head does not get caught, and medicine bottles must be fitted with child-proof caps. Standards also ensure the safety of electric trains, bicycles, and some children's toys.

The Consumer Product Safety Commission's toll-free hotline — (800) 638-CPSC — is not very good, but it's better than nothing. If you call between 8:30 and 5:30 eastern time, Monday through Friday, you get a prerecorded voice instructing you to push a button on your Touch-Tone telephone to learn about specific products that have been recalled. If you push enough buttons, you'll eventually get to a real person with whom you can either register a complaint or find out whether the product that concerns you is on the commission's list. The National Highway Traffic Safety Administration has a similar hotline for information about recalls of children's car seats. Its number is (800) 424-9393.

Private organizations have chosen to fill the gap left by the government. *Consumer Reports* compares products for safety, effectiveness, and cost. If you call (914) 378-2000, an operator will tell you which issue contains the information you want. The Consumer Federation of America, an advocacy and public education group, also provides information. Contact it at 1424 16th Street, Washington, DC 20036, (202) 387-6121.

Hazardous Substances
Each year, more than 22 billion tons of hazardous chemicals are released into the air you breathe, the water you drink, and the land you live on, according to the Environmental Action Foundation. These chemicals, along with radiation, toxic gases, and deadly substances, can cause cancers, respiratory diseases, birth defects,

reproductive problems, and brain damage, among other illnesses. Consider the following depressing statistics:

- At least 40 million Americans drink water with potentially dangerous levels of lead, according to Environmental Protection Agency estimates.
- Nine out of ten toxic chemical dumps are located directly above groundwater supplies. The cost of cleaning up toxic chemical sites may run to $20 billion by the end of the decade.
- Twenty-five states report groundwater contaminated by pesticides.

The U.S. Congress and state legislatures have passed thousands of laws aimed at making the air breathable, the water drinkable, and hazardous substances less dangerous to people. In 1969, Congress created the Environmental Protection Agency (EPA) to monitor and enforce the laws, a task carried out at state and local levels by health and environmental protection departments. Federal and state consumer protection, health, and occupational health and safety departments also play a role in protecting people from hazardous substances.

Despite this legislative and regulatory assault, we remain vulnerable. "To protect yourself, read the warning labels required by law," says Columbia University law professor Frank Grad, an expert in environmental law. "Get as much information as you can and take appropriate precautions." Environmental organizations, both government and private, provide help to concerned consumers, often through toll-free hotlines. Take advantage of them.

Lead, Asbestos, and Radon
Your home is not a haven when it comes to environmental hazards. In particular, lead, asbestos, and radon can ruin your health and that of your family. Lead poisoning can cause kidney failure and hypertension in adults and memory loss, lower intelligence, slow reaction time, and short attention span in children. In fact, it is now considered the number-one environmental threat to children, who are particularly vulnerable because their neurological systems are still developing. According to the U.S. Agency for

Toxic Substances and Disease Registry, more than 3 million children — one in six — have a high enough level of lead in their blood to impair their development.

The two main sources are lead-based paint and water. When lead-based paint chips or peels, it turns into dust. If your children breathe enough dust or eat enough paint chips, they will be poisoned. Three quarters of all houses and apartments built before 1950 contain lead-based paint. Lead also enters the water supply through lead pipes, soldering, or faucets.

During the 1970s and 1980s, Congress banned the use of leaded gasoline, lead-based paints, and lead-based solder in plumbing systems. If you live in an old house, are renovating one, or your children go to a school built before 1950 whose paint is peeling, you'll probably find lead.

Asbestos, once believed to be a miracle mineral, is considered a health menace. A natural substance, asbestos can perform amazing feats. It can insulate against heat and cold, muffle noise, and is virtually indestructible. Because of these virtues, massive quantities of asbestos were used between the 1920s and 1970s in more than three thousand products, including insulation for heating pipes and air-conditioning systems, ceiling and floor tiles, incubators, cigarette holders, and drapes. It is used today in automobile brake linings and sand for children's sandboxes, among other products.

Asbestos can also kill. When asbestos products deteriorate or are damaged, microscopic fibers are released into the air. If you breathe sufficient amounts, you can come down with asbestosis, a scarring of the lung tissue that makes it difficult or impossible to breathe, mesothelioma, a cancer of the lung lining or abdominal cavity, or lung cancer. These potentially fatal diseases often do not show up until fifteen to twenty years after exposure.

The EPA estimates that asbestos can be found in over seven hundred thousand public and commercial buildings, thirty thousand schools, and countless millions of homes. Although asbestos is rarely used in buildings anymore, and will be totally banned as a building material by 1997, if your home, workplace, or child's school was constructed before 1970, you're probably living with asbestos. According to the American Lung Association, asbestos is a health hazard only when fibers are released into the air, for example, by deteriorating or crumbling insulation or during extensive home renovation.

If you think you have an asbestos or lead problem or are buying or renovating an old house, you would be wise to order an inspection by an environmental engineer or contractor. If you *know* you have a problem, you would be a fool not to contact one. But how can you find somebody reliable? Your best bet is to look for an industrial hygienist certified by the American Board of Industrial Hygiene. This does not guarantee quality (nothing does), but it does assure you that the inspector has experience in the field, has passed rigorous exams, and has kept up to date. For a nominal charge, you can get a list of board-certified industrial hygienists from the American Board of Industrial Hygiene, 4600 West Saginaw, Lansing, MI 48917, (517) 321-2638.

Another source of names is the membership list of the American Industrial Hygiene Association. Although its members do not have to pass exams for board certification in order to join, membership implies that a person is an expert who keeps up with the field. Contact the American Industrial Hygiene Association, 345 White Pond Drive, Akron, OH 44311, (216) 873-2442.

The EPA hotlines listed in the "Where to Turn for Help" section of this chapter and state and local health departments can also provide names of companies that can inspect your home for environmental hazards. Since most states do not license lead contractors, that is, do not require them to pass an exam or meet minimum standards, they list companies in the field, not necessarily ones they recommend. On the other hand, asbestos contractors in all but three states are required to complete a course that meets the standards of the Environmental Protection Agency. When they have completed it, they are licensed or certified by their state government. Ask the health department for a list of state-licensed or certified asbestos contractors. You can also get the names by requesting *The Asbestos List* from the Consumer Product Safety Commission, Washington, DC 20207, (301) 492-6580.

Ask the contractor you hire whether the lead and asbestos samples will be analyzed at a lab certified by the state or by the American Industrial Hygiene Association. If the tests turn out to be positive, you have a number of options, ranging from doing nothing to removal. In the case of asbestos, for example, the EPA recommends removal only as a last resort.

Another silent domestic killer is the radioactive gas radon, a natural by-product of uranium found in the earth's crust, which you cannot see, touch, or smell. It seeps into basements and, if breathed in sufficient quantities, can cause lung cancer. Every year an estimated sixteen thousand people die from radon, making it the second leading cause of lung cancer deaths after cigarettes.

Radon is easy to detect and get rid of. You can get a testing kit at hardware or department stores or, in some states, from the health department. If you buy one on your own, make certain it is EPA certified or approved. This assures that the company participated in the EPA's Radon Measurement Proficiency program. You can also hire a private contractor. For information on radon detection and abatement, call the EPA's radon hotline, (800) 767-7236, or the radon office in your state. The telephone numbers are listed below.

STATE RADON OFFICES

Alabama (205) 261-5315	**Delaware** (800) 554-4636	**Indiana** (800) 272-9723
Alaska (907) 465-3019	**District of Columbia** (202) 727-7728	**Iowa** (515) 281-7781
Arizona (602) 255-4845	**Florida** (800) 543-8279	**Kansas** (913) 296-1560
Arkansas (501) 661-2301	**Georgia** (404) 894-6644	**Kentucky** (502) 564-3700
California (415) 540-2134	**Hawaii** (808) 548-4383	**Louisiana** (504) 925-4518
Colorado (303) 331-4812	**Idaho** (208) 334-5933	**Maine** (207) 289-3826
Connecticut (203) 566-3122	**Illinois** (217) 786-6384	**Maryland** (800) 872-3666

Massachusetts
(413) 586-7525
or in Boston
(617) 727-6214

Michigan
(517) 335-8190

Minnesota
(612) 623-5341

Mississippi
(601) 354-6657

Missouri
(800) 669-7236

Montana
(406) 444-3671

Nebraska
(402) 471-2168

Nevada
(702) 885-5394

New Hampshire
(603) 271-4674

New Jersey
(800) 648-0394

New Mexico
(505) 827-2940

New York
(800) 458-1158

North Carolina
(919) 733-4283

North Dakota
(701) 224-2348

Ohio
(800) 523-4439

Oklahoma
(405) 271-5221

Oregon
(503) 229-5797

Pennsylvania
(800) 23-RADON

Rhode Island
(401) 277-2438

South Carolina
(803) 734-4631

South Dakota
(605) 773-3153

Tennessee
(615) 741-4634

Texas
(512) 835-7000

Utah
(801) 538-6734

Vermont
(802) 828-2886

Virginia
(800) 468-0138

Virgin Islands
(809) 774-3320

Washington
(800) 323-9727

West Virginia
(304) 348-3526

Wisconsin
(608) 273-5180

Wyoming
(307) 777-7956

Where to Turn for Help

Devotees of *Alice in Wonderland* know all about the Mad Hatter, the character who poured hot tea on the sleeping Dormouse's nose at Alice's tea party and later sang "Twinkle, twinkle, little bat." What Alice's fans probably didn't realize was that the Mad Hatter was most likely suffering from mercury poisoning, which can cause neurological damage characterized by bizarre behavior. In those days, mercury was commonly used in the hatmaking process.

With more than seventy thousand chemicals in use, not to mention heavy metals and radiation, the list of potentially harmful substances appears inexhaustible. A number of organizations provide information and help to people wanting to know what to look out for, what to do in case of exposure, how to bring a citizen's suit against a company violating environmental laws, how to force cleanup of a toxic waste site, and where to get further help. Contact one or more of them for assistance.

Lead

- EPA Lead Hotline, (202) 554-1404
- The Alliance to End Childhood Lead Poisoning, 600 Pennsylvania Avenue, SE, Washington, DC 20003, (202) 543-1147

Asbestos

- EPA Asbestos Information Hotline, (800) 835-6700
- Asbestos Victims of America, P.O. Box 559, Capitola, CA 95010, (408) 476-3646
- White Lung Association, P.O. Box 1483, Baltimore, MD 21203-1483, (301) 243-5864

Pesticides

- EPA Pesticide Hotline, (800) 858-PEST
- National Coalition Against the Misuse of Pesticides, 701 E Street, SE, Washington, DC 20003, (202) 543-5450

Toxic Wastes

- EPA Toxic Waste Hotline, (800) 424-9346
- Citizen's Clearinghouse for Hazardous Waste, P.O. Box 926, Arlington, VA 22216, (703) 276-7070

Indoor Air

- National Center for Environmental Health Strategies, 1100 Rural Avenue, Voorhees, NJ 08043, (609) 429-5358
- American Lung Association, 1740 Broadway, New York, NY 10019, (212) 315-8700

Tobacco Smoke

- Action on Smoking and Health, 2013 H Street, NW, Washington, DC 20006, (202) 659-4130
- American Cancer Society, 19 West 56th Street, New York, NY 10001, (212) 586-8700

Water

- Clean Water Action Project, 1320 18th Street, NW, Washington, DC 20003, (202) 457-1286
- EPA Safe Drinking Water Hotline, (800) 426-4791

Art Equipment and Supplies

- Center for Safety in the Arts, 5 Beekman Street, New York, NY 10038, (212) 227-6220
- Arts, Crafts and Theater Safety, 181 Thompson Street, New York, NY 10012, (212) 777-0062

Environmental Advocacy Groups, General

- The Audubon Society, 666 Pennsylvania Avenue, SE, Washington, DC 20003, (202) 547-9009
- Environmental Action Foundation, 6930 Carroll Avenue, Tacoma Park, MD 20719, (301) 891-1100
- Environmental Defense Fund, 257 Park Avenue South, New York, NY 10010, (212) 505-2100
- EPA Watch, Government Accountability Project, 25 E Street, NW, Washington, DC 20001, (202) 408-0034
- Natural Resources Defense Council, 40 West 20th Street, New York, NY 10011, (212) 727-2700

If You Get Hurt

It can happen to anybody from almost any product — a deodorant soap causes blisters; a can of tuna fish contains a tack; foam insulation for a house is found to cause cancer. The list is almost endless. Every year dangerous products injure more than 33 million Americans and kill over twenty-eight thousand. Here's what you can do if you are affected:

Get Treatment
Should a bottle of beer explode in your hand, you'd obviously get help. But what about the dizziness and nausea you felt after taking a strong cough medicine or the upset stomach and diarrhea you got after taking an antibiotic your doctor prescribed for an infection? Or the uncharacteristically low test scores that suddenly appeared on your children's school reports around the time you were renovating your old house?

If you or your child has developed *any* side effects while on medication, assume that the drug is the culprit, advises the Public Citizen Health Research Group. For other symptoms, such as the drop in your child's reading scores, the cause may be harder to identify. The point is that you should consult a health professional if you *think* a product is the culprit or if you've developed unusual or inexplicable symptoms.

Report an Injury or Illness
While few people think about reporting injuries, your written complaint can alert government authorities about potentially dangerous products and help you if you decide to sue. Moreover, if it gets enough complaints, a government agency may investigate and require a warning label or even recall the product.

As a start, write to the manufacturer and the store where you bought the product in question and send a copy to the appropriate government consumer protection agency. Depending on the kind of product, notify the following:

- **Drugs and medical devices:** the Food and Drug Administration
- **Food (other than meat or poultry) and cosmetics:** the Food and Drug Administration, or if the problem is one of false or misleading advertising, the Federal Trade Commission
- **Meat, eggs, and poultry:** the Department of Agriculture
- **Water:** if it comes from a bottle, the FDA; if it comes from the tap, the Environmental Protection Agency.

- **Children's car seats:** the National Highway Traffic Safety Administration
- **Other consumer products:**
    the Consumer Product Safety Commission
    the state or local consumer protection agency
    the Better Business Bureau — call national headquarters, (703) 276-0100, for the nearest state or city branch
- **Chemicals and toxic substances:** the Environmental Protection Agency or your local health department

The addresses and phone numbers of government agencies, except health departments, are listed at the end of this chapter. State health departments are found at the end of Chapter 2.

Last Resort: A Product Liability Lawsuit

If you are seriously injured by a product, you can bring a product liability lawsuit against the manufacturer and those involved in its sale. For a long time, it was difficult for an injured consumer to get on the court docket, much less win a lawsuit against the manufacturer of a harmful product. Unless you bought the product directly from the manufacturer, the courts did not want to hear about it. Since almost everybody buys products from a retail outlet, the requirement of direct purchase from the manufacturer essentially shut out consumers, no matter how badly they may have been hurt. Courts finally did away with this requirement, which they quaintly called privity of contract.

Negligence and Breach of Warranty

Even though injured consumers were finally allowed into court, winning remained tough. For the most part, they had to prove negligence — that the manufacturer made the product in a careless or substandard manner — or breach of warranty — that the company guaranteed the product was safe and it wasn't. Both were very difficult to prove.

Strict Liability

Because of this basic inequity, the law evolved so that a person injured by a harmful product did *not* have to prove that the manufacturer was negligent or at fault in any way. This is known as strict liability. It began in 1963 with the case of William Greenman. When the Californian tried out the combination power tool his wife bought him for his birthday as a lathe, a piece of wood flew out of the machine and struck him in the eye. Mr. Greenman sued Yuba Products, the manufacturer, and won on the basis of strict liability, even though he could not prove that the manufacturer was negligent. "A manufacturer is strictly liable," wrote Judge Roger Traynor of the California Supreme Court, "when an article he places on the market, knowing that it is to be used without inspection for defects, proves to have a defect that causes injury."

All states now permit people injured by harmful products to bring lawsuits under a strict liability theory. To win, you must prove that you were injured by a defective product that was unreasonably dangerous. Remember, however, that it is not enough to show that you used and were injured by a product. You must prove to the satisfaction of a judge or jury that there was a defect in the manufacture of the product, that the design was faulty and led to danger, that you were not told about the product's risks, or that the packaging was inadequate or unsafe.

Manufacturing Defects
A manufacturing defect may be a power saw without a safety protector or that tack in the can of tuna fish.

Design Defects
The classic case of a design defect is the old Ford Pinto. The car was designed in such a way that when it was hit from behind, the gas tank would explode. In May 1972, thirteen-year-old Richard Grimshaw was a passenger in a Pinto that stalled on Interstate 15 near San Bernardino, California. Another car hit the Pinto from the rear. The gas tank exploded, and Grimshaw was badly burned when the car burst into flames. He sued Ford Motor Company. During the course of the trial, his lawyer introduced a memorandum from Ford's files showing that the company knew the gas tank could cause injuries or death but reckoned it was cheaper to pay damages resulting from lawsuits than to fix the problem. A jury awarded Grimshaw $2.8 million in compensatory damages

and $125 million in punitive damages. The latter amount was later reduced by the judge to $3.5 million.

Failure to Warn

Aside from obvious dangers — for example, that a knife is sharp and may cut you — a manufacturer has a duty to warn about the known or reasonably foreseeable dangers of its products. What this means in practice is left to a judge or jury to decide. Two similar examples involved women injured by their deodorant.

In a Massachusetts case, Florence Wright sued the Carter company, the makers of Arrid, after the deodorant, advertised as "harmless," caused her skin to erupt and blister. The judge found for the plaintiff, ruling that the manufacturer had a duty to "warn those few persons who it knows cannot apply its product without serious injury."

In a New York case, nineteen-year-old Inga Kaempfe of the Bronx was not so fortunate. She, too, developed a severe skin rash with burning and blistering after using Etiquet Spray-On Deodorant and sued the manufacturer. Although the label on the deodorant read "safe for normal skin," Ms. Kaempfe lost when the judge ruled that the company did not have to warn her since she was one of "a microscopic fraction of potential users who may suffer some allergic reaction."

Failure to Package Safely

Finally, you have a case if you can prove that a product was inadequately packaged. A company that sold liquid drain cleaner in a bottle that could easily be opened by children would be liable for injuries that result from its packaging.

CHECKLIST: TIPS ON PRODUCT LIABILITY LAWSUITS

- If you have been seriously injured by a product and believe you may have grounds for a lawsuit, contact a lawyer with experience in product liability cases. For advice on how to find one, see Chapter 14.
- Most lawyers who handle product liability cases bill on a contingency basis; namely, they take a percentage — often

a third — of any damages you are awarded. If you lose, you pay no fee for their time, but you may have to pay for the expenses incurred in bringing the case. Watch out — these can add up quickly.

- You can sue the manufacturer of the product as well as wholesalers, distributors, and retailers. Many lawyers prefer to bring them all in.

- You can sue on several grounds simultaneously. Many lawyers choose to sue under theories of negligence, strict liability, breach of warranty, and any other grounds that might produce a winning verdict.

- You can ask for two different kinds of damages: *compensatory*, which reimburses you for medical expenses, rehabilitation costs, lost wages, and pain and suffering, and *punitive*, which are occasionally levied against companies to punish them for intentionally or recklessly causing harm.

- Manufacturers can defend themselves by showing that you misused the product, tampered with it, failed to follow directions, bought it used, or knew it was dangerous but continued using it anyway. Whether these defenses succeed depends on state law, the specific facts, and the quality of the lawyers for both sides.

- A key piece of evidence is likely to be the harmful product itself. Save it if possible.

- You have only a limited time to bring a product liability lawsuit after being injured — usually two to three years — although, as we point out in the discussion of "A Note on Toxic Torts," many states delay the start of their statute of limitations for injuries or illnesses that do not show up immediately.

- Even in cases brought under strict liability, you still have to prove that the product itself, or its instructions or packaging, was defective. Being injured by a product is not enough.

- Many states have taken steps to reduce the number of, and high awards in, product liability cases. These include placing caps on damages; limiting the contingency fees that lawyers can charge; and eliminating the "deep pockets" system in which wealthy defendants pay a disproportionately large share of damages.

A Note on Toxic Torts

If you become ill from exposure to chemicals or other toxic products and are considering suing the manufacturer, you should be aware of some of the unique problems you are likely to face.

The first is proving that the product "caused" the injury. Since fifteen to forty years may elapse between the time of exposure and onset of an illness, cause and effect may be difficult to prove. In addition, you may have been exposed to other hazardous substances, including self-inflicted ones such as cigarette smoke, that contributed to the condition. In practice, toxic tort lawsuits often turn into battles of the experts, with each side producing doctors, epidemiologists, and statisticians to testify that the product did, or did not, cause the harm charged.

The second problem is identifying the manufacturer. Who of us knows for certain who made the chemicals we were exposed to years ago? In some cases, the courts have eased this problem by hauling in all the manufacturers and assigning them liability on the basis of their market share at the time of exposure. That's what happened to the daughters of women who took DES and developed cancer. The women did not know who manufactured the product that their mothers had taken many years ago. Rather than denying them legal recourse, courts assessed damages on the basis of share of the market held by the DES manufacturers at the time the mothers took the drug.

The third is bringing a case within the time limits set by the statute of limitations, often two or three years after exposure. Since the latency period for environmentally caused diseases may be fifteen years or more, strict adherence to statutes of limitations would mean that virtually nobody could bring a lawsuit. Legislatures and courts have attempted to remedy the problem by ruling that the statute of limitations does not begin running until a person discovers, or should have discovered, an illness. Some states have set outside limits, such as ten or twelve years after exposure, within which a lawsuit must be brought.

Despite these hurdles, plaintiffs do bring and win toxic tort lawsuits. Asbestos victims, for example, have brought successful lawsuits against companies that manufactured the product. "Over three hundred thousand lawsuits against asbestos manufacturers are pending," says Paul Safchuck, president of the White Lung Association, a nonprofit asbestos victims' association. One attempt to cope with this massive litigation saw twenty-six thousand cases brought in federal courts consolidated into one large lawsuit in 1991, to be heard before a single judge in Philadelphia.

If you believe that you have been harmed by exposure to a hazardous product, contact a lawyer experienced in toxic tort litigation.

Key Government Agencies

FOOD AND DRUG ADMINISTRATION

Consumer Affairs Offices

Northeast Region
(*Connecticut, Maine,*
  Massachusetts, New Hampshire,
  Rhode Island, Vermont)
One Montvale Avenue
Stoneham, MA 02180
(617) 279-1479

(*New York City and Suburbs*)
850 Third Avenue
Brooklyn, NY 11232
(718) 965-5043

(*Upstate New York*)
599 Delaware Avenue
Buffalo, NY 14202
(716) 846-4483

Mid-Atlantic Region
(*Delaware, Pennsylvania*)
U.S. Courthouse
2nd and Chestnut Streets
Philadelphia, PA 19106
(215) 597-0837

(*New Jersey*)
61 Main Street
West Orange, NJ 07052
(201) 645-6365

(*Maryland*)
900 Madison Avenue
Baltimore, MD 21201
(301) 962-3731

(*Virginia, West Virginia, District of*
  Columbia)
1110 N. Glebe Road
Arlington, VA 22201
(703) 285-2578

(*Ohio*)
1141 Central Parkway
Cincinnati, OH 45202
(513) 684-3501

(*Ohio*)
3820 Central Road
Brunswick, OH 44212
(216) 273-1038

Southeast Region
*(Alabama, Georgia, North
  Carolina, South Carolina)*
60 Eighth Street, NE
Atlanta, GA 30309
(404) 347-7355

(Florida)
6601 N.W. 25th Street
P.O. Box 59-2256
Miami, FL 33159-2256
(305) 526-2919

(Florida)
7200 Lake Ellenor Drive
Orlando, FL 32809
(407) 855-0900

(Kentucky, Mississippi, Tennessee)
297 Plus Park Boulevard
Nashville, TN 37217
(615) 736-2088

(Arkansas, Louisiana)
4298 Elysian Fields Avenue
New Orleans, LA 70122
(504) 589-2420

Midwest
(Illinois)
433 West Van Buren Street
1222 Main Post Office Building
Chicago, IL 60607
(312) 353-7126

(Michigan)
1560 East Jefferson Avenue
Detroit, MI 48207
(313) 226-6260

(Minnesota, Wisconsin)
240 Hennepin Avenue
Minneapolis, MN 55401
(612) 334-4103

(Indiana)
675 N. Pennsylvania
Indianapolis, IN 46204
(317) 269-6500

(Texas)
3032 Bryan Street
Dallas, TX 75204
(214) 655-5310

(Texas)
1445 N. Loop West
Houston, TX 77008
(713) 220-2322

(Texas)
727 E. Durango
San Antonio, TX 78206
(512) 229-6737

(Iowa, Kansas, Missouri, Nebraska)
1009 Cherry Street
Kansas City, MO 64106
(816) 374-6366

(Missouri)
Laciede's Landing
808 North Collins Street
St. Louis, MO 63102
(314) 425-5021

*(Colorado, Montana, North Dakota,
  South Dakota, Utah, Wyoming)*
P.O. Box 25087
6th and Kipling
Denver, CO 80225-0087
(303) 236-3000

Pacific Region
*(Northern California, Hawaii,
  Nevada)*
50 United Nations Plaza
San Francisco, CA 94102
(415) 556-1364

(*Arizona, Southern California*)
1521 West Pico Boulevard
Los Angeles, CA 90015
(213) 252-7597

(*Alaska, Idaho, Oregon,*
  Washington)
22201 23rd Drive, SE
Bothell, WA 98021-4421
(206) 483-4953

CONSUMER PRODUCT SAFETY COMMISSION

Eastern Regional Center
(*Connecticut, Delaware, Washington, DC, Florida, Maine, Maryland,*
  Massachusetts, New Hampshire, New Jersey, New York, North Carolina,
  Pennsylvania, Puerto Rico, Rhode Island, South Carolina, Vermont,
  Virgin Islands, Virginia, West Virginia)
6 World Trade Center
New York, NY 10048-0950
(212) 264-1125

Central Regional Center
(*Alabama, Georgia, Illinois, Indiana, Iowa, Kansas, Kentucky, Michigan,*
  Minnesota, Mississippi, Missouri, Nebraska, North Dakota, Ohio, South
  Dakota, Tennessee, Wisconsin)
230 South Dearborn Street
Chicago, IL 60604-1601
(312) 353-8260

Western Regional Center
(*Alaska, Arizona, Arkansas, California, Colorado, Guam, Hawaii, Idaho,*
  Louisiana, Montana, Nevada, New Mexico, Oklahoma, Oregon, Texas,
  Utah, Washington, Wyoming)
555 Battery Street
San Francisco, CA 94111-2390
(415) 556-1816

FEDERAL TRADE COMMISSION

Regional Offices

Atlanta Region
(Alabama, Florida, Georgia,
Mississippi, North Carolina,
Tennessee, Virginia, except
metropolitan D.C. area)
1718 Peachtree Street, NW
Atlanta, GA 30367
(404) 347-4836

Boston Region
(Connecticut, Maine,
Massachusetts, New Hampshire,
Rhode Island, Vermont)
10 Causeway Street
Boston, MA 02222
(617) 565-7240

Chicago Region
(Illinois, Indiana, Iowa, Kentucky,
Minnesota, Missouri, Wisconsin)
55 East Monroe Street
Chicago, IL 60603
(312) 353-4423

Cleveland Region
(Delaware, Maryland, except
metropolitan D.C. area,
Michigan, Ohio, Pennsylvania,
West Virginia)
668 Euclid Avenue
Cleveland, OH 44114
(216) 522-4210

Dallas Region
(Arkansas, Louisiana, New Mexico,
Oklahoma, Texas)
100 N. Central Expressway
Dallas, TX 75201
(214) 767-5503

Denver Region
(Colorado, Kansas, Montana,
Nebraska, North Dakota, South
Dakota, Utah, Wyoming)
1405 Curtis Street
Denver, CO 80202
(303) 844-2271

Los Angeles Region
(Arizona, Southern California)
11000 Wilshire Boulevard
Los Angeles, CA 90024
(213) 575-7890

New York Region
(New Jersey, New York)
150 William Street
New York, NY 10038
(212) 264-1207

San Francisco Region
(Northern California, Hawaii,
Nevada)
901 Market Street
San Francisco, CA 94103
(415) 744-7920

Seattle Region
(Alaska, Idaho, Oregon,
Washington)
915 Second Avenue
Seattle, WA 98174
(206) 553-4656

ENVIRONMENTAL PROTECTION AGENCY

Regional Offices

Region 1
(*Connecticut, Maine,
Massachusetts, New Hampshire,
Rhode Island, Vermont*)
J. F. Kennedy Federal Building
1 Congress Street
Boston, MA 02203
(617) 565-3400

Region 2
(*New Jersey, New York, Puerto Rico,
Virgin Islands*)
26 Federal Plaza
New York, NY 10278
(212) 264-2525

Region 3
(*Delaware, Washington, DC,
Maryland, Pennsylvania,
Virginia, West Virginia*)
841 Chestnut Street
Philadelphia, PA 19107
(215) 597-9814

Region 4
(*Alabama, Florida, Georgia,
Kentucky, Mississippi, North
Carolina, South Carolina,
Tennessee*)
345 Courtland Street, NE
Atlanta, GA 30365
(404) 347-4727

Region 5
(*Illinois, Indiana, Michigan,
Minnesota, Ohio, Wisconsin*)
230 South Dearborn Street
J. C. Kluczynski Federal Building
Chicago, IL 60604
(312) 353-2000

Region 6
(*Arkansas, Louisiana, New Mexico,
Oklahoma, Texas*)
1445 Ross Avenue
Dallas, TX 75202-2405
(214) 655-2100

Region 7
(*Iowa, Kansas, Missouri, Nebraska*)
726 Minnesota Avenue
Kansas City, KS 66101
(913) 551-7006

Region 8
(*Colorado, Montana, North Dakota,
South Dakota, Utah, Wyoming*)
999 Eighteenth Street
Denver, CO 80202-2405
(303) 293-1603

Region 9
(*Arizona, California, Guam,
Hawaii, Nevada, Trust Territory
of the Pacific Islands — Caroline
Islands, Mariana Islands,
Marshall Islands*)
75 Hawthorne Street
San Francisco, CA 94105
(415) 744-1001

Region 10
(*Alaska, Idaho, Oregon,
Washington*)
1200 Sixth Avenue
Seattle, WA 98101
(206) 442-0479

STATE CONSUMER PROTECTION OFFICES

Alabama
Consumer Protection Division
Office of Attorney General
11 South Union Street
Montgomery, AL 36130
(205) 261-7334
toll free in state:
(800) 392-5658

Alaska
Consumer Protection Section
Office of Attorney General
1031 West Fourth Avenue
Anchorage, AK 99701
(907) 456-8588

Arizona
Financial Fraud Division
Office of Attorney General
1275 W. Washington Street
Phoenix, AZ 85007
(602) 542-3702 (fraud only)
toll free in state:
(800) 352-8431

Financial Fraud Division
Office of Attorney General
402 W. Congress Street
Tucson, AZ 85701
(602) 628-5501

Arkansas
Office of Attorney General
200 Tower Building
4th and Center Streets
Little Rock, AR 72201
(501) 682-2007
toll free in state:
(800) 482-8982

California
California Department of
    Consumer Affairs
1020 "N" Street
Sacramento, CA 95814
(916) 445-0660
(complaint assistance)
(916) 445-1254
(consumer information)

Public Inquiry Unit
Office of Attorney General
1515 "K" Street
P.O. Box 944255
Sacramento, CA 94244-2550
(916) 322-3360
toll free in state:
(800) 952-5225

Colorado
Consumer Protection Unit
Office of Attorney General
1525 Sherman Street
Denver, CO 80203
(303) 866-5167

Connecticut
Department of Consumer
    Protection
State Office Building
165 Capitol Avenue
Hartford, CT 06105
(203) 566-5374

Delaware
Division of Consumer Affairs
Department of Community Affairs
820 North French Street
Wilmington, DE 19801
(302) 577-3250

Office of Attorney General
Economic Crime and Consumer
 Protection Division
820 North French Street
Wilmington, DE 19801
(302) 577-3250

District of Columbia
Department of Consumer and
 Regulatory Affairs
614 H Street, NW
Washington, DC 20001
(202) 727-7000

Florida
Department of Agriculture and
 Consumer Services
Division of Consumer Services
218 Mayo Building
Tallahassee, FL 32399
(904) 488-2226
toll free in state:
(800) 342-2176

Georgia
Governor's Office of Consumer
 Affairs
2 Martin Luther King, Jr., Drive,
 Southeast
Atlanta, GA 30334
(404) 656-3790
toll free in state:
(800) 282-5808

Hawaii
Office of Consumer Protection
Department of Commerce and
 Consumer Affairs

828 Fort Street Mall
P.O. Box 3767
Honolulu, HI 96812-3767
(808) 548-2560
(administration and legal)
(808) 548-2540
(complaints and investigations)

Idaho
Office of the Attorney General
Consumer Protection Unit
Statehouse
Boise, ID 83720-1000
(208) 334-2424
toll free in state:
(800) 432-3545

Illinois
Governor's Office of Citizens
 Assistance
201 West Monroe Street
Springfield, IL 62706
(217) 782-0244
toll free in state:
(800) 642-3112

Consumer Protection Division
Office of Attorney General
100 West Randolph
Chicago, IL 60601
(312) 917-3580
(312) 793-2852

Indiana
Consumer Protection Division
Office of Attorney General
219 State House
Indianapolis, IN 46204
(317) 232-6330
toll free in state:
(800) 382-5516

Iowa

Iowa Citizen's Aide/Ombudsman
215 East Seventh Street
Capitol Complex
Des Moines, IA 50319
(515) 281-3592
toll free in state:
(800) 358-5510

Consumer Protection Division
Office of Attorney General
1300 East Walnut Street
Des Moines, IA 50319
(515) 281-5926

Kansas

Consumer Protection Division
Office of Attorney General
Kansas Judicial Center
Topeka, KS 66612
(913) 296-3751
toll free in state:
(800) 432-2310

Kentucky

Consumer Protection Division
Office of Attorney General
209 Saint Clair Street
Frankfort, KY 40601
(502) 564-2200
toll free in state:
(800) 432-9257

Louisiana

Consumer Protection Section
Office of Attorney General
State Capitol Building
P.O. Box 94005
Baton Rouge, LA 70804
(504) 342-7013

Maine

Consumer and Antitrust Division
Office of Attorney General
State House Station No. 6
Augusta, ME 04333
(207) 289-3716
(9 A.M.–1 P.M.)

Maryland

Consumer Protection Division
Office of Attorney General
Seven North Calvert Street
Baltimore, MD 21202
(301) 528-8662
toll free in state:
(800) 492-2114

Massachusetts

Consumer Protection Division
Department of Attorney General
131 Tremont Street
Boston, MA 02111
(617) 727-8400

Michigan

Consumer Protection Division
Office of Attorney General
670 Law Building
Lansing, MI 48913
(517) 373-1140

Michigan Consumers Council
414 Hollister Building
106 West Allegan Street
Lansing, MI 48933
(517) 373-0947

Minnesota

Office of Consumer Services
Office of Attorney General
117 University Avenue
St. Paul, MN 55155
(612) 296-2331

Mississippi
Chief, Consumer Protection
  Division
Office of Attorney General
P.O. Box 220
Jackson, MS 39205
(601) 354-6018

Missouri
Department of Economic
  Development
P.O. Box 1157
Jefferson City, MO 65102
(314) 751-4962

Trade Offense Division
Office of Attorney General
P.O. Box 899
Jefferson City, MO 65102
(314) 751-2616
toll free in state:
(800) 392-8222

Montana
Consumer Affairs Unit
Department of Commerce
1424 Ninth Avenue
Helena, MT 59620
(406) 444-4312

Nebraska
Consumer Protection General
Department of Justice
2115 State Capitol
P.O. Box 98920
Lincoln, NE 68509
(402) 471-4723

Nevada
Consumers Affairs Commission
Department of Commerce
State Mail Room Complex
Las Vegas, NV 89158
(702) 486-4150

New Hampshire
Consumer Protection and Antitrust
  Division
Office of Attorney General
State House Annex
Concord, NH 03301
(603) 271-3541

New Jersey
Division of Consumer Affairs
1100 Raymond Boulevard
Newark, NJ 07102
(201) 648-4010

New Mexico
Consumer and Economic Crime
  Division
Office of Attorney General
P.O. Drawer 1508
Santa Fe, NM 87504
(505) 872-6910
toll free in state:
(800) 432-2070

New York
New York State Consumer
  Protection Board
99 Washington Avenue
Albany, NY 12210
(518) 474-8583

Bureau of Consumer Frauds and
  Protection
Office of Attorney General
State Capitol
Albany, NY 12224
(518) 474-5481

North Carolina
Consumer Protection Section
Office of Attorney General
Department of Justice Building
P.O. Box 629
Raleigh, NC 27602
(919) 733-7741

North Dakota
Consumer Fraud Division
Office of Attorney General
600 East Boulevard
Bismarck, ND 58505
(701) 224-3404
toll free in state:
(800) 472-2600

Ohio
Consumer Frauds and Crimes
   Section
Office of Attorney General
30 East Broad Street
State Office Tower
Columbus, OH 43266-0410
(614) 466-4986 (complaints)
toll free in state:
(800) 282-0515

Consumer Counsel
77 South High Street
Columbus, OH 43266
(voice/TDD)
(614) 466-9605
toll free in state:
(800) 282-9448

Oklahoma
Consumer Affairs Section
Office of Attorney General
112 State Capitol Building
Oklahoma City, OK 73105
(405) 521-3921

Oregon
Financial Fraud Section
Department of Justice
Justice Building
Salem, OR 97310
(503) 378-4320

Pennsylvania
Bureau of Consumer Protection
Office of Attorney General
Strawberry Square
Harrisburg, PA 17120
(717) 787-9707
toll free in state:
(800) 441-2555

Rhode Island
Consumer Protection Division
Department of Attorney General
72 Pine Street
Providence, RI 02903
(401) 277-2104
toll free in state:
(800) 852-7776

South Carolina
Consumer Fraud and Antitrust
   Section
Office of Attorney General
P.O. Box 11549
Columbia, SC 29211
(803) 734-3970

Department of Consumer Affairs
P.O. Box 5757
Columbia, SC 29250
(803) 734-9452
toll free in state:
(800) 922-1594

South Dakota
Division of Consumer Affairs
Office of Attorney General
State Capitol Building
Pierre, SD 57501
(605) 773-4400

Tennessee
Antitrust and Consumer Protection
  Division
Office of Attorney General
450 James Robertson Parkway
Nashville, TN 37219
(615) 741-2672

Division of Consumer Affairs
Department of Commerce and
  Insurance
500 James Robertson Parkway
Nashville, TN 37219
(615) 741-4737
toll free in state:
(800) 342-8385

Texas
Consumer Protection Division
Office of Attorney General
Capitol Station
P.O. Box 12548
Austin, TX 78711
(512) 463-2070

Office of Consumer Protection
State Board of Insurance
One Republic Plaza
333 Guadalupe, Box 144
Austin, TX 78701
(512) 495-6448

Utah
Division of Consumer Protection
Department of Commerce
160 East 3rd South
P.O. Box 45802
Salt Lake City, UT 84145
(801) 530-6601

Vermont
Public Protection Division
Office of Attorney General
109 State Street
Montpelier, VT 05602
(802) 828-3171

Virginia
Antitrust and Consumer Litigation
  Section
Office of Attorney General
Supreme Court Building
101 North Eighth Street
Richmond, VA 23210
(804) 786-2116
toll free in state:
(800) 451-1525

Washington
Consumer and Business Fair
  Practices Division
Office of Attorney General
North 122 Capitol Way
Olympia, WA 98501
(206) 753-6210

West Virginia
Consumer Protection Division
Office of Attorney General
812 Quarrier Street
Charleston, WV 25301
(304) 348-8986
toll free in state:
(800) 268-8808

Wisconsin
Division of Trade and Consumer
  Protection
Department of Agriculture, Trade,
  and Consumer Protection
801 West Badger Road
P.O. Box 8911
Madison, WI 53708
(608) 266-9836
toll free in state:
(800) 362-3020

Office of Consumer Protection and
   Citizen Advocacy
Department of Justice
P.O. Box 7856
Madison, WI 53707
(608) 266-1852
toll free in state:
(800) 362-8189

Wyoming
Office of Attorney General
123 State Capitol Building
Cheyenne, WY 82002
(307) 777-7841

7

CONTRACEPTION AND ABORTION

CONTENTS

IN 1873, a muttonchop-whiskered, avuncular ball of a man, one Anthony Comstock, set up an office just off the floor of the U.S. Senate. His mission was to lobby the U.S. Congress into passing a law banning contraceptives, abortifacients, and similar "obscene" items. Charged with a religious fervor, Comstock succeeded beyond his wildest dreams. That year Congress passed a law making it a crime to import contraceptives or abortifacients or to transport them from one state to another. New York and Massachusetts quickly followed, passing their own bans on contraception. Connecticut went so far as to forbid the *use* of contraceptives. Comstock's reward was an appointment as a U.S. postal inspector. From that vantage point, he placed ads in newspapers, luring unsuspecting women to order contraceptives by mail, which, armed with an arrest warrant, Comstock himself often delivered. He once bragged of jailing enough people to fill a train stretching from Washington to Baltimore.

There's no telling what Comstock would do if he were alive today and saw condoms openly displayed on drugstore counters, realized that the Pill is used by more than 16 million women, or learned that nearly two thirds of married women between the ages of thirty-five and forty-four have chosen to be sterilized. No doubt he would be an active member of a right-to-life group, trying once again to make abortion illegal and to ban the sale of contraceptives.

From Comstock's time to the present, the government has been involved in decisions about "bearing and begetting" children, to quote former Supreme Court Justice William Brennan. Congress and nearly every state have passed legislation concerning abortion, and decisions of the Supreme Court determine whether millions of women will be allowed to terminate unwanted pregnancies legally. Birth control is not far behind as a controversial topic. When Norplant, a long-acting contraceptive was first introduced in 1991, proposals by a few judges and lawmakers to forcibly implant it in poor women who refused to stop having babies aroused the anger of women's rights and civil liberties groups. The legal problems faced by teenagers who want contraceptives is another time bomb. Just look at the furor any time a school district suggests making condoms available to high school students or offering birth control information as part of a school health program.

Controversy often leads to ignorance and misinformation. Many people simply do not know what their rights are, partly because the law changes rapidly and partly because it's hard to get a straight answer. Yet in these intimate areas of sexuality and reproduction, it is important to be fully informed before making decisions. In this chapter, we tell you what your rights are to contraception, voluntary sterilization, and abortion; what to ask your doctor so that you can make an informed choice; what to do should something go wrong; and whom to call for the latest information or advice.

Contraception

Contraception and the Right of Privacy

When Estelle Griswold, director of the New Haven, Connecticut, Planned Parenthood organization, and Dr. Lee Buxton, director of obstetrics and gynecology at Yale Medical School, met thirty years ago with other members of the state's medical elite to plan the opening of a new birth control clinic, they knew that what they were doing was against the law. At the opening of the facility, colleagues from the medical establishment showed up — along with the police. The latter arrested Ms. Griswold, Dr. Buxton, and assorted guests and charged them with violating Connecticut's Comstock law. The case made its way to the Supreme Court. In a landmark decision, *Griswold v. Connecticut,* Justice William O. Douglas wrote that the right to use contraceptives was protected by the U.S. Constitution. Decided in 1965, *Griswold* became the first of many cases which concluded that the distribution, advertising, and use of contraceptives fell within a constitutional right of privacy. In other words, as an adult, you have a constitutional right to buy and use contraceptives.

Informed Consent: What You Should Know about Contraceptives

Before a birth control pill or device is allowed on the market, the U.S. Food and Drug Administration (FDA) must certify that it is safe and effective. The FDA also tells the manufacturer what it can claim about the drug or device. If necessary, the FDA has the power to recall a harmful contraceptive. While the contraceptive is on the market, the manufacturer must monitor it and report harmful side effects to the FDA.

Although FDA approval of a contraceptive is reassuring, it does not guarantee safety or effectiveness, only that the manufacturer successfully passed the tests showing that, on the whole, the benefits outweigh the risks.

However, no drug — contraceptive or otherwise — is perfectly safe. You may be allergic to it or be among the people who shouldn't take it for medical reasons. Or tests may have raised questions about a drug's safety. One example is Depo-Provera, a three-month injectable contraceptive manufactured by the Upjohn pharmaceutical company. Tests on beagles and monkeys indicated a higher-than-expected rate of cancer. Although thousands of women in European and Third World countries used Depo-Provera without developing abnormal rates of cancer, the FDA, basing its decision on the animal studies, turned down the manufacturer's request to approve the injectable for contraceptive use in this country. Even extensive testing may not uncover long-term risks of cancers that do not show up for twenty years — as the tragedy of women who took DES (diethylstilbestrol) reveals. Perhaps 2 million women in the 1950s, 1960s, and 1970s took it to prevent miscarriages. DES was found to cause cervical and vaginal abnormalities, including cancer, in the daughters of many women who took it. Cases of cancer and other illnesses appearing in their granddaughters are now being reported.

Don't rely solely on FDA approval. Instead, ask your doctor and pharmacist for the latest information about your contraceptive choices, including the risks, side effects, and benefits of each. "Most women choose their contraceptive method on the basis of what their friends tell them or what they read in magazines or see on television. That information is often wrong," says Dr. Louise Tyrer, former vice president for medical affairs of the Planned Parenthood Federation of America.

"There are many rumors and fears about contraceptives," adds Dr. Allan Rosenfield, dean of Columbia University's School of Public Health and a leading expert on birth control. "Studies have shown that any reported bad news travels fast, while positive findings receive little public attention."

If you have questions, contact the nearest Planned Parenthood office (if you have trouble finding it, call the national headquarters, (212) 541-7800), the National Women's Health Network, 1325 G Street, NW, Washington, DC 20005, (202) 347-1140, or the Women's Information Center, 240A Elm Street, Somerville, MA 02144, (617) 625-0271.

Birth Control Pills

> "Diaphragms and condoms are, well, just not aesthetic. But the Pill isn't messy. I prescribe it to most of my young patients. Side effects? Crossing the street can be dangerous, you know."
> — Gynecologist to a twenty-four-year-old patient

When the Pill came on the market in the halcyon days of the 1960s, it was heralded as the answer to the dreams of every woman who didn't want to get pregnant. It remains the most popular temporary means of birth control in the United States today. In theory, if you take the Pill, you won't become pregnant. In fact, about 7 percent of the women using oral contraception do get pregnant every year, usually because they use it incorrectly or forget to take it at all. As a symbol, the Pill represents the days when medicine seemed to have most, if not all, of the answers.

By now the Pill is probably the most thoroughly investigated drug in the history of medicine. "Current research indicates that the Pill can cause blood clots and strokes in a very small percentage of users, particularly among women over thirty-five who are heavy smokers," says Dr. Rosenfield. "On the other hand, it protects women against ovarian and endometrial cancers, pelvic inflammatory disease, and ectopic pregnancies and avoids pregnancy, which itself can present substantial risks to a woman's health."

New evidence about oral contraception and women's health emerges all the time. The association between the Pill and breast cancer, for example, is currently under intensive scrutiny. Because the Pill affects millions of healthy women and because there was so much concern and publicity about its side effects, the Food and Drug Administration took the unusual step of requiring manufacturers to include an insert with every package. The insert, which contains a great deal of information about risks and benefits, is written to FDA specifications and updated periodically to reflect current medical knowledge.

Intrauterine Devices

Centuries ago, camel drivers crossing the Arabian desert inserted stones into the uterus of their camels to keep them from becoming pregnant on the journey. Over the years, gynecologists built on this idea and found that placing a foreign body in a woman's uterus would prevent her from becoming pregnant. In the early 1900s, new forms of intrauterine devices (IUDs) were developed in Germany and Japan. By the 1960s, intrauterine devices were considered the perfect method of contraception — they worked, and once inserted, they stayed in place.

That was before the Dalkon Shield, a hideous example of corporate greed. Beginning in 1971, the A. H. Robins Company, makers of Robitussen cough medicine and Chapstick lip balm, manufactured and promoted an IUD called the Dalkon Shield. It was used by an estimated 2.2 million women in this country and another 2 million overseas. Soon after its introduction, evidence mounted that the Dalkon Shield caused severe infections, sterility, dangerous ectopic pregnancies, and even death. Although it knew its IUD was potentially deadly, A. H. Robins continued to promote the product. Only in 1974, under pressure from the Food and Drug Administration, did the company stop selling the IUD (Congress did not give the FDA legal authority to force the recall of harmful devices until 1976; the legislation was passed largely as a result of the Dalkon Shield debacle).

One victim of the Dalkon Shield was described by Susan Perry and Jim Dawson in their book *Nightmare*. Linda Towle was a twenty-year-old secretary at a Baltimore life insurance company when she had a Dalkon Shield inserted. When Ms. Towle got her period, she had searing cramps and heavy bleeding. A year later, she had the IUD removed. Five years later, she developed severe stomach pains; afterward, the pain kept coming back. Then, during a sightseeing trip to New York with her husband and stepchildren, she doubled over with agonizing cramps. Her temperature rose dramatically. She was rushed to a hospital for exploratory surgery, and the truth emerged. She had bands of scar tissue all over her uterus.

She tried to get pregnant without success. She went to fertility specialists. She had eight operations, including one to reconstruct her fallopian tubes. Finally, unlike the tales of thousands of women who used the shield, this story ended happily when Ms. Towle gave birth to a healthy baby boy.

Ms. Towle and over three hundred thousand women injured by the Dalkon Shield sued A. H. Robins. Many of the cases were consolidated into one huge lawsuit that was settled in 1989. Under the settlement, $2.3 billion was set aside to pay the claims of women injured by the Dalkon Shield. Most women received less than $725. As a footnote, A. H. Robins, which had filed for bankruptcy, was bought by American Home Products, a large drug conglomerate that paid a handsome price for the company. Who says crime doesn't pay?

The Robins litigation led to lawsuits against the G. D. Searle and Ortho Pharmaceutical companies, the other large manufacturers of IUDs. Although these companies won or settled almost all the suits against them, they decided to withdraw their products from the market in the mid-1980s because the cost of fighting lawsuits was too high.

As a result, IUDs have almost disappeared from the market. Only two small companies manufacture them. "The new copper-bearing devices are the safest and most effective IUDs developed to date," says Dr. Rosenfield. "For women in stable relationships they are a very good method of contraception." To reduce their potential liability, the two manufacturers require potential IUD users to sign every paragraph of a detailed consent form that runs more than ten pages. It is one of the rare cases in which informed consent is virtually forced upon patients.

If You're Injured
If you are seriously injured by a contraceptive, you can sue the manufacturer, even though the chances for success are slim. Assuming you can prove that the contraceptive caused your injury, the main question for a judge or jury is whether you were ade-

quately warned about its risks. If the warning was adequate — if you knew that there was a risk to your health but decided to take it anyway — you are likely to lose the lawsuit. But if you can prove that you were not given sufficient information, you might be successful.

Usually, the manufacturer of a drug must warn doctors about potential health hazards, and the doctors are supposed to communicate this information to their patients. Special rules apply to prescription contraceptives, however. The manufacturer must let you, the consumer, know about the risks and benefits directly through a package insert. Some courts have ruled that you don't have a case if the FDA approved the contraceptive and the insert followed its guidelines. Other courts contend that the insert does not give the manufacturer blanket protection from injured users, particularly if the company did not reveal damaging new information about the contraceptive's adverse side effects or the package insert was written to minimize the risks.

Carole MacDonald of Massachusetts brought one of the early cases against a manufacturer of birth control pills. Ms. MacDonald was twenty-six years old when she first took Ortho-Novum in 1973. The package insert, which was prepared in accordance with FDA regulations, warned about side effects, the most serious being "abnormal blood clotting which can be fatal." What the insert and a booklet aimed at patients did not mention was that the Pill might cause a stroke — which is exactly what Ms. MacDonald experienced in 1976. Permanently disabled, she successfully sued the Ortho Pharmaceutical Corporation. On appeal, the Massachusetts Supreme Court upheld the verdict, saying that Ortho's failure to state that the Pill could cause strokes downplayed the risks.

Lawsuits against manufacturers are something like a lottery. The vast majority of injured plaintiffs receive nothing or the cases are settled out of court. Occasionally somebody wins big, encouraging other potential plaintiffs and raising threats by manufacturers that they will be forced to withdraw their products.

Esther Kociemba won more than $7 million from G. D. Searle & Company for the company's failure to disclose that its Copper-7 IUD could cause pelvic inflammatory disease. The decision is being appealed. Roberta Baroody was awarded $1.5 million from

Ortho Pharmaceutical Corporation because it did not reveal that its All-Flex diaphragm could cause toxic shock syndrome.

Then there was the unusual case of Mary Maihafer, a thirty-two-year-old college instructor from Georgia. Ms. Maihafer used Ortho-Gynol, a popular spermicide, for four weeks before discovering that she was pregnant. The package insert said that the spermicide might cause irritation, that it was not 100 percent effective, and that it should be kept away from children. It did not mention the risk of birth defects, and according to current medical evidence, there was none. In fact, an advisory committee of the FDA had, a short time previously, found that nonoxynol-9, the effective ingredient in the spermicide, did not cause birth defects.

When Ms. Maihafer gave birth, her daughter, Katie Wells, was born without a left arm and had only a stub for a left shoulder, a deformed right hand, a cleft lip, and an optic nerve defect in one eye. Ms. Maihafer sued the manufacturer, Ortho Pharmaceutical Corporation, a subsidiary of Johnson & Johnson. During the trial, a parade of expert witnesses testified that the spermicide either did or did not (depending on whose side they were testifying) cause Katie's birth defects. The judge found Katie Wells's witnesses believable and, on the basis of their testimony, awarded Ms. Maihafer $5 million. Several months after the trial, the FDA's advisory panel studied new evidence and repeated its conclusion that spermicides do not cause birth defects.

Voluntary Sterilization

Informed Consent for Sterilization
Sterilization is the most popular method of contraception in the United States. More than 23 million women have opted for tubal ligation, and more than 11 million men have had a vasectomy, a fifteen-minute operation that can be done in a clinic or a doctor's office. Although there is a lot of talk about reversal, the Association for Voluntary Surgical Contraception, a New York group that monitors and sets standards for sterilization, cautions that it should be considered permanent.

Sterilization in this country has a curious history. During the first half of the century, at least thirty states passed laws authoriz-

ing compulsory sterilization of criminals and the mentally retarded. More than seventy thousand people were sterilized under
these now-discredited "eugenic sterilization" laws. In the 1970s,
coerced sterilization of poor women was widely reported. Even
today, an occasional judge will order that a sex offender or a pregnant woman on welfare be sterilized.

Although some people have been sterilized against their will,
others have found it nearly impossible to get the operation. Until
the early 1970s, many doctors followed the "120 rule," by which a
physician would not sterilize a woman unless the number of her
living children times her age equaled 120 or more. Under this
formula, a thirty-year-old woman with four children could be
sterilized (30 × 4 = 120), but a twenty-two-year-old woman with
five children could not (22 × 5 = 110). Although the 120 rule has
withered away and sterilization is widely available, some women
still have difficulty finding a doctor willing to perform the procedure.

An adult has the same right to sterilization as to any other
means of birth control — with some limitations designed to prevent abuse. U.S. government regulations ensure that anyone sterilized under a federally funded program has given his or her informed consent. California and New York City have issued similar
guidelines for sterilizations performed within their borders.

The key to the guidelines is a requirement that anyone planning
to be sterilized must sign a written consent form at least thirty
days before the operation. Thus a person has a month to think
about the operation and change his or her mind. The guidelines
also prohibit the sterilization of people under twenty-one years of
age and those who are mentally incompetent. By the same token,
a woman who is in active labor or having an abortion cannot
consent to be sterilized. Hysterectomy for family planning purposes is also forbidden. These guidelines offer protections that
make sense for anybody considering permanent contraception.
They should be a normal part of the process of informed consent
before contraceptive surgery.

"Surprise, You're Pregnant!"
For many years, the courts threw out cases brought by new parents
who had been "sterilized." The birth of a healthy child, even an

unexpected and unwanted one, is a blessed event, they said. What possible grounds could there be for suing over the birth of a healthy child?

Today, lawsuits brought by couples who were sterilized and then find themselves pregnant are permitted in nearly every state. Called wrongful pregnancy or wrongful conception suits, they are a branch of medical malpractice. To win, parents must prove to the satisfaction of a jury or judge that the doctor performed the operation negligently, namely, that he or she did something wrong. It is not enough simply to show that a doctor performed a sterilization and afterward a baby was born. Tubes can reconnect on their own or, in the case of female sterilization, a woman could already have been pregnant.

Even if a doctor is found liable, there is the tricky question of damages. Should a negligent doctor pay for the expenses of prenatal care and delivery? For raising the child to adulthood? For college? The states are divided on this issue. The majority allow parents to recover costs associated with pregnancy and delivery, including prenatal and postpartum care, but not the full cost of raising a normal, healthy child. Damages may also be awarded for the physical and mental pain suffered as a result of the pregnancy, for lost wages, and for loss of companionship.

Sterilization of the Mentally Retarded

Parents of a mentally retarded daughter, concerned that she will not be able to raise her own child, may want to have her sterilized. Many doctors, fearing lawsuits, will not perform the operation unless it is authorized by a judge or state law. It presents agonizing choices for parents, doctors, lawmakers, and judges. On the one hand, sterilization permanently takes away a person's right to have a child, a right protected by the Constitution. On the other hand, if a mentally retarded woman is incapable of rearing a child, it is not in her best interest to have one. (The same choice is present when permission is sought to sterilize a mentally retarded male, although that happens far less often.) Two old cases, still read by law students, illustrate the ways courts react when asked to approve the sterilization of a mentally retarded young woman.

In 1978, Dianne Tully, a twenty-year-old Californian with cerebral palsy and brain damage, had the mental capacity of a three-year-old and could neither understand nor cope with her normal menstrual cycles. Since California law was silent about sterilization of the mentally retarded at the time, the parents asked a judge to authorize the operation. Medical testimony that she would never improve, that pregnancy would cause her psychiatric harm, and that she was incapable of raising a child was undisputed. Everyone agreed that sterilization would be in her best interest, yet the judge refused to authorize it. Only the state legislature has the power to decide whether mentally retarded people can be sterilized on their parents' say-so, he ruled.

Then there was the case of Linda Sparkman, a De Kalb, Ohio, teenager. Although she was moderately retarded, she attended public school and was promoted with her class. When Linda was fifteen, her mother, Ora McFarlin, decided that her daughter ought to be sterilized. The doctor refused to perform the operation without a court order, and a judge promptly authorized it. Ms. McFarlin told Linda that she had to go to the hospital to have her appendix removed. Unbeknown to Linda, she was sterilized. Several days later, Linda went home, appendix intact but tubes severed. Only when she married and could not become pregnant did she learn the truth. She sued her parents, the doctor, the hospital, and the judge. The case made it all the way to the U.S. Supreme Court, which, in 1978, ruled that the judge could not be sued for a decision he made. There is no record of what happened in the lawsuits against the other parties involved.

Parents considering the sterilization of a mentally retarded child should contact a lawyer or the Association for Voluntary Surgical Contraception, 79 Madison Avenue, New York, NY 10016, (212) 561-8000, before going ahead with the procedure. Find out whether state law authorizes sterilization of the mentally retarded and what steps must be taken. The laws vary widely. By 1992, nineteen states had laws authorizing such sterilization. In general, they allow a judge or an administrative panel to authorize sterilization based on convincing evidence that it would be in the person's best interest.

If there is no state law, find out whether judges are willing to intervene. In almost every state where it has come up recently, judges have approved sterilization of mentally retarded children if it was clearly in their best interest and if procedural safeguards to protect against abuse were followed.

Abortion

The Legality of Abortion

Norma McCorvey was an unmarried, pregnant twenty-year-old Texan whose search for an abortion changed the law of the land. Under Texas law, abortion was allowed only to protect the life of a pregnant woman. Using a pseudonym to protect her anonymity, Ms. McCorvey sued to have the Texas law declared unconstitutional in a case that worked its way up to the Supreme Court. In January 1973, well after Ms. McCorvey's baby was born, the Supreme Court announced its opinion in *Roe v. Wade.*

In its decision, the Court ruled that abortion is protected under the constitutional right of privacy. During the first trimester — to about the thirteenth week of pregnancy — a woman has the right to terminate her pregnancy without any obstacles imposed by state or local government. After the first trimester, a state or local government can restrict abortion as long as the laws are aimed at protecting the pregnant woman's health — for example, by requiring that clinics have a hospital backup. Once a fetus is viable, that is, able to live outside the womb, state and local governments can pass laws designed to protect the fetus. They can ban abortions, except those necessary to save the life or protect the health of a pregnant woman.

Roe v. Wade is probably the most controversial decision in Supreme Court history. It gave women a new constitutional right, overturned the law of every state, and spawned a right-to-life movement devoted to making abortion illegal again. Abortion has become a critical political issue — sometimes *the* critical issue — in everything from federal court appointments to local mayor's races.

The Supreme Court itself has gradually chipped away at *Roe v. Wade,* upholding the constitutionality of laws that restrict abortion. In 1980, it decided that a law cutting off federal funding of abortions, even medically necessary ones, for poor women was constitutional. In 1989, it upheld a Missouri law that, among its other restrictions, prohibited public hospitals from providing abortions. In 1991, it ruled that a federal regulation preventing doctors who practice family planning in federally funded settings from discussing abortion with their patients was constitutional.

Many people believe the Supreme Court will overturn *Roe v. Wade.* Whether it does or simply continues to erode the 1973 landmark decision, the practical implications for women wanting to terminate a pregnancy remain the same. Many conservative state legislatures will pass restrictive laws, secure in the knowledge that federal courts are not likely to strike them down. But these laws may violate *state* constitutions. As a result, supporters of the right to choose will look increasingly to state rather than federal courts for protection.

Among the issues likely to arise in the future are: Must a husband be told about his wife's decision to have an abortion? Can he exercise veto power? Can states make a woman wait, say, twenty-four hours, before getting an abortion? Can states limit abortions to those performed during the first or early second trimester? Can governments require doctors, as part of the consent process, to give women graphic descriptions of abortion designed to scare them away? These issues will be decided on a case-by-case basis by state and federal courts and perhaps the Supreme Court.

Where to Turn for Help
To find out about the law in your state or to get assistance, contact one of the following organizations:

- National Abortion Federation, (800) 772-9100
- Planned Parenthood offices. If you run into difficulty finding one, contact the national headquarters, 810 Seventh Avenue, New York, NY 10019, (212) 541-7800.
- National Abortion Rights Action League, 1101 14th Street, NW, Washington, DC 20005, (202) 408-4600
- National Women's Law Center, 1616 P Street, NW, Washington, DC 20036, (202) 328-5160
- American Civil Liberties Union. If you cannot locate a nearby chapter, contact the ACLU's headquarters, 132 West 43rd Street, New York, NY 10036, (212) 944-9800.

Adolescents

When New York City school chancellor Joseph Fernandez proposed that schools distribute condoms to students without parental consent, angry opponents charged that he was destroying the sanctity of the family, fostering immorality, and trying to usurp the role of parents. Fernandez's supporters responded that dramatic solutions were needed to attack the devastation of AIDS, that distributing condoms promoted safe sex, and that students had a right to obtain contraceptives without their parents' knowledge.

Although a closely divided board of education gave Fernandez the green light, the antagonism that characterized the board's deliberations illustrates the depth of feeling that adolescent sexuality arouses. While everybody agrees that teenage pregnancy is a national tragedy, there is bitter disagreement about how to prevent it or what to do when it occurs.

The legal issue can be stated very simply: Do one or both parents of an adolescent have the right to consent to, or even know about, their child's decision to use contraception or have an abortion? The answer is not so simple. Although the policy of all family planning organizations and clinics is to involve parents whenever possible, teenagers often want to keep them in the dark. People on both sides of the issue are haunted by the death of Becky Bell, the Indiana teenager who couldn't bring herself to tell her parents she was pregnant and died during a botched abortion in 1988. The law, reflecting society's lack of consensus, varies from state to state and is subject to rapid change as the composition of courts, particularly the Supreme Court, shifts.

The key to understanding the law is to recognize that courts and legislatures must strike a balance between the rights of adolescents and the rights of their parents. As we point out in Chapter 10, children have constitutional rights, including a right of privacy, that grow stronger with age until they reach adulthood at eighteen or twenty-one. Parents have a constitutional right to bring up their children without government interference. When the rights of the two conflict, courts and legislatures must decide whose should prevail.

The Supreme Court has established emancipation and maturity as the points at which the balance tends to shift in favor of adolescents. As a general rule, when teenagers are emancipated — living away from home, married, or serving in the military — they can consent to their own reproductive health care. This is also true if they are mature enough to understand the risks and benefits of contraception or to grasp the implications of abortion and its alternatives.

Contraception
Under current constitutional law, mature and emancipated minors can probably obtain over-the-counter contraceptives without their parents' consent or knowledge. Although it did not face the issue directly, the Supreme Court indicated in 1977 that a state law requiring parental consent or notification for nonprescription methods would be unconstitutional.

Whether the same logic would apply to contraceptives that must be prescribed is unclear. Whether a state or local government could constitutionally require doctors to obtain the consent of, or to notify, parents about a daughter's use of prescription contraceptives has not been tested in the courts. The only relevant case, also decided in 1977, involved Michigan parents who sued a birth control clinic for allegedly dispensing the Pill to their teenage daughter without their knowledge or permission. A federal appeals court, finding that the daughter's rights outweighed those of the parents, ruled that the clinic could keep information about the girl confidential.

Twenty-four states and the District of Columbia have laws allowing teenagers, usually emancipated or mature ones, to obtain contraceptives without their parents' consent, according to a survey conducted by the Alan Guttmacher Institute, a public policy group specializing in reproductive health issues. Some of the laws prohibit notification of parents. Others allow parents to be informed, either before or after the fact.

Abortion
The Supreme Court has returned to the issue of parental consent and notification for abortion in half a dozen cases beginning in 1976, one indication of the difficulty of writing clear guidelines. Although the rules are still somewhat murky and may change with the next decision of the Court, the current law can be sum-

marized as follows. Parental *consent* requirements are unconstitutional. Parental *notification* requirements are constitutional as long as they do not unduly burden access to abortion. While a state government has no obligation to require parental notification, if it decides to do so, it must also give a pregnant teenager an opportunity to go to court and ask a judge to authorize an abortion without her parents being told. A judge *must* grant the young woman's request for an abortion if she is emancipated or mature. Even if she fails to convince a judge of her maturity, the abortion must be authorized if the judge believes it would be in her best interest to have one.

State laws on parental consent and notification are a hodgepodge. In some states, a pregnant teenager can get an abortion on her own, without any parental involvement whatsoever. In others, one or both parents must be notified and the pregnant teenager is given the alternative of having the abortion confidentially authorized by a judge. In still others, old laws requiring parental consent or notification remain on the books, usually unenforced. To learn the law in your state and obtain assistance if necessary, contact one of the organizations listed in the "Where to Turn for Help" section of this chapter.

8

INFERTILITY AND NEW
REPRODUCTIVE TECHNOLOGIES

CONTENTS

Infertility

Eight years ago, my husband and I decided that we wanted to have a baby and assumed that when we stopped using birth control we would get pregnant. However, after two years it hadn't happened. My doctor suggested that I take my temperature every day and keep a chart of my cycle. I did it for the next five years, and sex for us became timed around that cycle chart. Not very romantic.

I spent the next two and a half years going to doctors who were gynecologists and claimed that they also did infertility. By the fifth year we were doing vaginal inseminations, which meant that I was racing to the doctor with my husband's sperm in a jar. That was pretty much what sex had become for us.

We began to wonder if the dream we shared — to have a baby — was going to kill our marriage. We did not know why we were not getting pregnant. No one could give us any answers or solutions, except to "relax and not think about it." By the sixth year I would cry every time I saw a mother and baby and felt angry and jealous when I saw a pregnant woman.

My sense of failure was so strong that I began to feel I must be guilty of something terrible, that I was being punished, but I did not know for what. That I could not do the very thing my body was designed to do — conceive and carry a child — must mean that I was not fully a woman, I felt. All my other accomplishments in life seemed to fade into the background in the face of this failure.

When I found this infertility specialist, I felt such relief. Four months later a miracle occurred — I became pregnant. My husband and I were ecstatic. At twelve weeks, during a routine sonogram, the radiologist informed us that the baby had died.

My infertility specialist sent me to an in vitro fertilization program in Los Angeles. We did the GIFT procedure, and to my surprise, I got pregnant again. But I was one of the unlucky one or two percent who had an ectopic pregnancy.

> After this second loss, we decided to adopt, and now we
> have a beautiful baby boy. However, we have decided we
> want another child, and we are planning to give GIFT or in
> vitro another try. The seed of hope never dies.
> — *Actress Jo Beth Williams, excerpts from testimony,*
> *Subcommittee on Regulation, Business Opportuni-*
> *ties, and Energy, U.S. House of Representatives,*
> *1989*

Infertility affects one out of every twelve couples in the United
States. This translates to 10 million people who are unable to have
a baby after a year of trying — the medical definition of infertility.
A couple may not be able to conceive or, perhaps, it may not be
possible to bring the pregnancy to term.

There are many causes of infertility. Some are men's problems,
such as an inability to produce enough sperm or sperm strong
enough to penetrate the egg. Others are women's problems, such
as endometriosis or blocked fallopian tubes. Often the difficulty
can be traced to the biology of both partners. Many couples who
delay childbearing until they are in their mid-thirties or early
forties find that the woman can get pregnant only with great difficulty, if at all. The biological clock is a reality, and it starts to tick
rapidly when a woman reaches her thirties.

Finding an Infertility Specialist

Couples desperate for a child are often willing to try anything —
and often do, only to end up with shattered hopes and depleted
savings. To spare yourself emotional, financial, and perhaps physical trauma, get as much information as you can *beforehand*. Investigate the cause of your infertility and what can be done. Find out
about alternative treatments and their risks, likelihood of success,
and cost. Many books available at libraries and bookstores can tell
you about infertility in nontechnical language. Two organizations
provide excellent information:

- RESOLVE, a national network of more than twenty thousand
  members and fifty-two chapters, can do everything from giving you the names of reliable infertility specialists in your area
  to putting you in touch with other couples. Contact the head-

quarters at 1310 Broadway, Somerville, MA 02144-1731, (617) 623-0744.

- The American Fertility Society is a professional organization for doctors and others interested in infertility. It publishes pamphlets on all aspects of infertility and can refer you to clinics and doctors who adhere to its standards. It is located at 2140 Eleventh Avenue, Birmingham, AL 35205, (205) 933-8494.

Since any doctor can hang out a shingle saying "Infertility Specialist," look for one who is board certified or board eligible in reproductive endocrinology and whose practice is devoted largely to couples with infertility problems.

Diagnosis and Treatment

The standard workup and treatment for infertility can be time-consuming, expensive, and embarrassing. Your bedroom may become a laboratory. Listen to Deborah Gerrity, president of RESOLVE's Washington, D.C., chapter.

> I have taken my basal body temperature approximately 1,260 times for about forty-five inconsecutive months. Imagine not being able to move a muscle in the morning until you reach for a thermometer. It is hard to relax and stop thinking about your infertility when it has to be the very first thought that enters your waking mind. And that is the easy part.
>
> During the diagnostic phase, I had three endometrial biopsies, which consist of taking tissue from the inside of the uterine wall to determine hormone levels, and two postcoital tests — removal of the cervical mucus to analyze sperm activity. I have also had two diagnostic laparoscopies — the navel surgery, done with general anesthesia, to look at the ovaries, tubes, and uterus. The second of these surgeries included a hysteroscopy — examination of the inside of the uterus — and a D and C. Both times I had minor complications and was forced to take a week off of work, although the average time for most women is three to four days. All of that comprised the diagnostic workup. My diagnosis was unexplained infertility. Medical treat-

ment for unexplained infertility involves trying a variety of things to see if anything will work. We did six months of artificial insemination by husband, a year of hormonal treatment, and an attempt at in vitro fertilization.

During the surgery, they found that I had moderate endometriosis — growth of the uterine lining outside of the uterus — which had not previously been detectable. Major surgery to remove the endometriosis required a month off work to recuperate.

During this time, my husband was tested a couple of times and the results came back as normal. With the updating of technology, he recently had a different type of test and was found to have a high percentage of antisperm antibodies in his semen. As this is a highly controversial diagnosis and not a well-documented cause of infertility, there are very few treatments available for us at this time.

To summarize this to a bare sentence, I have accumulated a total of ninety-two failures — ninety-two months of trying with no children to show for it. During those months I had three miscarriages, the longest pregnancy lasting six weeks. The grief and depression that I felt after those losses changed me as a person. Considering the present state of medical technology and research in infertility, I will probably never have a biological offspring. I won't be able to produce a child who will have my husband's smile and his wonderful eyes. And that thought is devastating to me and my family.

> — *Excerpts from testimony, Subcommittee on Regulation, Business Opportunities, and Energy, U.S. House of Representatives, 1989*

Standard medical treatment, such as drugs to induce ovulation or surgery to clear obstructions of the fallopian tubes, succeeds in about two thirds of cases, meaning that two out of three couples have a pregnancy within eighteen months. When you ask your doctor about the risks of drug treatment, be sure to discuss the likelihood of having twins or triplets or an ectopic pregnancy, and of bearing a child with birth defects.

If drugs or surgery do not work, in vitro fertilization, artificial insemination, and surrogate motherhood are available to help Mother Nature along. With these reproductive technologies, babies can be created in glass dishes and women can give birth to children who have no genetic relation to them. They make it possible for a child to have up to five people claiming to be parents — a sperm donor, an ovum (egg) donor, a woman providing a womb for gestation, and a couple rearing the child — and raise legal and ethical problems that would perplex King Solomon if he were alive today.

In Vitro Fertilization (IVF)

When Louise Brown was born in England in 1978, she became known as the world's first test-tube baby, although no test tube was involved. It was the first time that fertilization took place outside a woman's body. Since 1978, more than five thousand IVF children have been born in the United States. The procedure is legal, has become standard medical practice, and is offered at nearly two hundred clinics throughout the country. Here's how it works: A woman is given a drug to stimulate the development of several eggs simultaneously, instead of the one that normally develops each month. When the eggs are mature, they are removed by a thin needle guided by ultrasound or the surgical procedure laparoscopy. The five to seven eggs that are retrieved are placed in a glass dish (hence the name in vitro, which means "in glass") and allowed to mature further for several hours. Then they are mixed with a man's sperm. About two days later, if fertilization has occurred, some — usually two or three — of the embryos, as they are now known, are transferred to the woman's uterus. The rest are frozen and stored for later use if necessary.

Offshoots of the in vitro method of uniting sperm and egg include GIFT and ZIFT. In GIFT (gamete intra-fallopian transfer), the eggs and sperm are mixed and immediately placed in a woman's fallopian tubes, where fertilization is supposed to take place naturally. ZIFT (zygote intra-fallopian transfer), an even newer procedure, is like GIFT except that the eggs are fertilized in a laboratory dish and then inserted into the woman's fallopian tubes. The technology is mind boggling. Ask your doctor about the latest developments.

The Right IVF Clinic: Getting Past the Hype

In vitro fertilization has become big business. Some IVF clinics hype their product and exaggerate their success rates, practices that some lawmakers feel border on the fraudulent. "Many infertile couples are desperate to have children. They are vulnerable to exploitation and to those who would unfairly try to rip them off," stated Congressman Ron Wyden in 1989 as he opened congressional subcommittee hearings on IVF clinics. Although federal legislation to set standards for IVF clinics has been introduced, they remain unregulated. Only two states, Louisiana and Pennsylvania, regulate these clinics, and their main purpose seems to be giving legal rights to the embryo.

With so little consumer protection offered by state and federal government, you must be your own watchdog. Before you sign on with any clinic, get as much information as you can about the facility, its personnel, and its success rates. Here is what you can do:

CHECKLIST: FINDING AN IVF CLINIC

- **Contact RESOLVE or the American Fertility Society for the names of IVF clinics.** RESOLVE recommends clinics and doctors. The American Fertility Society sends a list of clinics that meet its standards. Their addresses and phone numbers appear earlier in this chapter. Both organizations have useful booklets for couples considering in vitro fertilization.
- **Ask about the success rates of the clinics you are considering.** Clinics give their rates in a number of different ways, some quite misleading. "The key question, the bottom line, is 'Over the past two years, how many women about the same age and with a similar problem have been treated at the clinic and how many have gone home with babies?'" says Joyce Zeitz, spokesperson for the American Fertility Society.
- **Ask about the risks of treatment, particularly the likelihood of multiple embryos, ectopic pregnancy, and bearing a child with birth defects.**

- **Find out how long the IVF team has worked together.** "The longer a team has been working together, the better the chances of success," says law professor Alta Charo, an IVF expert at the University of Wisconsin. "All things being equal, choose the place with the most experience."
- **Get a feeling for how comfortable you are with the team.** You will spend a lot of time with them and share some very private moments. It's important to have a good fit. Make sure you can reach a team member day or night.
- **Ask how much it will cost.** In vitro fertilization can be expensive. The cost runs between $6,000 and $10,000 per *attempt*. Find out whether IVF is covered by insurance. Although some insurance companies and health mainte- nance organizations cover it, most do not. Currently, ten states — Arkansas, California, Connecticut, Hawaii, Illi- nois, Maryland, Massachusetts, New York, Rhode Island, and Texas — have laws requiring insurance companies to include IVF in the plans they offer employers. In some states, employers must provide coverage of IVF treatment as a health benefit to their employees. In others, employers are free to decline to offer that coverage. Even if the proce- dure is not included, the clinic may be able to write the bill so that legitimate items, such as laparoscopy, will be paid by insurance. Your insurance company or the state insur- ance commission should have information about coverage of IVF.

Unimplanted Embryos

Recall that five to seven eggs are normally retrieved from a woman during IVF. Normally, all are mixed with sperm in the hope of their being fertilized, but only two or three are inserted in a woman's uterus or fallopian tubes. The remainder are usually frozen. If another IVF cycle is necessary, they can be thawed and inserted. Profound ethical problems arise when the unimplanted embryos are no longer needed. Can they ethically be destroyed? Can they be used for research? Should they be stored indefinitely? The argu- ments are similar to those heard in the abortion debate.

Some, including the Catholic church, believe that life begins at the moment of conception and equate the destruction of these embryos with murder. Others contend that life does not begin at conception and that it makes little sense to consider a three- or four-cell embryo as a human being; they argue that excess embryos can ethically be used for research purposes or destroyed. At the moment, the federal government prohibits research on such embryos, and any decision on keeping or destroying them must be consistent with the law on abortion.

The moral questions raised sometimes shade into legal issues. Give some thought to them beforehand. You don't want to be in the position of Junior and Mary Sue Davis, a Tennessee couple whose divorce and reproductive history became news in 1989 when they wrangled publicly over possession of their frozen embryos. Newspaper accounts told of their unsuccessful attempts to have children. Married in 1980, Ms. Davis had five ectopic pregnancies, one of her fallopian tubes ruptured, and she nearly died. She had the other tube tied. In vitro fertilization offered some hope, and between 1982 and 1988, the Davises spent almost $50,000 on five unsuccessful attempts. On the seventh attempt in early 1988, nine eggs were removed and fertilized; two were implanted and the remaining seven were frozen and stored at the Fertility Center of Eastern Tennessee in Knoxville.

In February 1989, the Davises began divorce proceedings. They agreed on everything but the fate of the fertilized eggs. Ms. Davis wanted to have them inserted in her uterus after the divorce. She argued that the embryos were her only chance at having a baby and that because she had gone through the surgery and the programs, she had a better right to them. Mr. Davis responded that because he no longer wanted her to be the mother of his children, he had the right to decide whether he wanted to become a father and asked the court to allow the embryos to be destroyed. A Tennessee judge awarded Ms. Davis custody of the seven embryos. On appeal, the decision was reversed. The Tennessee Court of Appeals ruled that the embryos were joint property and that both parties must agree about what becomes of them. They remain in cold storage.

Before you decide on this procedure, consider the legal implications should you divorce or die. Like many couples who blithely sign prenuptial agreements thinking divorce will never happen to *them*, those who embark on the financial drain and emotional roller coaster of in vitro fertilization rarely think about the dread *D* words. Think about them. Try to agree in advance on the disposition of the embryos. The contract with an IVF clinic should include a clause setting forth the couple's decision on how long to keep the embryos frozen and what disposition to make of the eggs should the couple separate, divorce, or if one or both of them dies.

Artificial Insemination

From California's Repository for Germinal Choice, which actively seeks semen from Nobel Prize winners and other geniuses, to more than one hundred sperm banks across the country that recruit less celestial donors, artificial insemination is a thriving business in America. More than 11,000 doctors offer it as a treatment for infertility. Each year, at least 172,000 women use artificial insemination, which results in about 65,000 births, according to a survey by the U.S. Congress Office of Technology Assessment.

When the California "genius" clinic opened in 1979, there was great concern that a brave new world was approaching. Years later, these fears have not been realized. A more realistic worry is sperm that is damaged, lost, or mixed up.

Julia Skolnick went to a Manhattan sperm bank to be inseminated by the sperm deposited by her husband, who was dying of cancer. Both she and her husband were white, so when Ms. Skolnick gave birth to a black daughter, she sued the sperm bank. In 1991, the case was settled out of court for $400,000.

Since sperm banks are regulated only loosely and mix-ups can occur despite precautionary measures, there is no way to be 100 percent sure that the same thing won't happen to you. One safeguard is to use a sperm bank affiliated with the American Association of Tissue Banks or one that follows the guidelines of the American Fertility Society. Contact the American Association of Tissue Banks, 1350 Beverly Road, McLean, VA 22101, (703) 827-9582 and the American Fertility Society at the address provided earlier in this chapter.

If you decide on this procedure, you probably already know that there are three types of artificial insemination. The first, artificial insemination by husband (AIH), which uses semen from a husband, is the most popular, accounting for about half the procedures done today. It was the procedure Ms. Skolnick used.

In artificial insemination-combined (AIC), a rarely used procedure, the husband's semen is mixed with that of a donor, thus offering the possibility of the husband's being the biological father.

The third is artificial insemination by donor (AID), or as it is increasingly called, therapeutic donor insemination (TDI), which uses the semen of a third person, usually an anonymous donor. Some early court decisions held that AID was adultery and that the resulting children were illegitimate. Today, AID is lawful in every state, although legal questions arise concerning the legitimacy of children, parental responsibilities, informed consent, and confidentiality of records.

Legitimacy of Children Born of Artificial Insemination

Artificial insemination is so simple that it can be done by a woman with a turkey baster. Despite its simplicity and accessibility, the law defines artificial insemination as a medical matter. The laws of thirty-five states specify that if insemination is done by a doctor with a husband's consent, the children are the legitimate offspring of the couple. Although the children of married parents would probably be declared legitimate in any case, it's best to have a physician perform the insemination, just to be sure and to avoid future legal headaches.

Bringing Up Baby

A husband who consents to his wife's insemination with another man's sperm is considered the legal father of the child, with all the rights and responsibilities of fatherhood. He is no different from a biological father. In case of divorce, he has the obligation to support his child and visitation rights if he does not have custody. Courts go to great lengths to assure that children are part of a family and that parents carry out their responsibilities in bringing up and supporting the child. This holds true even for nontraditional families that stretch the definition of "parent" to its limits.

Consider the truly bizarre case of Karin versus Michael/Marlene. When she was in her twenties, Marlene tried to shed her female identity and live like a man. Changing her name to Michael, she dressed in men's clothing and worked on construction gangs. Michael and Karin started living together and shortly thereafter obtained a marriage license (nobody bothered to ask for a birth certificate) and were married. They had two children through artificial insemination. After the birth of their second child, Karin and Michael split up. In the divorce proceedings, Karin sued for child support. Michael argued that, as a woman, she obviously couldn't be the children's father. A New York court found that Michael, aka Marlene, was the legal parent and therefore could not dodge child support.

The other side of the equation is that the donor is free and clear of any responsibility to the child. He donates his sperm, is paid, and moves on — no responsibility, no rights. About the only exception is the rare case in which a donor is selected by a woman and acts as a father to the child.

Consent: What You Should Know about Artificial Insemination

As with any medical procedure, you should be fully informed about artificial insemination before undergoing it. This means knowing about the benefits, risks, and other considerations discussed in Chapter 2. The most significant risk appears to be that of being inseminated with infected semen.

Semen that is not properly tested may carry a sexually transmitted disease such as gonorrhea, a genetically transmitted disease such as cystic fibrosis, or AIDS. In 1985, before screening tests for the AIDS virus were developed, a man whose sperm was used to inseminate nineteen women was later found to be HIV positive. More recently, infected semen was inadvertently used in at least two instances, although no cases of AIDS from this source have been reported in the United States. By following two simple rules, you can help protect yourself against being given infected semen:

- Use only *frozen* semen that has been quarantined for at least six months and came from a man who, six months after donating it, was tested for the AIDS virus. These procedures do not eliminate the risk of AIDS entirely — nothing does — but they certainly reduce it.
- Use semen that comes from a sperm bank affiliated with the American Association of Tissue Banks or follows the guide-

lines of the American Fertility Society. Although this does not guarantee that a clinic does adequate screening, says attorney Lori Andrews, a research fellow with the American Bar Foundation and expert on infertility law, it increases the likelihood that the bank tests donors for sexually and genetically transmitted diseases, analyzes sperm to make sure it is fertile, and eliminates drug addicts and alcoholics as donors.

Confidentiality and Access to Records

Some children of artificial insemination contend that they should be able to learn the identity of their biological father. Like adopted children, they have met with little success. Donors who know that their anonymity is in danger would no longer donate, goes a common line of reasoning. Records about artificial insemination are considered confidential. If they can be inspected at all, it is only under court order.

Children of artificial insemination may, however, need a complete family medical history, for example, to find out about a genetic disorder inherited from the donor. Many states have passed laws permitting adopted children to learn about the health and ethnic background of their biological parents without revealing their identity. These laws may be extended to include children of artificial insemination donors.

Surrogate Motherhood

In 1987, Americans were captivated by the Baby M case. William Stern, a forty-two-year-old biochemist, and his wife, Elizabeth Stern, a forty-one-year-old pediatrician unwilling to have children because of her multiple sclerosis, wrote a contract with Mary Beth Whitehead, the twenty-nine-year-old mother of two children of her own, to bear their child. Ms. Whitehead was artificially inseminated with Mr. Stern's semen and paid $10,000. When the baby, named Melissa by the Sterns and Sara by Ms. Whitehead, was born on March 27, 1986, Ms. Whitehead could not bear to part with her.

Three days after the birth, Ms. Whitehead visited the Sterns, told them how much she was suffering, and begged to have the child for a last visit, if only for a week. Afraid that Ms. Whitehead would commit suicide, the Sterns turned the baby over to her. Then Ms. Whitehead refused to give up the baby. When the Sterns obtained a court order for the baby's return, Ms. Whitehead and her husband fled to Florida with the baby, where they lived as fugitives at about twenty different motels for the next three months. Eventually, a private detective tracked down the Whiteheads, and the child was brought back and turned over to the Sterns.

A two-month trial followed. The lower court judge ruled that the surrogacy contract was valid, determined that the baby's best interests were with the Sterns, and awarded them custody. Then the New Jersey Supreme Court struck down the lower court's decision, ruling that, in New Jersey, surrogate mother contracts for pay were illegal, unenforceable, and possibly criminal. This made the surrogate contract that Mr. Stern and Ms. Whitehead had signed at the Infertility Center of New York null and void. Once the contract was invalidated, the case became a custody dispute. Like the lower court, the New Jersey Supreme Court determined that the Sterns would provide a better home environment for Melissa than Mary Beth Whitehead. It awarded them custody with liberal visiting rights to Ms. Whitehead.

Although the personal anguish and moral concerns generate great publicity when a surrogate mother goes to court to keep a baby, very few people are affected. "About fifteen hundred surrogate mothers have given birth. Fewer than one percent have changed their mind and mounted a court challenge," says Ms. Andrews.

A typical surrogate motherhood arrangement involves an infertile couple wealthy enough to afford the high costs — up to $30,000, of which $10,000 to $12,000 is paid to the surrogate, the balance of $18,000 to $20,000 going to cover medical costs and to a surrogacy center, which serves as the middleman. Usually a surrogate mother responds to an ad placed by a surrogacy center. The surrogate is artificially inseminated, carries the baby to term, and turns it over to the couple for adoption. The problem occurs when the surrogate changes her mind and wants to keep the baby.

To its critics, surrogate motherhood threatens the very nature of the family, smacks of baby selling, which is illegal everywhere, and exploits women, particularly poor ones. They argue that surrogate motherhood has so much potential for creating legal and ethical problems that it should be banned. Others contend that surrogate motherhood benefits couples who otherwise could not have a baby, that making it illegal would only drive the practice underground, and that women have the right to be surrogates as long as they are not coerced. They argue that surrogacy should be permitted, but regulated to prevent abuse.

Two cases that stretch the limits of law and technology illustrate some of the pitfalls and potential benefits of surrogate motherhood. Both involve a surrogate carrying a baby that is the product of others' sperm and egg. Crispina Calvert, a thirty-six-year-old nurse, was unable to bear a child because of a partial hysterectomy. (She still had her ovaries.) She and her husband, Mark, a thirty-four-year-old insurance underwriter, arranged for Anna Johnson, twenty-nine, a nurse working in the same California hospital as Ms. Calvert, to carry their baby. Their contract called for Ms. Johnson to be paid $10,000 after handing the infant over to the Calverts.

Since Ms. Calvert could still produce eggs, she and her husband conceived a child through in vitro fertilization. The embryo was transferred to Ms. Johnson, who had a complicated pregnancy and was hospitalized several times. Toward the end of her pregnancy, Ms. Johnson changed her mind. She tried to invalidate the contract, claiming that she had bonded with the baby, that the Calverts had shown little interest during her difficult pregnancy, and that because she had carried the baby, she was really its mother.

Christopher Michael was born on September 19, 1990, amid a bitter court battle to establish whether his parents were the woman who carried him for nine months or the couple whose sperm and egg created him. An Orange County judge ruled that the contract was valid and awarded custody to the Calverts. Unlike the Baby M case, in which Melissa came from the union of Mary Beth Whitehead's egg and William Stern's sperm, Michael had no genetic relation to Anna Johnson. "Anna has no parental rights, contractually or other," wrote Judge Richard Parslow. "I think a two-natural-mom claim is ripe for crazy making." The decision was affirmed by a California appeals court in 1991.

In the second case, which gave the press a field day, Arlette Schweitzer, forty-two, an Aberdeen, South Dakota, schoolteacher, carried and gave birth to her own grandchildren. Mrs. Schweitzer's daughter, Crista Uchytila, who was born without a uterus, could not bear children. An embryo created of Mrs. Uchytila's egg and the sperm of her husband, Kevin, was implanted in Mrs. Schweitzer. No money changed hands, no contract was signed. It was a pure labor of love. "You do what you do for your children because you love them," Mrs. Schweitzer told the *New York Times*. "If you can do something to help your children, you do it." On October 11, 1991, she gave birth to twins.

State laws reflect the lack of agreement about how to handle surrogate motherhood. Fourteen states have passed laws on surrogacy, according to the National Conference of State Legislatures, which keeps track of the latest developments. They are all over the lot. Michigan makes it a crime to enter into or assist a surrogate motherhood contract in which money changes hands and the surrogate must surrender the baby. Louisiana law considers surrogacy contracts, whether for pay or not, to be unenforceable. Florida allows surrogacy contracts but gives the surrogate mother seven days to change her mind.

If you are considering entering into a surrogate motherhood arrangement, consult a lawyer. Whether you are volunteering to be a surrogate mother or are a couple that wants a baby, you must protect yourself. Remember that surrogacy centers are profit-making businesses whose lawyers are paid to protect their interests, not yours.

Here are some of the issues to consider before entering into a surrogacy arrangement:

- **Payment.** How much will the surrogate receive and when will she be paid? What happens in the event of a miscarriage or stillbirth? Who is responsible for payment for prenatal care, delivery, life insurance, maternity clothes, and the like?
- **Physical and emotional testing.** A potential surrogate mother should undergo both physical and psychological tests. Most surrogacy centers do this as a matter of course, and many screen both sets of husbands and wives.
- **Counseling.** A physician should make sure the surrogate understands the physical risks of the insemination, pregnancy, and delivery. The contract should call for counseling of the

surrogate and her husband, if applicable, and about the potential psychological consequences of giving up the baby. No doubt should remain that the surrogate mother is psychologically capable of releasing the newborn.

- **Prenatal screening and restrictions.** Will the surrogate smoke or drink? Take medication? What tests will be done during the course of the pregnancy? It is probably unconstitutional to require an abortion if testing reveals a genetic defect, but this possibility should be discussed.
- **Surrogate's continued involvement.** What rights, if any, does the surrogate mother have to receive information about the child? To have continued contact?
- **Birth defects.** Does the birth of a handicapped child affect the agreement? About the worst scenario imaginable is the birth of a handicapped child whom nobody wants. In 1983, Judy Stiver entered into a contract to bear a child for Alexander Malahoff. The child was born retarded, and neither Ms. Stiver nor Mr. Malahoff wanted the baby. Eventually a blood test for paternity was performed with the results announced, believe it or not, on the *Donahue* show. The blood test revealed that Mr. Malahoff was not the father. The father turned out to be none other than Ms. Stiver's husand.

A Note on Adoption

For many infertile couples who are desperate to have a child genetically related to at least one of the parents, adoption is not an easy option to consider. Added to this is the shrinking pool of adoptable babies. The combination of effective birth control, legal abortion, and increasing numbers of single women who keep and raise their babies has dramatically decreased the number of available infants. The National Committee on Adoption estimates that two million couples compete to adopt the forty thousand babies who are placed for adoption every year. The scarcity of healthy white infants is particularly acute. The wait may be six to eight years and the cost up to $50,000 (normally the cost is between $8,000 and $15,000). Couples willing to adopt a nonwhite baby, an older child, or a handicapped youngster find the road much smoother.

Bob and Katherine H., both forty-year-old New Yorkers, tried for two years to have a baby before looking into adoption. "First we talked to the licensed adoption agencies, but they were very discouraging," recounts Mr. H., an investment banker. "They had a waiting list of more than five years for white infants, which is what we wanted. Besides, we were both over their cutoff age. We knew of couples who had adopted children from Colombia and Korea, so we thought about international adoption. But we felt it was too risky — there were just too many unknowns.

"That put us into the private adoption market, which meant finding a lawyer who would learn about a pregnant woman willing to give up her baby for adoption. We weren't happy about this option because many of the lawyers we talked to seemed sleazy, and we were worried about violating state laws against baby selling. We checked and found that private adoption is legal in most states. We were set to pursue that option when, through some miracle, Katherine became pregnant."

Many organizations can help couples considering adoption. Among them are the following:

- RESOLVE, 1310 Broadway, Somerville, MA 02144-1731, (617) 623-0744
- National Adoption Hotline, (202) 328-8072
- Adoptive Families of America, 3333 Highway 100 North, Minneapolis, MN 55422, (612) 535-4829
- National Committee for Adoption, 1930 17th Street, NW, Washington, DC 20009-6207, (202) 328-1200
- North American Council on Adoptable Children, P.O. Box 14808, Minneapolis, MN 55414, (612) 625-0330
- National Adoption Information Clearinghouse, 11426 Rockville Pike, Suite 410, Rockville, MD 20852, (301) 231-6512.

9

AIDS AND THE LAW

CONTENTS

AIDS: What It Is and How It's Spread

Except by readers of the gay press or scientific journals, the 1981 report of the death of five otherwise healthy homosexual men from a rare form of pneumonia went unnoticed. A month later, the announcement of twenty-six additional deaths attracted more interest — and signaled a growing concern in the gay community. Soon the disease known as AIDS (*A*cquired *I*mmune *D*eficiency *S*yndrome) spread its cloud of death over entire populations.

By 1982, it was reported in intravenous drug users, people who had received blood transfusions, hemophiliacs, heterosexual women, and young children. By the following year, two thousand cases had been reported in the United States. As of 1992, more than two hundred thousand people in the U.S. had developed AIDS. Nearly two thirds have died, most within two years after the symptoms first appeared. It has become the nation's worst epidemic.

Cases of AIDS have been reported in every state, although more than half have occurred in California and New York State. Already it is threatening to exhaust the emergency rooms and hospitals of the two hardest hit cities, San Francisco and New York City, where it is the leading cause of death of men aged thirty to thirty-four and women twenty-five to twenty-nine.

AIDS is caused by the *h*uman *i*mmunodeficiency *v*irus (HIV), which causes a breakdown in the body's immune system, increasing its susceptibility to diseases and infections. As a result of the body's inability to fight disease, people carrying the virus often contract such rare diseases as pneumocystis carinii pneumonia and Kaposi's sarcoma. The federal Centers for Disease Control (CDC) defines AIDS in terms of these and other rare diseases and has proposed expanding the definition to include HIV-positive people whose immune systems are very weak. A person who is HIV positive — carrying the virus — does not always come down with AIDS. Since it can take ten years or more for the AIDS virus carrier to develop symptoms of the disease, nobody is sure what percentage of HIV-positive people will eventually contract AIDS. Estimates range from 50 to 100 percent. Many people — perhaps more than a million — who have the virus are still walking around with no symptoms; the danger is that these people can spread the virus to others.

In 1985, the federal Food and Drug Administration approved the use of the *enzyme-linked immunosorbent assay* (ELISA) blood test, which reveals whether a person has developed antibodies to the AIDS virus. The test is quite effective in identifying people infected with the virus — indeed, too much so. ELISA sometimes wrongly identifies virus-free people as being infected with HIV. Because of this tendency, public health officials recommend a second ELISA for anybody who tests positive. If two ELISAs reveal antibodies to the AIDS virus, another, more accurate and more expensive test, usually the Western Blot, is given to confirm those results.

Remember these three important points:

- A single positive ELISA is not proof that a person has the AIDS virus. It takes two positive ELISAs confirmed by a Western Blot or similar test.
- Although a negative test is reassuring, it doesn't offer 100 percent certainty that a person is free of the AIDS virus. It can take six months after infection for antibodies to the AIDS virus to develop.
- People who are carrying the human immunodeficiency virus — who are HIV positive — do not necessarily have AIDS. Most, but perhaps not all, HIV-positive persons will eventually develop sicknesses that characterize AIDS, but all HIV-positive people can transmit the virus to others.

As of this writing, there is no cure for AIDS, which is considered fatal. It appears that if the HIV is detected early enough, AIDS can be delayed with use of medications such as azidothymidine (AZT) and dideoxynosine (DDI).

One of the keys to understanding the law, described below, is to appreciate the difficulty of catching the AIDS virus. The human immunodeficiency virus is very fragile. It can, for example, be killed by ordinary soap and water or household bleach. According to the CDC, there are only four ways that the AIDS virus can be transmitted:

- Sexually. Sexual contact, particularly with many partners, is highly risky. Homosexual transmission accounts for over 60 percent of AIDS cases, a proportion that has decreased as the gay community has adopted "safe sex" practices of abstinence and condom use. Although AIDS is often perceived as a disease afflicting homosexuals, it can also be transmitted from men to women. And, as Magic Johnson's 1991 announcement that he was HIV positive made clear, from women to men. About one in every ten AIDS victims is a woman, largely as a result of contact with bisexual men or intravenous drug use. The percentage is rising rapidly — in 1990 the number of women with AIDS grew by 29 percent, compared with an 18 percent increase in men.
- Through sharing infected needles. Needle sharing among intravenous drug users accounts for 25 percent of the reported cases of AIDS. As AIDS among the gay population decreases, it is becoming increasingly a disease of poor, drug-abusing, minority men and women.
- Through infected blood. Although tests in use since 1985 have made today's blood supply almost completely safe, there is still a small possibility — estimated at one in 250,000 — of getting the AIDS virus from a blood transfusion.
- Through pregnant women or lactating mothers. The chances of a woman with the AIDS virus transmitting it to her baby, during pregnancy or through infected breast milk, are thought to be between 25 and 30 percent.

Just as important as understanding how the AIDS virus is spread is knowing how it is *not* transmitted. The surgeon general of the United States wrote every family in the United States to assure them that:

- The AIDS virus is *not* spread through casual contact or touching.
- It is *not* spread through saliva, sweat, tears, or kissing, although the virus has been found in saliva and tears.
- It is *not* spread from clothing, telephones, or toilet seats, by being on a crowded bus or elevator, or by working next to a person who has AIDS.

Every state and the District of Columbia have enacted AIDS-related laws. More than five hundred laws directly related to AIDS have been passed since 1981. The laws reflect a tension between public health needs and individual privacy rights. Public health officials, likening AIDS to syphilis and other sexually transmitted diseases, often call for measures that traditionally have been used to control communicable diseases, for example, widespread testing and reporting of people who are HIV positive; locating and notifying sexual or needle-sharing partners that they are at risk; and sometimes quarantining infected persons who place others at risk by their behavior. Civil libertarians and those at risk for the infection often doubt that information can be kept confidential, fear discrimination, and say they do not want government snooping into their private lives. Each state, and many counties and cities, resolve these tensions differently.

In this chapter, we inform you of your rights — whether you have AIDS, work with, employ, or know someone who is HIV positive, or are a worried patient or health professional. We also tell you where to find information should you need it.

Reporting, Confidentiality, and Contact Tracing

Reporting

Cases of AIDS must be reported by health professionals to the health department of every state. Some states require that the name of the person with AIDS be given; others require only demographic information, such as age and sex. In all states, the health departments treat the names as confidential.

What about reporting the names of people who are infected with HIV but have not developed AIDS? Here a policy debate rages. Some health experts, such as Dr. Stephen Joseph, the former New York City health commissioner, argue that the names of people testing positively for the virus should be reported to the health department, which can then contact and notify their sexual or needle-sharing partners that they are at risk. Since drugs such as AZT and pentamidine prolong life if taken early enough, Dr. Joseph reasons, there is a moral obligation to notify people who might be at risk. On the other side, public health authorities such as Mark Barnes, former policy director of the New York State AIDS Institute, argue that reporting by name will scare many people away from seeking medical care and lead to discrimination by employers or insurance companies. Mr. Barnes also contends that tracing the partners of a sexually active adult over the past, say, five years may prove a Herculean, expensive, and perhaps impossible task.

The variety of state laws concerning reporting of people carrying the AIDS virus reflects the lack of consensus. According to Kate Cauley of the AIDS Policy Center of George Washington University, five states require reporting of the names of people who test positive. Another nineteen require reporting by name but allow people to be tested anonymously as well. Nineteen other states do not require the names of people infected with the virus to be revealed, although four states allow exceptions to this rule under certain circumstances. The remaining states and the District of Columbia have no reporting requirements. If you have a question about reporting requirements in your state, call the National AIDS hotline, (800) 342-AIDS.

Notifying Partners and Others at Risk
Notifying the sexual partners of an infected person is a standard public health practice to control communicable diseases. Although gay and civil liberties groups have opposed efforts to locate and warn partners, their position is changing, according to Professor Ronald Bayer of the Columbia University School of Public Health. Thirty-three states have laws authorizing health authorities to find and notify the sexual or needle-sharing partners of HIV-positive people that they may be at risk of contracting the disease. All partner notification programs depend on the willingness of infected persons to reveal the names of their partners. The laws require that the name of the HIV-infected person not be revealed to the persons contacted, and the record of the public health authorities in maintaining confidentiality is very good.

A doctor who warns the sexual or needle-sharing partner of a patient would generally be violating a confidential relationship. Fear of lawsuits by angry patients keeps physicians from warning people at risk. To overcome this fear, thirty states have passed laws shielding doctors from liability.

The most common approach is that adopted by the New York State legislature. Doctors are encouraged to urge HIV-positive patients to inform their partners about their condition. If a patient refuses to do so, a doctor, without fear of a lawsuit for breaching the doctor-patient relationship, can warn the partner or inform the health department which, in turn, can notify the partner. In states that have no legislation on the matter, it appears that the health benefits of warning a person at risk of getting the virus are likely to outweigh the importance of doctor-patient confidentiality.

In some states, doctors may have a duty to warn the known partner of an infected patient. A physician who failed to do so might be endangering the life of an innocent person. In the influential case cited in Chapter 2, a California psychotherapist did not warn a woman that his patient, her former boyfriend, had threatened to kill her. After the patient murdered the young woman, her parents sued the therapist for failing to warn their daughter about the danger she faced. They won. The same reasoning might apply to a doctor who failed to warn the known partner of an HIV-positive patient.

Infected people probably have a legal duty to tell their partners. People with communicable diseases such as herpes have been successfully sued for failing to warn their partners. Some states make it an offense for HIV-positive people not to disclose their condition to their partners. A few years ago the tabloids were filled with details of a lawsuit brought by Marc Christian, the longtime lover of Rock Hudson, who died of AIDS. Although free of the virus, Christian won $21 million from the actor's estate because Hudson did not reveal that he was infected.

Confidentiality of Test Results

Generally, test results are confidential. Some states, such as Massachusetts, have passed laws prohibiting the disclosure of HIV test results without the written consent of the person tested. California and New York, the two states with the most AIDS cases, also have strict laws to guard the confidentiality of test results. In states with no specific legislation regarding confidentiality of HIV test results, AIDS-related medical records are protected by general public health confidentiality laws.

Exceptions to Confidentiality

Although the duty, in some states, to warn people at risk is the most important exception to the confidentiality of HIV test results, it is not the only one. For example, Wisconsin and other states allow health professionals to disclose the HIV status of a patient, without his or her consent, to organ transplant services, blood banks, and hospital staff committees. Illinois is one of a number of states that authorize the disclosure of test results when a health professional, police officer, or firefighter has come in contact with potentially infected blood. Insurance companies have the right to know the results of an HIV test taken by an applicant for a policy.

Even though the confidentiality of AIDS-related information is protected by law in many states and the number of leaks has been negligible, a surprisingly large group of people may have access to it. If you are concerned about leaks, get tested at a place that does not require your name. Anonymous testing sites exist in most states. Or use a pseudonym. You'd be amazed at how many times "Donald Duck" has been tested.

Informed Consent

In about twenty states, the law mandates that a person must consent before having the test for the AIDS virus. Testing without prior authorization would be illegal in them. Even in states without specific legislation, a doctor probably cannot order an AIDS virus test without first obtaining a patient's consent. In ordinary circumstances, you don't have to be told all the diseases your blood is being tested for. But testing for the AIDS virus is different, given the profound impact of a positive result, including the increased risk of suicide. Many state laws require that HIV testing be accompanied by counseling on the disease and its prevention and transmission.

Testing Without Consent

Most public health officials advocate a voluntary system of testing with results being held in confidence except when there is an overriding need to know. There are, however, some circumstances under which testing is required by law.

At one time there was a movement to require premarital testing of couples for HIV, just as they were tested for syphilis. Lawmakers in almost every state proposed legislation, although only Illinois and Louisiana passed a law. In both states, the testing program was a costly and ineffective bust. Illinois, for example, found only twenty-six positive results out of 155,000 people tested — at an estimated cost of more than $100,000 for each one identified. Both states repealed their mandatory testing laws, although they, like many others, require premarital AIDS counseling.

The federal government demands HIV testing of the military, foreign service personnel, Peace Corps volunteers, and Job Corps recruits. Some states mandate testing, without their consent, of people who may have exposed others to the virus. These include suspects who bite police officers, bleeding patients treated by emergency technicians and other health care workers, and victims resuscitated by the police and firefighters. In addition, aliens can be tested without their consent.

Quarantine and Criminalization
Fear of AIDS has led to suggestions that people carrying the virus be quarantined, isolated, and even tattooed. It probably would be unconstitutional to put somebody away just because he or she has the virus. Sickness is not a crime. However, when a person poses a risk to the health of others, public health officials can order him or her to be quarantined, as is frequently done in cases of communicable diseases such as tuberculosis or typhoid. It is within the traditional powers of a health department to isolate a person who threatens the well-being of others.

A person with the AIDS virus who simply refuses to stop having sex or sharing needles would certainly be included in this category. Gaetan Dugas, the notorious Patient Zero, was a former airline steward who, knowing he had AIDS, continued to have almost nonstop unprotected sex. According to Randy Shilts, author of the best-selling *And the Band Played On*, Dugas had sexual relations with 40 of the first 250 people reported to have AIDS in the United States. Patient Zero was never quarantined, but others have been. In Florida, when a female prostitute with AIDS refused to stop walking the streets, a court confined her to her home and ordered her to carry an electronic beeper that signaled the police if she went farther than two hundred feet from her telephone.

Several states have passed laws specifically authorizing public health authorities to isolate people with the AIDS virus who continue to pose a risk to others. Since quarantine is such a drastic measure, the laws usually require a health department to show that nothing else has worked and that isolation is the last resort.

Twenty-four states make it a crime for a person to knowingly transmit, or attempt to transmit, the virus to another person. Even without a specific law, local prosecutors have brought criminal cases against those whose behavior could transmit the virus to an unsuspecting individual. Most prosecutors have failed, partly because the AIDS virus is so hard to spread and partly because it is so difficult to prove intent to transmit.

Insurance

Screening Applicants

The critical factor that determines if you can get insurance is whether you are eligible for a group insurance policy, which usually comes through an employer. As a member of a group, you can probably buy health insurance even though you have AIDS. There is a hitch: AIDS treatment may not be covered for a period of six months to two years if the disease is considered to be a pre-existing condition.

If you apply for an individual policy and have AIDS or the AIDS virus, you're in for a tough time. With a few exceptions, such as Blue Cross–Blue Shield plans in about a dozen states, insurance companies routinely turn down applicants for individual health policies — as well as applicants for life insurance — who are HIV positive, just as they reject people with tuberculosis, cancer, and other illnesses. "You don't insure a burning building" is an old insurance industry adage.

Always remember that insurance companies are businesses. As such, they are extremely leery of covering people with AIDS, particularly now that AZT and other treatments can extend their life span. Insurance companies routinely require applicants to take an

AIDS test as one way to deny coverage. It is legal in all states. Although California, Massachusetts, New York, and Washington, D.C., passed laws in the mid-1980s prohibiting insurers from requiring applicants to take HIV tests, these laws were struck down by the courts or, in the case of the nation's capital, by the U.S. Congress.

An insurance company can ask applicants directly whether they have been diagnosed as having the AIDS virus or, indirectly, whether applicants have symptoms, such as swollen glands, night sweats, or sudden weight loss, that can indicate an HIV infection.

All these questions are legal, and an insurance company could turn you down for refusing to answer them. What is not legal in most states is asking applicants to guess whether they are HIV positive ("Do you have any reason to believe you are carrying the virus?") or denying them insurance because of sexual orientation. Under most state laws and guidelines of the National Association of Insurance Commissioners, insurance companies are not permitted to inquire about sexual orientation.

Insurance companies are not supposed to turn you down because you live in an area populated by "high-risk" groups, because you work in an industry that employs many gays, or because you are a mature, unmarried male who lives with his male roommate. It is a violation of state insurance and human rights laws, yet discrimination on the basis of sexual orientation is an everyday occurrence. Young blacks and Hispanics also suffer from the same practice, known as redlining.

If you believe that you have been discriminated against, contact one of the advocacy groups listed at the end of this chapter.

Canceling Policies and Raising Premiums

Some people believe their insurance policy can be canceled if AIDS or HIV infection is diagnosed. Wrong. Mark Scherzer, a New York City attorney who is a specialist in AIDS law, says, "A diagnosis of AIDS is not a legitimate basis for cancellation of an insurance policy. The policy should continue as long as the premiums are paid when due and the other terms of the policy are complied with."

An insurance company is more likely to raise premiums than to cancel, which hits employees of small companies hardest. Many such businesses have been forced to drop health coverage altogether because their premiums rose astronomically after an employee contracted AIDS.

Limiting Coverage

Some insurance companies have begun to limit the amount they pay for AIDS treatment. While this violates the law of some states, it may be legal in others and for companies that self-insure. John McGann, for example, who worked for the H & H Music Company in Houston, Texas, found out the hard way. The company's health plan had a maximum of one million dollars in lifetime benefits. Shortly after McGann discovered he had AIDS, the company dropped its old plan and acted as its own insurance carrier, placing a $5,000 cap on AIDS benefits. McGann went to court, claiming that the change discriminated against him. The company countered that it would go broke under the old plan; it either had to limit coverage of AIDS or cancel its insurance for all its employees. McGann lost. The court ruled that since the company insured itself, it was not subject to a state insurance law under which a cap on benefits might be illegal. Under federal law, said the judge, a cap on benefits for people with AIDS would be legal.

Continuing Insurance Coverage

At some point, most people with AIDS have to quit their jobs. Their health insurance coverage can also end. However, under the federal COBRA law (see Chapter 3), an employee with AIDS working for a company with twenty or more employees can continue a group health policy, at his or her own expense, for up to twenty-nine months.

Many health plans permit a person leaving a company to convert from a group to an individual health policy. The period for doing so expires after a short time (one to three months), so former employees have to act quickly. Some states have set up risk pools (see Chapter 3) to enable otherwise uninsurable people to obtain some health insurance coverage.

Experimental Drugs

Life-threatening illnesses such as cancer or AIDS lead desperate people to desperate measures. As likely as not, new or experimental treatments won't be covered by insurance. Under the terms of most policies, the company is required to pay the reasonable cost of medical treatment approved by the U.S. Food and Drug Administration. Unusual or experimental treatment may be, and usually is, excluded from coverage.

Under new policies of the federal Food and Drug Administration, many people with AIDS can have access to drugs that are still being tested for safety and effectiveness. However, many insurance companies refuse to pay for these drugs because they are still experimental. As one bewildered person with AIDS asked, "What am I supposed to do? I'm allowed to use a drug that may prolong my life, but I can't afford to pay for it."

Government Programs

The federal government provides benefits for disabled people. The most important for those with AIDS are:

- **Social Security Disability Insurance.** To claim benefits, an individual must have a condition that prevents or is expected to prevent him from working for at least twelve months. AIDS is automatically considered a disability. Benefits, which are tied to earnings, can begin six months after the onset of the disease. The program is administered by the federal Social Security Administration.
- **Supplemental Security Income** is a welfare program for poor people who are disabled, blind, or elderly. It, too, is administered by the federal Social Security Administration.
- **Medicare,** the federal health insurance program for the elderly, also covers people with disabilities. The problem for people with AIDS is that there is a two-year waiting period, which is beyond the life expectancy of many who have the disease. Individuals receiving Social Security Disability Insurance benefits are automatically enrolled when the two-year waiting period is up.
- **Medicaid** is the joint federal-state health program for people with low income. Many people with AIDS spend so much

money on doctors, home care, and drugs that they become poor enough to qualify for Medicaid. The program is administered by state social services departments.

- **AZT Program.** In 1988 Congress allocated money to help low-income AIDS patients pay for the drug AZT and has continued to fund the AZT program every year. The program, which is administered by the states, can cover the cost of AZT, alpha interferon, aerosolized pentamidine, and other specified drugs.

In addition, many states have enacted their own programs to help people with AIDS cope with the costs of fighting the disease. The result is a dizzying array of benefit programs, each of which has its own cumbersome bureaucracy. Thomas McCormick, author of *The AIDS Benefits Handbook,* cautions patience and persistence as you try to locate a person who can even *understand* your problem, much less be responsible for handling it.

Employment

Questions about AIDS in the workplace usually fall into two camps: employer and coworker. Both are motivated by fear. An employer, who is worried about the cost of health insurance or losing customers, may try to bar people with AIDS or fire them once their condition is discovered. Frightened coworkers may refuse to work with an HIV-positive fellow employee, afraid they will catch the deadly virus. Are these legal? What rights does an HIV-positive worker have? What are the rights of his or her coworkers? The company?

The answers, which have not yet been wholly determined, depend on the interpretation of state laws and two federal laws: the 1973 Rehabilitation Act and the 1990 Americans with Disabilities Act. Although the law of AIDS in the workplace is still emerging, two principles should help you understand the rights of people with the virus, their fellow workers, and their employers:

- People with AIDS and those who are HIV positive are legally considered handicapped or disabled under federal laws. The federal laws, and the laws of just about every state and many large cities, protect people with the AIDS virus against discrimination.

- The AIDS virus is extremely hard to transmit and cannot be spread by the casual contact associated with a normal workplace.

Employees with the AIDS Virus

When Vincent Chalk, a teacher of hearing-impaired students in Orange County, California, told his supervisor he had AIDS, the school transferred him to an administrative position. But Mr. Chalk wanted to teach. He brought a lawsuit, claiming that, as a person with AIDS, he was handicapped. Since he was still able to teach and the disease was not contagious, he argued that he was the victim of discrimination in violation of the federal Rehabilitation Act. A federal court in California agreed and in 1988 ordered the school to reinstate him. When Mr. Chalk returned to his classroom, he was greeted with acceptance, homemade gifts, and hugs from the students and their parents. He continued to receive enthusiastic support until, a few years later, the illness forced him to take disability leave.

The Americans with Disabilities Act of 1990 bans discrimination against disabled employees or job applicants, including those who have AIDS, are HIV-positive, or are perceived as being in one of these categories. The act, which we discuss in Chapter 4, currently applies to employers of twenty-five or more workers, which will drop to fifteen or more employees in 1994. (Smaller companies will continue to be bound by state and local law.) Even if an employee is disabled, he or she must, as the law states, be "qualified," that is, able to perform the essential tasks of the job. New York Law School professor Arthur Leonard, an AIDS expert, says that there are two tests to determine whether a person is so qualified:

- Does the person have the mental and physical ability to do the job? In the case of an HIV-positive person showing no signs of AIDS, this is easy to resolve in favor of the individual. If a person does have some of the symptoms of AIDS — for example, excessive fatigue — the opinion of one or more doctors will probably be needed. If he or she cannot do the job, the employee can be let go or placed on disability.

• Does this HIV-positive individual pose an unacceptably high danger to others? With the possible exception of some health care workers, the answer is very likely to be no. Because the AIDS virus is extremely difficult to transmit, few people who carry it present a threat to the health of others.

Unless an employer can prove it would cause undue hardship, it must try to make a "reasonable accommodation" (to quote federal law again) so that a disabled employee can continue working. This could mean restructuring a job, reassigning an employee, or modifying the work schedule. Exactly what "reasonable accommodation" means and when it imposes an "undue hardship" are still being defined through government regulations and lawsuits and is apt to differ according to the individual case.

Pre-employment Testing

The federal Disabilities Act also prohibits pre-employment testing to screen out people with AIDS or the AIDS virus. This is a major shift from the past, when each state determined the legality of testing job applicants for the AIDS virus. Here's how the new law works.

Once a conditional job offer has been made, the law permits an employer to require a physical examination, but only to determine whether an applicant is able to perform the required tasks. To justify HIV testing, a company must show that the test is for the purpose of determining job fitness, a potentially impossible task, since many HIV-positive people have no symptoms at all. "Simply being infected with HIV does not impair a person's ability to perform a job," says Evan Wolfson, an attorney with the Lambda Legal Defense and Education Fund.

For most companies, there is no advantage to requiring HIV testing. A positive result reveals little about a worker's ability to perform a job and places the company at risk of a lawsuit for violating the federal Disabilities Act or state civil rights laws. If an applicant's positive test result leaks out, a company could be sued for invasion of privacy. Despite this, some businesses, worried about crippling hikes in insurance premiums or not wanting to hire people who might have AIDS, order HIV tests for job applicants or as part of current employees' normal physical checkups.

Transferring away from a Coworker with AIDS

Given the fear of AIDS, many people do not want to work next to a person who has the disease. Understandable as these fears may be, they do not provide a legal or medical basis for transferring away from a coworker with the AIDS virus. According to the surgeon general of the United States, "You won't just catch AIDS like a cold or flu or through everyday contact with the people around you in school, in the workplace, or in stores."

Because the AIDS virus is not passed on through casual contact at the workplace, there is no legal right to transfer. Under the Occupational Safety and Health Act and federal labor laws, an employee has the right to refuse to perform a task because of a reasonable fear of death or serious illness. The key word is "reasonable." Attorney Mark Barnes concludes that refusal to work with a coworker who has AIDS will not be protected under federal law because the employee's fear, while real, is not reasonable.

AIDS and the Blood Supply

When a doctor told Howard D. that he needed surgery, he thought, "What happens if I need a transfusion? Is the blood supply safe? Can I get AIDS from it?" This is a normal reaction, given the widespread knowledge that the virus can be transmitted by contaminated blood. According to an article in the *Journal of Legal Medicine,* 10,000 hemophiliacs, out of a total of 14,000, and 29,000 transfusion recipients have received blood infected with HIV, almost all of them before 1985.

Prior to 1985, there was no way to tell whether or not donated blood was infected. Then, in that year, the Food and Drug Administration approved the ELISA test, which accurately screens out HIV-infected blood. All suppliers of blood for transfusions and blood-clotting factors for hemophiliacs screen donated blood for the AIDS virus. In addition, blood banks tell high-risk donors to stay away.

The blood supply, although considered safe, is not wholly free from risk. Experts estimate the chances of getting the AIDS virus from a blood transfusion at about one in 250,000, but nobody knows for sure. Although Red Cross officials say the blood supply is as safe as modern technology can make it, fears about its safety continue to grow. If you are scheduled to have an operation that may require blood transfusions, investigate the options available to you. One is donating your own blood beforehand, which is held for you and used if necessary. Another, directed donation, is to have a person whose blood is compatible with yours and is likely to be free of the AIDS virus donate blood for you. Make sure to discuss these options with the surgeon and your doctor well before the date of the operation.

People who develop AIDS through contaminated blood are left with little legal recourse. "Blood shield" statutes in nearly every state and Washington, D.C., designed to protect the supply of blood, make it difficult to win a lawsuit. To be successful, you must prove that the blood bank was negligent in that it failed to use reasonable care in screening donated blood. Since blood banks follow federal government standards and industry guidelines, they are, almost by definition, using reasonable care. The chances of a successful suit by anybody who contracted AIDS from the blood supply after 1985, when the ELISA test was approved, are slim.

Doctors, Dentists, and AIDS

Patients everywhere shuddered when the media reported that David Acer, a forty-year-old Florida dentist who died of AIDS in 1990, had somehow infected five of his patients, among them Kimberly Bergalis, who was twenty-three when she died in December 1991. Since needle sharing and sex were ruled out as sources, how the five got the virus remains a mystery to this day. Dr. Acer is the only health professional known to have transmitted the AIDS virus to a patient out of more than 200,000 reported cases of AIDS.

Yet the possibility of contracting AIDS continues to frighten patients. The key question is whether infected health care workers should stop performing procedures that put patients at risk of getting the virus or tell patients about their condition. (Surgeons, operating room nurses, and dentists are the people who really cause the concern. Their hands are inside you when the risk of a needle prick could result in their infected blood mixing with yours.)

In a 1991 New Jersey case, a court ruled that a surgeon with the AIDS virus must disclose his condition to his patients. "The ultimate risk to the patient is so absolute, so devastating, that it is untenable to argue against informed consent," wrote Superior Court Judge Philip S. Carchman.

The New York State Health Department took exactly the opposite approach. In 1991, it issued guidelines stating that infected health care workers do not have to inform patients about their condition and can continue practicing, including surgery, for as long as they are able. The rationale behind the New York guidelines, which are the law in that state, is that the risk of transmission is nearly infinitesimal and that health professionals, fearful of losing their livelihood, will refuse to treat HIV-positive patients. Supporters of the New York guidelines argue that a system of mandatory testing of health professionals, perhaps as often as every six months, would be nearly impossible to implement and cost billions of dollars, may be unconstitutional, and might violate state and federal laws prohibiting discrimination against disabled people.

In 1991, the federal Centers for Disease Control, issued guidelines adopting a middle course. Although rejecting the call for mandatory testing, the CDC urged health care workers who perform "exposure-prone" invasive procedures to be tested for the AIDS virus and, if they tested positive, to stop unless they received permission from an expert panel and informed their patients of their condition. The CDC called on professional medical and dental societies to develop a list of high-risk invasive procedures. To date, the response to the CDC guidelines has been mostly negative. Medical, dental, and nursing associations charged that such a list is unscientific and would be impossible to draw up. The New York State Health Department rejected the guidelines outright. In response, CDC dropped the proposal.

Besides that of Dr. Acer, no case of an infected doctor or dentist transmitting the virus to a patient has been reported. More important than learning whether your doctor or dentist is HIV positive is knowing whether he or she follows standard infection control procedures, the "universal precautions" developed by the U.S. Centers for Disease Control. They include:

- Wearing gloves and a mask during invasive procedures
- Changing gloves after each patient
- Washing hands thoroughly
- Proper disposal and sterilization of needles, scalpels, and other sharp instruments
- Using resuscitation bags or other ventilation devices to minimize the need for mouth-to-mouth resuscitation

Far more likely than a doctor's giving the virus to a patient is a patient's transmitting it to a physician. By the end of 1991, forty health workers were known to have been infected by patients. Given these facts, can a health worker refuse to treat a person who is HIV positive?

Although some doctors — particularly surgeons facing the possibility of being splashed with infected blood — have refused to treat people with AIDS, this violates the ethical standards of every professional society that has considered the matter, including the American Medical Association, the American Dental Association, and the American Nursing Association.

Refusal to treat an AIDS patient may also violate federal and state laws. Although a doctor can turn away a new patient for just about any reason, the federal Disabilities Act specifically includes doctors' offices among the sites covered by its antidiscrimination provisions. The federal law, as well as many state disabilities laws, prohibit a doctor from refusing to accept a new patient because he or she has AIDS.

Children with AIDS

Ryan White, the Indiana boy who contracted the AIDS virus through a blood transfusion and whose parents fought successfully for his right to attend school, made Americans aware of the plight of children with AIDS. What are their rights? And what are the rights of their classmates whose parents fear a virus that could lead to death? The answer to these questions depends on disability law and the current state of medical knowledge, which indicates that the AIDS virus is extremely hard to transmit.

Laws prohibiting discrimination against people with the AIDS virus apply to children as well as to adults. In addition, the Education for All Handicapped Children Act, a federal law that requires public schools to place handicapped children into regular classrooms whenever possible, may give special protection to schoolchildren with the AIDS virus. Under these laws, a child who does not pose a threat to the health of his or her classmates has a right to attend public school.

But is there a danger to the other children? This is where the current state of medical knowledge enters. In 1989, the National Association of State Boards of Education (NASBE) convened an expert panel to review the medical evidence and develop policies to guide school boards throughout the country. It concluded:

- Infected children do not pose a threat to the health of their classmates, except in the special circumstances of a child who has a secondary infection, such as tuberculosis, that can be transmitted to others.
- Barring a child's having tuberculosis or another communicable disease, children with the AIDS virus should be admitted to or remain in school.
- The risk of transmitting the AIDS virus through bites, urine, feces, tears, or kisses is extremely low or nonexistent.
- Each case should be reviewed by the superintendent of schools, the child's doctor, and a public health official.

Parents of HIV-positive children who have sued to keep their youngsters in school have won every case that has gone to court. In one influential case, the parents of Ryan Thomas, who was five when he was infected with the AIDS virus, challenged the decision of the Atascadero, California, school district to remove him from kindergarten after he had bitten a classmate. Following a thorough examination of the medical evidence, the judge found: "There are no reported cases of the transmission of the AIDS virus in a school setting. The overwhelming weight of medical evidence is that the

AIDS virus is not transmitted by human bites." Concluding that Ryan posed no risk to his classmates or teachers, the judge ordered the school district to keep him in school. When he died in 1991, he had not passed on the virus to anyone.

Even when an HIV-positive child is permitted to enter or stay in school, questions of confidentiality arise. NASBE advises that only one person in a school system, the superintendent, has to know the identity of the child. Others who could be told that a student with HIV will be attending school — without identifying the child — include the principal, the school nurse, and the homeroom teacher. The policies issued by school districts about who can be told the name of an HIV-positive student vary widely. In the Ryan White controversy, the court said that the principal and teachers should be told. In a New York City case, nobody but the superintendent was allowed to know. Other school districts allow teachers and even a child's classmates to know. The law concerning the identity of an HIV-positive schoolchild and at what point confidentiality is breached has not been settled.

Where to Turn for Help

A wide network of organizations offer information, advice, and referrals about AIDS. Some of the key ones are:

- The National AIDS Hotline — (800) 342-AIDS — provides information and referrals to advocacy organizations in your state.
- The National AIDS Clearinghouse — (800) 458-5231 — run by the Centers for Disease Control can send you publications on just about anything having to do with AIDS.
- The Lambda Legal Defense and Education Fund, 666 Broadway, 12th Floor, New York, NY 10012-9996, (212) 995-8585, and the Lesbian/Gay Rights and AIDS Project of the American Civil Liberties Union, 132 West 43rd Street, New York, NY 10036, (212) 944-9800, represent clients in lawsuits and have a profound understanding about the law and its workings.
- Two regional groups knowledgeable about AIDS law are the Gay Men's Health Crisis, 129 West 20th Street, New York, NY

10011, (212) 807-6655, and the AIDS Legal Referral Panel, 11 Sansome Street, San Francisco, CA 94104, (415) 291-5454.

- The National Association of People with AIDS, 1413 K Street, NW, Washington, DC 20005, (202) 429-2856, is an advocacy and service organization for people with AIDS.
- The AIDS Action Council, 2033 M Street, NW, Washington, DC 20003, (202) 293-2886, is an umbrella organization of nearly four hundred AIDS service providers.
- The AIDS Policy Center of the Intergovernmental Health Policy Project, 2021 K Street, NW, Washington, DC 20006, (202) 872-1445, keeps track of federal and state legislation on AIDS.

10

PARENTS AND CHILDREN

CONTENTS

When the fever started, Darci was eight months old. When it persisted, her mother, Linda F., took her to the pediatrician. Suspecting an infection, he did a urine culture, then ordered a set of X rays of the urinary system. "He said this is a urinary tract infection and she has to have the X rays," says Ms. F., a thirty-two-year-old researcher. "He didn't say how they would do them — if they would use a local or general anesthetic or if she would have to be catheterized. I was really upset, but I didn't question him."

When Ms. F. got home, she pulled out a popular book on baby care, which recommended the X-ray series only after two infections. "When I asked him about that, he wouldn't budge," says Ms. F., still angry at the recollection. "He said if there was something anatomically wrong, they could correct it. I asked to talk to somebody else, but he never gave me the name of another physician." Instead, he sent her to a pediatric urologist. "He hardly examined her," says Ms. F. "His attitude was that doctors are gods and she needs the X rays."

Then Darci woke up screaming one night with a bulge in her groin. It turned out she also had a hernia. That was when Ms. F. decided to make one last attempt to get another opinion. Her pediatrician gave her the name of a pediatric surgeon. "The next day I went to see him. He took one look at Darci and said, 'This baby has fused labia. She doesn't need X rays. Anybody could have discovered this.' It turned out that this is part of a routine examination of newborn girls."

A few days later, Darci had corrective surgery on an outpatient basis and was home that night. "If I hadn't found another doctor, I don't know what would have happened," says Ms. F. "The experience made me believe even more that, as a parent, you always have to be vigilant."

Parents are considered to be the protectors of their children and to know what is best for them. As a parent, it is your legal right to be fully involved in your children's care and your duty to make decisions in their best interest. This means that you have a right to be fully informed about the medical options for your child.

Don't be afraid to ask your doctor if you don't understand something. Ask again and again if it remains unclear. Remember, it's *your* child and *your* right.

Although many hospitals still restrict parents' visits to their sick children, you have a right to be with your child in a doctor's office or a hospital. "You must be prepared to be assertive if you want to participate fully in your children's care," says Michael Rooney of the Pennsylvania-based People's Medical Society.

However, there are some exceptions to parents' rights:

- Sometimes the rights of children and their parents may conflict, as when decisions about whether to treat a handicapped newborn can lead either to the child's death or to its living a short, painful life. Such life-and-death decisions arise even before birth. Increasingly, fetuses are considered to have rights of their own, to be balanced against those of the parents.
- As children approach adulthood and become old enough to understand what is going to happen to them, they are allowed to make medical decisions on their own.
- Certain kinds of care, like treatment of sexually transmitted diseases, involve a degree of embarrassment that teenagers may not wish to share with their parents.

In this chapter, we examine the health rights of children and parents from embryo through adolescence.

Genetic Testing and Counseling

Say you're twenty-eight, riding the crest of yuppiedom with a career as an interior designer, a husband in investment banking, and an entire brownstone on a soon-to-skyrocket New York City block. You're also pregnant. Amniocentesis? Isn't that for the over-thirty-five set? Then the impossible happens. With no history in your family, your daughter is born with Down's syndrome. What do you do?

If you're Elizabeth Goodwin, you go into shock, grieve, listen, then get mad. "There was a lot of pressure not to keep her," says Ms. Goodwin, who now lives in Connecticut with her family, which includes two normal sons. "I was told later that I was the first person at the hospital from a private practice who went home with her baby. But I couldn't give her up." Nor could she cope with the dismal prediction of the hospital's geneticists. With seed money from a benefactor and friend, Ms. Goodwin organized a conference of top scientists, leading to the founding of the National Downs Syndrome Society, which has a mailing list of over fifty thousand.

That was more than thirteen years ago. While current thinking over the wisdom of institutionalizing all Down's syndrome babies has shifted dramatically, many parents are still lost when confronted with the alien world of genetics. They struggle to find out what tests are available, where to get genetic screening, and what to ask a genetics counselor.

Dr. Dorothy Warburton, professor of clinical genetics at New York's Columbia-Presbyterian Medical Center, warns that many doctors know very little about genetics. "You should be wary of getting genetic advice from anyone other than a person specially trained in the field or a team of people including an ob-gyn, a geneticist, and a genetics counselor," she says. This is likely to take you to a major medical center or one of its satellite programs and may turn you into a medical detective.

Birth Defects and Testing
We are on the brink of a golden age of genetics. Scientists have tracked down the gene that causes cystic fibrosis, which affects one in twenty-five hundred Caucasian children. They have devised tests that identify people who will develop Huntington's disease, the debilitating illness that killed Woody Guthrie, and are on the verge of identifying the genetic markers for certain cancers and for Alzheimer's disease. But identifying is a long way from finding a cure. "We are in a period when we can diagnose but not treat genetic disease," says attorney Lori Andrews, an expert on law and genetics. More secrets locked in the complexities of DNA are sure to come to light. Over $15 billion is to be spent through 2005 on the truly awesome Human Genome Project, whose goal is to identify every one of the fifty to one hundred thousand human genes.

Genetic testing can identify many fetuses that will be born with birth defects and adults who carry genes that may lead to birth defects in their children. Genetic counseling can help parents understand the choices they face. Available genetic tests include the following:

Before Pregnancy: Testing Carriers

Blood tests can identify carriers of genes that cause diseases like Tay-Sachs, sickle cell anemia, and thalassemia. These people do not have the diseases but can pass them on to their children.

During Pregnancy: Fetal Testing

- A blood test for *alpha fetoprotein*, found in mothers' blood, can be done at around fourteen weeks of pregnancy. It identifies fetuses that have brain or spinal column damage, found in one out of five hundred pregnancies, and can screen for (although not very accurately) women who may be carrying a Down's syndrome baby.
- *Amniocentesis.* Between the twelfth and eighteenth weeks of pregnancy, a physician inserts a needle through the abdomen into the uterus and extracts a small amount of amniotic fluid. Amniocentesis can reveal all recognizable chromosomal disorders such as Down's syndrome, about one hundred genetic disorders, and brain and spinal defects with nearly 100 percent accuracy. Common practice is to recommend amniocentesis for women thirty-five years and older.
- *Chorionic villus sampling.* In this relatively new procedure, done during the ninth through twelfth weeks of pregnancy, the physician guides a thin tube through the cervix and suctions cells from the developing placenta. Except for brain and spine defects, it identifies the same genetic abnormalities as amniocentesis. The advantage is that the test can be done early in pregnancy, and the results are ready within days rather than the several weeks it takes for amniocentesis. In comparing amniocentesis and chorionic villus sampling, make sure to inquire about the risk of miscarriage and deformities from each.
- *Ultrasound,* which examines a fetus through a computerized picture created by high-frequency sound waves, is used routinely to determine the age and sex of the fetus and measure

head size and circumference; it can also detect many birth defects. The accuracy depends on the technology and the skill of the person doing the sonogram.

- *Fetoscopy.* By inserting a fetoscope, a long, slim instrument with a light attached, into the amniotic sac, a physician can observe the fetus for birth defects such as cleft palate or club foot and take blood and tissue samples. A delicate and relatively rare procedure that carries some degree of risk, fetoscopy should be performed by a highly skilled specialist.

After Childbirth: Newborn Testing
In the afterglow of childbirth, most parents of healthy babies are too relieved to think about tests. Yet, in all states, a drop of blood is routinely taken from the heels of newborns to test for birth defects that can cause brain damage, growth complication, and even death. All states test for PKU (phenylketonuria), which affects one in fifteen thousand babies and can cause brain damage if untreated, and congenital hypothyroidism, which affects one in five thousand babies and can lead to mental growth retardation if not caught early. Some states require testing for up to six more diseases. "Early diagnosis and proper treatment can make the difference between lifelong impairment and healthy development," writes Dr. Richard Morton, vice president of the March of Dimes Birth Defect Foundation.

Resources
For information about birth defects, tests to screen for them, and genetic counseling, contact one of the following:

- The March of Dimes Birth Defects Foundation, 1275 Mamaroneck Avenue, White Plains, NY 10605, (914) 428-7100
- The National Center for Education in Maternal and Child Health, 38th and R Streets, NW, Washington, DC 20057, (202) 625-8400
- The American Board of Medical Genetics, 950 Rockville Pike, Bethesda, MD 20814, (301) 571-1825
- The Alliance of Genetic Support Groups, 1001 22nd Street, NW, Washington, DC 20037, (800) 336-GENE

Genetic Negligence: Lawsuits

Nobody wants to have a baby with a birth defect. Parents who learn that their baby will be born with a handicap often face deep moral and ethical choices. Is the defect so severe that the baby will lead a life of pain and suffering? Can we handle the emotional trauma and financial burden? What about our other children? How do we feel about abortion? Some parents decide to terminate the pregnancy, while others have the emotional, and often the financial resources to raise a child with birth defects.

Whatever the decision, the parents must have sufficient information to understand and consider their options. They rely on their physician and genetic counseling team to advise them. They want to know the risk of bearing a handicapped child, the likelihood of its happening, and whether they need tests. If testing is recommended, what are the major risks and benefits of the different kinds of tests? If there is a birth defect, they count on their team to explain its gravity, treatment options, what the life of their child will be like, and what their choices are.

Even with sophisticated prenatal tests, parents are sometimes given the wrong information. Cathy M., a thirty-five-year-old high school teacher in the first trimester of her second pregnancy, received a call from her obstetrician late one Friday evening. The doctor reported that the results of a blood test showed that Cathy had tested positive for toxoplasmosis. The prognosis for her baby was devastating: blindness, mental retardation. Ms. M. and her husband, George, were numb with shock. Although they did not own a cat, one of the common transmitters of the disease, they remembered that their daughter played with a neighbor's animal. On the advice of her doctor, Ms. M. was retested at a much more specialized lab in California, which used a more sensitive test. The results came back borderline, but not enough to cause alarm. Seven months later, Cathy and George were the proud parents of Cynthia, a healthy, normal, seven-pound baby girl. Unfortunately, other stories do not turn out so happily.

Parents who bring a lawsuit for "wrongful birth" charge that they had a baby based on incorrect information negligently given them by a doctor, hospital, or genetics specialist. Almost every state allows parents to bring a wrongful birth action and permits them to recover at least the extraordinary expenses of raising a handicapped child. The Siemieniec family of Chicago had such a case.

If the baby she was carrying was afflicted with the hemophilia that had killed two of her cousins, said Janice Siemieniec and her husband in court papers, she would have had an abortion. At Lutheran General Hospital, Dr. Carol Booth, director of the department of genetics, told Ms. Siemieniec about amniocentesis and fetal blood sampling, then referred her to Dr. Juan Chediak in the division of hematology and oncology at another hospital. Dr. Chediak promised to examine her deceased cousins' birth certificates to see if they were registered hemophiliacs. He subsequently wrote a letter to Dr. Booth stating that the risk of classic hemophilia was "very low." Reassured by his letter, Ms. Siemieniec continued her pregnancy. Adam Siemieniec was born on October 17, 1980, and shortly thereafter had a bleeding episode. The diagnosis? Hemophilia. The Siemieniecs sued both physicians and the hospital for wrongful birth, based on the allegedly negligent diagnosis. The court ruled that the parents could be compensated for the extraordinary expenses they would incur in raising a child they would have aborted but for negligent medical advice.

Wrongful birth lawsuits may be accompanied by "wrongful life" actions brought on behalf of a child. One example is that of James and Donna Turpin, a Fresno, California, couple who, on the advice of their pediatrician, took their only daughter, Hope, to a community hospital for evaluation of a possible hearing problem. In their complaint, the Turpins alleged that Dr. Adam Soriano, the specialist who examined her, found that Hope's hearing was within normal limits and that based on this report, the Turpins had another baby, Joy. They also claimed that both Hope and Joy were "stone deaf" as the result of a hereditary ailment. Mr. and Mrs. Turpin sued for wrongful birth.

In addition, baby Joy herself brought a lawsuit for wrongful life. She claimed, through her attorneys, that she would have been better off never having been born than being born with a severe handicap. Although judges in most states feel uncomfortable making this choice, Joy was allowed to bring her case, making California one of the few states — with Louisiana, New Jersey, and Washington — that permit children to claim damages for being born disabled.

Brave New World: Your Genes Can Betray You

A few years ago, Harvard geneticist Paul Billings placed an unusual ad in a genetics trade journal. Now director of genetics at Pacific Presbyterian Medical Center in San Francisco and a visiting scientist to the Human Genome Project, Dr. Billings was searching for victims of genetic discrimination. He documented at least fifty cases. "All of them are asymptomatic or so mild that it doesn't affect their job," says Dr. Billings. Yet they have been turned down by health and life insurers, mortgage companies, and for automobile insurance. "Once turned down, even if Jonas Salk intervened, it wouldn't make a difference," he says. Nor are children exempt. In some instances, insurance companies have refused to pay for the special diet required for infants diagnosed with PKU, a biochemical disorder. Unless the infant is given this diet, the disorder can lead to mental retardation. "There's a huge push to reduce benefits to families," says Dr. Billings. "The result is that the whole family, including the healthy children, is affected."

The Human Genome Project has targeted $3 million to examine the ethical implications of its huge genetic mapping task. Just whom does the information belong to and how can it be used? These are questions that geneticists, lawyers, insurance companies, and ethicists are just beginning to address.

Until they are answered, make sure that any genetic tests you undergo are absolutely necessary. Nobel laureate James Watson, former director of the Genome project, cautioned a House of Representatives subcommittee in 1991 that genetic discrimination could cause people to lose employment and insurance benefits. In the past, insurance companies raised the premiums of American blacks carrying sickle cell anemia. Although these people did not have the disease, they might have borne children who did. Today, eight states have laws forbidding discrimination against carriers of sickle cell and Tay-Sachs diseases. Some of these laws contain even broader protection against discrimination.

Divided Loyalties

Maternal-Fetal Conflicts

We consistently advise that medical decisions are yours to make. It is your body, and your right as a patient, to choose or refuse treatment. But once a fetus enters the picture, the situation becomes complicated. Obstetricians, following the conclusion reached by the ethics committee of the American College of Obstetricians and Gynecologists, the ob-gyn professional society, have loyalties toward two patients: the pregnant woman and the baby she's carrying.

Most pregnant women are fiercely protective of the life growing inside them. Judy S., at forty, pregnant with her first child, had severe allergies during her pregnancy, yet refused to take any medication for fear it would affect her baby. Susan B., thirty, suffered from near-migraine headaches during her pregnancy rather than take even an aspirin.

Occasionally, a woman behaves in a way that doctors believe will damage her fetus. She may refuse a medically necessary Caesarean section out of personal conviction or religious belief or insist on smoking. Alcoholic and drug-addicted mothers fill hospital wards with the tiniest victims. Some are born prematurely and spend their first days connected to a maze of tubes, trembling from withdrawal symptoms. They may be permanently and profoundly handicapped because of their mothers' behavior during pregnancy.

While the law tends to favor the mother in situations of maternal-fetal conflict, it is uncertain about weighing the rights of the pregnant woman against the health of the fetus she is carrying. The issues have aroused fierce controversy. Dawn Johnsen, an attorney specializing in reproductive health issues, argues that government intrusion into the life of a pregnant woman violates her constitutional right of personal privacy, a right so fundamental that it justifies her decision to have an abortion. Would it be acceptable, Ms. Johnsen asks, for pregnant women to be charged with drinking too much wine, failing to get prenatal care, or carrying heavy groceries? Certainly not, she answers.

University of Texas law professor John Robertson, who takes the opposite view, would support laws that prohibit pregnant women from drinking, smoking, and taking drugs. A baby, in his opinion, has the right to be born of sound body and mind. Once a woman decides to forgo abortion, she loses the liberty to act in ways that may harm the fetus.

As a general rule, a woman's right to make decisions about her own health care remains paramount, but there are exceptions when the law attempts to protect a fetus. This has been true in two situations — substance abuse and forced Caesareans, but it certainly could be extended to others.

Substance Abuse and Pregnancy

At least one in ten new mothers use illegal drugs during their pregnancy, according to a survey by the National Association of Perinatal Addiction Research and Education (NAPARE). This could affect approximately 375,000 newborns who are exposed to crack and other illegal and dangerous drugs each year.

Alcohol, too, can damage a fetus. "Every year five thousand to seven thousand babies are born with fetal alcohol syndrome, which causes prematurity or severe physical and mental handicaps," says Luvon Roberson, director of public information of the Children of Alcoholics Foundation. Heavy cigarette smoking can also cause birth defects and low-birthweight babies.

To protect babies who might suffer the effects of drug and alcohol abuse, state legislators and prosecutors have resorted to child abuse and criminal statutes. "In eleven states, if a woman or her baby has a positive urine toxicology at the time of delivery, or if both the mother's and the baby's urines are negative but the mother admits to using drugs during pregnancy, it's a mandated report for child abuse," Dr. Ira J. Chasnoff, president of NAPARE, told the organization's annual meeting in 1991.

In some states, women have been charged with crimes for taking drugs while pregnant. One was Pamela Rae Stewart, twenty-six, of San Diego. Well into a dangerous pregnancy, Ms. Stewart was told by her doctor to stay off street drugs, avoid sex, and call for help if necessary. Ignoring the doctor's advice, she allegedly took amphetamines, had intercourse with her husband, and delayed going to a hospital for several hours after she began bleeding. Her baby was born brain damaged and died less than two months later. In October 1986, she was charged with violating the California child abuse law. A judge dismissed the charges, reasoning that the statute was not intended to penalize women for conduct during pregnancy. Because fetuses are not considered persons for the purpose of these laws, almost all the cases against drug-abusing mothers have been lost.

To get around this problem, prosecutors devised a novel legal strategy — charging women with delivering drugs to a minor through the umbilical cord. In the case of Kimberly Hardy, the strategy failed. Ms. Hardy was a twenty-four-year-old factory worker when she gave birth to her son in August 1989. After noticing that the baby was small and not eating well, a doctor ordered him tested for drugs. The baby's urine was found to contain traces of cocaine, and Ms. Hardy later admitted to the police that she had smoked crack thirteen hours before the baby was delivered. Prosecutors charged her with delivering drugs to a minor via her umbilical cord. A Michigan appeals court threw the case out, saying that the drug trafficking law was not written for this kind of situation.

While this unusual application of the law has sparked the imagination of prosecutors and the public, health professionals and civil liberties lawyers argue that it is bad policy, and perhaps unconstitutional, to criminalize drug addiction, which is a health problem. Moreover, pregnant women who cannot trust their doctors will not seek health care.

The real problem, says Dr. Wendy Chavkin, an expert in maternal-fetal conflict, is that women are not getting the drug treatment they need before their babies are born. Drug treatment facilities for pregnant women are not readily available. Dr. Chavkin found that 54 percent of the drug treatment programs in New York City categorically exclude pregnant women.

Court-ordered Caesarean Sections
Nothing illustrates the potential conflict between a pregnant woman and a fetus more dramatically than forced Caesarean sections. A doctor who performs a C-section on an unwilling patient, and the hospital in which it is performed, could be liable for assault and battery. To avoid that liability, hospitals sometimes ask a court to authorize a Caesarean the doctor believes is neces-

sary to save the life of a fetus. In all but a few of the approximately fifty such cases, the C-section was ordered by the court.

Almost all the cases were heard before that of Angela Carder in 1990. Ms. Carder, twenty-eight, of Washington, D.C., was twenty-six weeks pregnant and dying of cancer. While she was at George Washington University Hospital, her condition began to deteriorate. The doctors told Ms. Carder that there was only a small chance she would live and that while there was a 50 to 60 percent chance the baby would survive an immediate Caesarean section, it would worsen her risk. Heavily sedated and filled with tubes, Ms. Carder appeared to refuse consent to the C-section in her last conversation with her doctors. It was not even clear whether she had the mental capacity to give consent. The hospital's lawyers requested a court hearing so that a judge could authorize the Caesarean. The judge granted the request to give the fetus "an opportunity to live." The baby lived for a few hours after the surgery; Ms. Carder died two days later.

A federal appeals court later concluded that the section should never have been ordered and that Ms. Carder's wishes should have governed. Since Ms. Carder was unable to express an opinion, the appeals court ruled that the judge should have heard testimony to determine what she would have wanted had she been competent. "It would be an extraordinary case indeed in which a court might ever be justified in overriding a patient's wishes and authorizing a major surgical procedure such as a Caesarean section," wrote the appeals court judges.

Guidelines for Resolving Maternal-Fetal Conflicts

Probably the last place a pregnant woman and her obstetrician want to be is a court of law. Even when they disagree, going to court "is almost never justified," according to the ethics committee of the American College of Obstetricians and Gynecologists. It has suggested three ways to resolve disputes. Although the college's advice was aimed at physicians, it makes sense for pregnant patients, too.

- Consult other doctors, including pediatricians, about the recommended treatment or procedure.

- Seek to clarify your position by talking with other medical professionals — perhaps a nurse or the hospital's patient rights representative — whose opinion you respect.
- Discuss it with the hospital's ethics committee.

If none of these succeed in resolving a conflict and the hospital is threatening to go to court, contact your local office of the American Civil Liberties Union. You can get the address and phone number from its New York headquarters, (212) 944-9800.

Fetal Research

When a procedure is intended to benefit a fetus, few legal issues arise. "An experimental procedure to treat a fetus is considered therapy and the research aspect is secondary," says law professor Bernard Dickens, past president of the American Society of Law and Medicine. But not all research benefits the fetus. The goal may be to benefit others. For example, patients with Parkinson's disease can be helped by fetal tissue transplants. Fetal studies led to the development of polio and rubella vaccines, which benefit humanity.

Since this research often involves examining or taking tissue from fetuses that have been aborted, it becomes entangled with the politics of abortion and is highly controversial. The U.S. government will not fund research that uses fetal tissue, and about half the states have laws regulating fetal research, usually as part of an abortion statute. If you are approached about participating in a nontherapeutic fetal research experiment, make sure that you are aware of the risks, benefits, and purpose of the research and that you believe its importance justifies the experimentation.

Fetal Protection Policies

A company can't force a woman to choose between her job and her unborn child — it's against the law. Even if a job exposes an employee to toxic chemicals that may cause miscarriages or birth defects, companies can't ban pregnant women or women of childbearing age from doing that work.

For years, a policy of the Johnson Control Company, a manufacturer of batteries, prohibited nonsterilized women of childbearing age from working at jobs that exposed them to lead. A lawsuit challenging the policy was brought on the grounds that it violated the federal Civil Rights Act by discriminating against women. "Women who worked at the Johnson Control Company's battery plant argued in court that the company had no right to ban them from the better-paying positions because of their sex and that the company was required to clean up the workplace rather than exclude women from it," says attorney Joan Bertin, associate director of the American Civil Liberties Union Women's Rights Project. The case went all the way to the Supreme Court. In 1991, the Court struck down the company's policy. "Decisions about the welfare of future children must be left to the parents who conceive, bear, support, and raise them rather than to the employers who hire parents," wrote Justice Harry A. Blackmun.

Treating Handicapped Newborns: Who Decides?

Renée Holt, a former pediatric nurse who is now a lawyer and public health specialist living in Seattle, Washington, tells the following story about one of the infants under her care when she worked in the neonatal intensive care unit of a major Philadelphia hospital:

"The unit had been busy the entire month. One baby received the special attention of the medical and nursing staff. It was a little boy who had been born with severe head trauma. He was profoundly retarded. Although he was alive, he could not do any of the things that normal babies do. He could not suck; he could not hold his head up. He just lay there, doing nothing, with tubes sticking out of his little body. The specialists doubted that his condition would ever improve.

"The little boy had been in the nursery for several months. Everything possible was being done to keep him alive. He was fed through tubes, and no therapy that might possibly help him was spared. His parents were loving and devoted and wanted their baby to survive.

"Then one day, the baby 'died.' He choked while feeding and

stopped breathing. We rushed him to the treatment room. The doctors and nurses worked feverishly to bring the little boy back to life. We put tubes in his body to administer lifesaving drugs; we suctioned the food out of his air passage so he could breathe; we injected medication directly down his trachea to stimulate his breathing; we did cardiopulmonary respiration (CPR), which is particularly violent on somebody so little.

"We succeeded. We brought him back. Flush with our victory over death, the team felt a tremendous elation. It is hard to describe how high we felt.

"Later I had second thoughts. Although I didn't discuss it with them, I know that my colleagues were also troubled. 'Had we been right to save the baby? What kind of a life could this profoundly retarded infant, who would probably never be able to hold his head up by himself, look forward to? Did his parents truly understand the enormous responsibility, emotional strain, and perhaps financial burden that caring for their child would involve?'

"A few weeks later, the baby stopped breathing again. This time, despite the same heroic efforts, we were unable to save him."

Six percent of all infants born are rushed to neonatal intensive care units. If a hospital doesn't have such a unit, babies are transferred to one that does. These babies may be premature, have labor-related problems, or suffer from conditions such as heart disease, brain damage, or congenital deformities. In an earlier age, many of them would have died. But advances in neonatal technology, such as the use of respirators and electronic monitors, the analysis of blood samples, and the development of highly skilled teams of pediatric specialists, have contributed to the survival of small, very sick infants.

With all this technology available, deciding whether infants born with severe birth disabilities should live or die raises profound issues of law, medicine, and ethics. If and when to "let go" becomes an agonizing decision. Who should make it? On what grounds? "Sometimes I just want to hold the babies in my arms, care for them, love them. Instead, I am sticking them with needles, forcing food down them, making them suffer. It makes me want to cry. This isn't why I became a nurse," said Susan Cieutat, a neonatal intensive care nurse and former student of mine.

Baby Doe brought the issue of who makes the decision into the glare of national publicity. In 1974, a baby born with Down's syndrome in Bloomington, Indiana, needed an operation to clear her obstructed esophagus. Without surgery, she could not feed. Her parents refused to consent to the operation. When the hospital sought a court order to force the surgery, the judge upheld the right of the parents to withhold their consent. Six days later, Baby Doe died. But her death was only a beginning. Right-to-lifers pushed furiously in the courts and in the press for redress. As a result, the Department of Health and Human Services issued regulations making it a violation of federal law to withhold treatment from a handicapped newborn and setting up a toll-free hotline to receive reports of handicapped newborns being denied food or customary medical care. The regulations were struck down by the U.S. Supreme Court.

In 1984, the U.S. Congress passed amendments to the federal child abuse and neglect law, setting forth standards for treating impaired newborns. Under these amendments, withholding life-saving treatment from an impaired newborn is a form of child neglect, which must be reported to and dealt with by the state's child protection agency. Lifesaving treatment must be furnished to handicapped newborns, except in three instances: (1) when the child is in an irreversible coma; (2) when the treatment would merely prolong dying or would be futile; or (3) when the treatment would be "virtually futile" and inhumane. Food, water, and medicine must be given to all newborns, even if they fall into one of the three categories. This is the law in all states but California, Indiana, and Pennsylvania, which have their own standards for treating handicapped newborns.

As a result, parents have less leeway than they once had to make life-or-death treatment decisions for their newborns. "Where once the hospital or physician could look the other way if a parent refused consent to necessary care, the law now imposes a duty to act," writes law professor Arthur Southwick in *The Law of Hospital and Health Care Administration*.

In practical terms, once a baby is born with a serious handicap or low birthweight, it is immediately whisked away to a high-tech neonatal intensive care unit. The physician comes out and talks to the parents when the baby's condition is sufficiently stabilized, and may let them see their baby in the intensive care unit. "Be prepared for Star Wars," cautions Renée Holt. "Lights flash, machines whirl, monitors beep, and people scurry."

"Can families in the shock resulting from the birth of a defective child understand what faces them?" asked Dr. Raymond Duff and Dr. A. G. M. Campbell in the *New England Journal of Medicine*. "Can they truly give informed consent for treatment or withholding treatment? Some of our colleagues answer no to both questions. In our opinion, if families are heard sympathetically and are given information and answers in words they understand, the problems as well as the expected benefits and limits of any proposed care can be understood clearly in practically all instances."

As a parent, it's your job to know what's going on and to make decisions. Ask the doctors and nurses what's wrong with the baby, what will happen next and why, what the baby's chances of survival are, what life is likely to be like if the baby survives, and the options for treatment or nontreatment. Prepare a list of questions. Discuss the situation and options with close friends, relatives, and trusted advisers. Remember, it's your baby.

Don't let yourself be intimidated by jargon or rushed by busy medical personnel. If you and the doctors don't agree, or if they aren't communicating with you, ask to meet with the hospital's infant care review committee or ethics committee. Almost all hospitals have one.

Consent and Confidentiality: When Do Parents Have a Right to Know?

The general rule that parents must give their consent before a child can get any medical treatment holds true in almost all cases involving young children. Older children, however, can consent to their own medical care in many cases, even without the knowledge of their parents.

Young Children

A physician isn't going to ask a four-year-old girl whether she wants an appendectomy. Obviously, this is a matter that parents decide on the basis of medical advice. A physician who treated a young child without first obtaining a parent's consent might be liable for assault and battery or malpractice. The only exception to the rule requiring parental consent for medical treatment of young children is in the event of an emergency.

Older Children

As children reach adolescence, many are allowed to consent to at least some of their own medical care. The law recognizes them as adults at age eighteen in all but four states: Alabama, Nebraska, and Wyoming, where the age is nineteen, and Mississippi, where it is twenty-one. Before reaching this magical age, they are referred to as minors.

Emancipated minors are adolescents who are independent of their parents. They include teenagers who are married, who serve in the military, or who have children of their own. Depending on state law, they may also include college students. Emancipated minors can consent to their own medical treatment without parental permission.

Mature minors are teenagers who are old enough, usually fifteen and over, and mature enough to understand the nature of a proposed treatment and its risks and consequences. If the treatment will be beneficial and does not involve serious risks, the mature young patient can consent to it without parental involvement. An element of judgment is obviously involved. The same teenager who could consent to treatment for a cut finger could not consent, without parental knowledge, to a course of chemotherapy.

Sensitive situations. Certain types of medical care are so sensitive that teenagers might not want their parents to know. State law sometimes takes this into consideration. Almost every state has a law that permits adolescents to be treated for drug and alcohol abuse and sexually transmitted diseases without their parents' knowledge. Contraception and abortion — two other sensitive issues often the subject of state laws — are discussed in Chapter 7.

Minor treatment statutes. Twenty-one states have laws that allow minors over a certain age to consent to medical treatment. For example, Oregon law permits adolescents fifteen years and older to obtain medical care on their own. In most states, medical services are confidential, although in some parents must be told that their children were treated.

Must Uninformed Parents Pay?
If nonemergency medical care is given to a minor without parental knowledge, the parents are not responsible for the bill. Adolescents who receive treatment are liable for their own bills if they have money.

When Can Parents Refuse to Authorize Treatment?
It all began on April 3, 1986, according to news reports. That was when two-year-old Robyn Twitchell of Boston, Massachusetts, began screaming with pain and vomiting up the light dinner he had eaten earlier. As devout Christian Scientists, his parents tried desperately to cure Robyn with prayer. Five days later, he died of a bowel obstruction doctors say could have been corrected. Although Massachusetts law — one of forty such state laws — exempts Christian Scientists who rely on prayer from being charged with child abuse or neglect, a jury convicted the Twitchells of a different offense, manslaughter, in 1990. Sentenced to probation and community service, they had to pledge to provide medical care for their remaining children.

Parents sometimes attempt to withhold consent to treat a sick child on religious grounds, such as Christian Scientists or, more commonly, Jehovah's Witnesses, who refuse blood transfusions. In other instances, they may disagree with a doctor about the kind of treatment; for example, some parents of children with cancer once sought laetrile cures, a controversial method generally unaccepted by the medical community, rather than the more conventional chemotherapy. Or they may wish to let their child die and spare him or her a life of pain and suffering.

When parents want to withhold treatment that doctors consider necessary, or when parents and doctors disagree, the courts may be asked to step in. Every state defines withholding necessary medical care from a child as a form of abuse or neglect. In order to authorize treatment, hospitals may ask a court to declare a child a temporary ward of the state. They routinely seek court orders authorizing blood transfusions when parents refuse consent for religious reasons. Almost as routinely, judges authorize this lifesaving treatment over the parents' objections.

Sometimes, as with the Twitchells, parents of sick children who die when their parents refuse medical treatment are charged with manslaughter, endangerment, or child abuse. As Supreme Court Justice Oliver Wendell Holmes said in 1923, "Parents are free to make martyrs of themselves, but it does not follow [that] they are free to make martyrs of their children."

Whether treatment is ordered depends on the facts, the nature and severity of the illness, the type of treatment, the likelihood of its success, and the age of the child. Consider two classic New York cases involving non-life-threatening situations that are still used as examples in law schools. In the first, the father of fourteen-year-old Martin Seiferth would not consent to an operation to repair a cleft lip and palate. Despite pleas of doctors and social workers, the court refused to overrule the father's decision. In the second, the mother of fifteen-year-old Kevin Sampson refused to authorize surgery to remove a massive tumor on the right side of the boy's face. Even though the six-hour operation posed a substantial risk, the court overruled the mother's refusal in order to give him a "chance for a normal, happy existence, without a disfigurement so gross as to overshadow all else in his life."

Adolescents who are emancipated or mature enough to consent to treatment presumably can also refuse to authorize treatment. It happens rarely. An Illinois court permitted a mature seventeen-year-old Jehovah's Witness to refuse treatment for leukemia, even though her refusal was virtually certain to lead to her death.

Immunization

When Cambridge, Massachusetts, passed an ordinance in 1904 requiring all residents to be vaccinated against smallpox, Henning Jacobson refused to get a shot. The federal case he made of it reached all the way to the U.S. Supreme Court. He lost. The court, ruling in favor of the Cambridge city government, found the state's interest in protecting the public's health was strong enough to overcome the objection of an individual. This decision established the principle, still valid today, that buttresses compulsory vaccination programs.

Every state requires children to be vaccinated before they attend school. They generally must be immunized against seven childhood diseases: diphtheria, pertussis (whooping cough), tetanus, polio, measles, mumps, and rubella. Unless they are vaccinated, children cannot go to school. Despite these laws, more than one in five American two-year-olds go unprotected against polio, measles, rubella, or mumps. Children whose health would be harmed by immunization can be excused from the vaccination requirement, but they must have a letter from a physician. This is most common when a child develops a severe reaction to the pertussis vaccine.

Religion is another justification for not vaccinating school-age children. In all states except Mississippi and West Virginia, parents can claim a religious exemption by proving they are active members of a religion that opposes immunization. But in a public health emergency, the rules change. In 1991, the children of Philadelphia's Faith Tabernacle Congregation came down with measles. To curtail the epidemic, a family court judge authorized the city to immunize six children thought to be at risk, whose parents were members of the faith-healing congregation. Parents in twenty-two states can also refuse consent for their children to be vaccinated for personal or philosophical reasons. The specific grounds vary from state to state. If you have a question, consult your health department.

Under the National Childhood Vaccine Act, parents of a child injured by a vaccine can claim damages under a no-fault system. Parents do not have to prove that the manufacturer was negligent or did anything wrong. Instead, they must demonstrate to a special master (a judge in the U.S. Claims Court) that the child was vaccinated for one of the seven childhood illnesses and suffered a vaccine-related injury or death.

The act provides compensation for future medical, rehabilitation, and custodial costs. It places limits on the amount that can be awarded: $250,000 if the child died and a total of $30,000 for pain and suffering, loss of earnings, and lawyers' fees. Parents who are dissatisfied with the award can reject it and bring a lawsuit directly against the manufacturer. However, Congress stacked the deck against the parents. If the vaccine met the standards of the federal Food and Drug Administration, was properly packaged and accompanied by proper warnings, the manufacturer is almost certain to win.

The no-fault system sounds simple. In practice, it has not worked smoothly. Although the law was supposed to eliminate disputes, most claims have been contested, according to Wendy Mariner, a professor at Boston University's Health Law Program. She also notes that the large number of claims threatens to overwhelm the system and that there may not be enough money from Congress to pay all the claimants fairly.

Research on Children

Suppose your six-year-old daughter's pediatrician tells you he has been awarded a grant for research that involves electrolyte balances, metabolic processes, and other elements you don't understand. He would like your daughter to participate. It involves her giving a urine sample once a week for six weeks and a blood sample at the beginning and the end. Should you agree? On what grounds should you make a decision?

The following questions, based on U.S. government guidelines for federally funded research and the recommendations of a blue-ribbon government panel, should provide guidance.

CHECKLIST: ALLOWING YOUR CHILD TO PARTICIPATE IN RESEARCH

- **Will the research benefit my child?**
- **If not, who will benefit by it?**
- **What will happen to my child?** Learn exactly what your child's participation will involve, how long it will last, and what procedures are experimental.
- **What are the risks?** If they are more than minimal, make sure that the expected benefits outweigh them and are at least as favorable as benefits promised by alternative approaches.

    If the research is likely to benefit humanity or someone other than your child, be very cautious. Make sure that any additional risk posed by the research is small, that the research won't expose your child to potentially traumatic conditions, and that the anticipated results are of vital importance.

- **If an experimental course of treatment or diagnosis is involved, what alternatives are available and what are the risks of each?**
- **Has the research been approved by an institutional review board (IRB)?** Most hospitals and universities have set up IRBs whose function is to approve research projects and protect participants in the studies. If IRB approval for research has not been obtained, say no.
- **Whom do I contact if something goes wrong? Is medical treatment provided? Is it free?**
- **How will confidentiality be maintained?**
- **What happens if I change my mind? How do I withdraw my child from the study?**
- **Will I learn about the results?** You do not have a legal right to be informed of the project's results. Find out beforehand if you will have access to your child's, or the project's, findings.

Finally, remember that participation is not mandatory. By law, neither you nor your child can be deprived of any benefits or be penalized in any way for refusing to participate in a research study or for withdrawing once it has started. If you decide to authorize your child's participation, explain to him or her what will happen and the nature of the investigation. Be sure that you understand the consent form, which is the key to protecting your child. From my work as a member of IRBs, I know that many consent forms are written in unintelligible gibberish. Don't agree to let your child participate until all your questions have been answered.

11

MEDICARE AND MEDICARE SUPPLEMENT INSURANCE

CONTENTS

OUR NEIGHBOR Daniel F., a New York accountant, has entertained us for years with the exploits of his feisty almost-eighty-year-old parents. When he recently returned from celebrating their fiftieth anniversary with them in California, we expected to hear more tales about the lifestyles of the aging and the infamous. But there were no stories about his father's sailing lessons or his mother's flirting with her Spanish teacher. Instead, Dan told us that his father didn't even drive a car much anymore and his mother had dropped her Spanish class. They were starting to get sick and Dan was scared. His mother was scheduled to enter a hospital for exploratory leg surgery in a few weeks and asked Dan, their son the accountant, to go over their health insurance policies.

Dan found that his parents — who thought twice before going to the movies — had three insurance policies in addition to Medicare. His parents told him that the three policies picked up what Medicare didn't cover. But why three? Dan first tried calling Medicare's 800 number to find out what they did cover. And tried and tried. When he finally got through, a jargon-spouting bureaucrat talked to Dan and left him even more confused than he already was. Then he tried to decipher the three additional policies, which seemed to cover the same items.

Finally, Dan told us, his parents had talked seriously about selling the beautiful Victorian home they cherished. All their children lived far away, and they were afraid they would not be able to cope. They had looked into nursing homes, but the better ones had long waiting lists and were incredibly expensive. If it came to that, how could they afford it, even on a pretty decent pension? Would they have to go broke? At his parents' urging, Dan called a couple of agents to talk about long-term-care insurance. The policies that he deemed worth looking into cost a fortune, and the less expensive ones didn't seem worth the cost of the premiums. Could we help in all of this?

Unfortunately, Dan's story is all too typical. Parents age, children fly far from the nest, and capable, intelligent people are forced to cope with bewildering laws, unresponsive officials and slick insurance agents. In this chapter, we cut through the jargon and sales pitches. In the sections that follow, we provide clear, under-standable guidance for the elderly and their children. The law guarantees older people many benefits and protects them against practices that play on their vulnerability. The trick is to under-stand how the laws work. By knowing your rights, and those of your parents, you can protect them, and yourself, in old age.

Medicare: How to Get What You're Entitled To

Medicare is the U.S. government program that pays much of the hospital and doctors' costs for people aged sixty-five and older. It also covers medical costs of certain disabled people and those needing kidney dialysis or transplantation.

When President Lyndon B. Johnson signed Medicare into law in 1965, he said, "No longer will older Americans be denied the healing miracle of modern medicine. No longer will illness crush and destroy the savings that they have so carefully put away over a lifetime." Today that fine sentiment falls short of reality. Although Medicare gives a great deal of protection to 33 million older Amer-icans, it pays *less than half* of the average older person's health costs, because of what is *not* covered. The most important omis-sion is payment for standard nursing home care, which amounts to more than $60 billion a year nationwide.

Medicare is one of the most complicated laws ever written. It changes almost every year and is subject to the potshots of budget-busting congressmen and government bureaucrats. To find out the latest changes on coverage and cost, consult the *Medicare Hand-book* published each year by the U.S. Department of Health and Human Services; contact the American Association of Retired Persons, (202) 434-2277 or one of the Medicare advocacy groups listed later in this chapter, or call the Social Security Administra-tion, the government agency responsible for providing information about the program, (800) 772-1213.

How to Enroll

You are eligible for Medicare once you have reached the age of sixty-five and are entitled to Social Security or railroad retirement benefits. Even if you postpone collecting on your Social Security, you are still eligible for Medicare; you don't have to be retired. If you take early retirement, you can sign up when you reach sixty-two, but benefits won't start until you turn sixty-five. And you don't have to be poor. Rich and poor alike are entitled to Medicare.

To get a Medicare card, which you need in order to receive benefits, call or visit the nearest office of the Social Security Administration. The best time to sign up is three months before your sixty-fifth birthday. The enrollment period begins three months before that birthday and ends four months after it, although you can sign up later. If you are applying for retirement benefits, you do not have to fill out a separate application for Medicare; you will be enrolled automatically.

Medicare is divided into two parts. Part A pays a portion of the cost of hospital, skilled nursing, home health, and hospice care. Part B covers a portion of doctors' bills, outpatient services, and medical equipment and supplies.

If you are eligible for Medicare, Part A (Hospital Insurance) won't cost you a penny; you and your employer have already paid for it through a payroll tax. Part B (Medical Insurance) is optional. You pay a monthly charge, called a premium, which is deducted from your Social Security check. The 1992 premium is $31.80 per month. Part B is a good deal: for less than $400 a year, you cover most of your doctors' bills. Only a fool or someone with excellent insurance elsewhere would not opt for it.

People who have not worked long enough to qualify for Medicare can buy it on their own by signing up during specified enrollment periods — the three months before and four months after their sixty-fifth birthday and the first three months of every year thereafter.

Hospital Coverage

Part A covers most basic hospital costs, including a semiprivate room, meals, regular nursing services, blood beyond the first three pints, drugs, lab tests and radiology work included in the hospital bill, and operating room charges. You should receive bills only for such extras as television, telephone, private nursing care — and a private room, unless you can prove that it is medically necessary.

Benefit Periods, Deductibles, and Coinsurance

Medicare does not pay for indefinite hospital stays. It places a cap on the length of time it covers and requires you to pay for part of your hospital care through a system of a deductible and coinsurance payments. In our discussion of Medicare below, we list the deductible and coinsurance amounts for 1992. They will probably be higher in subsequent years.

Medicare covers up to 90 days of hospitalization for each *benefit period* or *spell of illness*. A benefit period or spell of illness begins when you are admitted to a hospital and ends when you have been out of the hospital, or a follow-up skilled nursing facility, for 60 consecutive days. You must pay the first $652 of your hospital expenses, which is your *deductible*. After you satisfy the deductible, Medicare pays almost all hospital expenses for the first 60 days.

Medicare covers the costs of an additional 30 days in the hospital during the same benefit period. However, for days 61 through 90, you must share the cost by paying $163 a day. This is the *coinsurance*.

Once you have been out of the hospital for 60 consecutive days, the old benefit period lapses and a new one begins. If you are hospitalized again, you are eligible for another 90 days of coverage once you have paid the deductible and coinsurance. There is no limit to the number of benefit periods you can have.

In addition, every person covered by Medicare has the right to an additional "lifetime reserve" of 60 days of hospital coverage. It will cost you $326 a day, and Medicare takes care of the rest. These 60 days are not replaceable. Once used, they are gone forever.

How does this work in practice? A few examples may make it easier to understand.

Let's say that on March 1 you are hospitalized for five days for removal of a benign tumor. You paid the deductible and Medicare paid the balance. On April 15, you slip on some ice, break your leg, and are readmitted to the hospital. Although you are hospitalized for a different condition, Medicare considers your broken leg to be treatment day 6 of this benefit period. Since 60 days had not elapsed, you do not have to pay another deductible.

In another scenario, let's say you entered the hospital for surgery in January. Five months later, you reentered the hospital to treat a recurrence of the problem. Since more than 60 days had elapsed, a new benefit period started, and you have to pay the deductible.

Or your aunt is afflicted with heart disease, circulatory problems, and a host of other illnesses that frequently land her in the hospital. During one particularly severe episode, she is hospitalized for 80 days. She returns to her nursing home, but two weeks later — still in the same benefit period — she is rushed to the hospital, where she stays for 75 days. Then she dies.

Her Medicare benefits ran out on the seventieth day of her second hospitalization. The calculation went like this. She was hospitalized for a total of 155 days (80 the first time, 75 the second) during the benefit period. She used up the 90 days to which she was entitled during the benefit period plus the 60 lifetime reserve on the 150th day. At her death, she owed the hospital five days that Medicare didn't cover. Table 2 illustrates what Medicare covers under Part A and what you can expect to pay for an extended hospital stay during a single benefit period.

DRGs: How to Avoid Being Sent Home When You're Still Sick

Who's Afraid of the DRG?
Say your eighty-year-old father is scheduled to be discharged from the hospital after being treated for pneumonia. When you go to pick him up, he looks as pale as the sheet and is shaky on his feet. You don't think he's in any condition to go home. Neither does he. You complain to his nurse, who directs you to his physician. After getting angrier by the hour, you finally talk to the doctor, who tells you that while your dad is no candidate for a marathon, he is not sick enough to stay in the hospital. "Anyway," says the doctor, "his DRG is up."

Variations on this scene are repeated, usually with more subtlety, in hospitals around the country every day. As hospitals, pushed by Medicare, try to hold down costs, they are releasing patients "sicker and quicker." If it happens to you, your spouse, or your parent, you can fight back. At the very least, you can buy a couple of days' time.

First, though, a little history about what's happened to Medicare over the past few years. When it began in 1965, hospitals were paid

Medicare Part A: Hospital Insurance — Covered Services per Benefit Period

Services	Benefit	Medicare Pays*	You Pay
Hospitalization Semiprivate room and board, general nursing, and miscellaneous hospital services and supplies	First 60 days	All but $652	$652
	61st to 90th day	All but $163 a day	$163 a day
	91st to 150th day†	All but $326 a day	$326 a day
	Beyond 150 days	Nothing	All costs
Posthospital skilled nursing facility care You must have been in a hospital for at least 3 days and enter a Medicare-approved facility, generally within 30 days after hospital discharge.	First 20 days	100% of approved amount	Nothing
	Additional 80 days	All but $81.50 a day	$81.50 a day
	Beyond 100 days	Nothing	All costs
Home health care	Medically necessary skilled care, home health aide services, medical supplies, etc.	Full cost of services; 80% of approved amount for durable medical equipment	Nothing for services; 20% of approved amount for durable medical equipment
Hospice care Available to terminally ill	As long as doctor certifies need	All but limited costs for outpatient drugs and inpatient respite care	Limited cost sharing for outpatient drugs and inpatient respite care
Blood	Blood	All but first 3 pints per calendar year	For first 3 pints‡

*The amounts are for 1992 and are subject to change each year.
†Sixty reserve days may be used only once; they are not renewable.
‡To the extent the blood deductible is met under one part of Medicare during the calendar year, it does not have to be met under the other part.

Source: National Association of Insurance Commissioners and Health Care Financing Administration.

on the basis of how much the services cost them. Somewhere along the line, health policy specialists realized that this system provided no incentive for hospitals to contain their costs. On the contrary, the more expensive, the better — and the more profitable.

So Congress set about scrapping the old system and devising a new one that would encourage, even force, hospitals to reduce their costs. It came up with a system based on "diagnostic related groups," or DRGs, and made it the law in 1982. The key features are:

- Hospitals are paid on the basis of a DRG: the illness or injury for which you are admitted. There are nearly five hundred categories. Your DRG is assigned when you become an inpatient.
- Each DRG specifies the number of days the average patient should be expected to stay, and the hospital is paid on the basis of this number.
- If the patient stays longer than the number of days allotted for the DRG, the hospital must absorb the additional costs from its own budget. If the patient is released early, the hospital is allowed to keep the money saved.

DRG 89 covers pneumonia, which is assigned a length of stay of eight days. That's what the hospital gets paid for. If your father remained in the hospital longer than that, the hospital would lose money. That is what the doctor meant when he said, "His DRG is up," and why they wanted Dad out of the hospital.

How to Fight Premature Discharge

Even though DRGs nudge hospitals to push patients out before they have fully recuperated, the Medicare law offers some protection. On admission, you should receive a sheet titled "An Important Message from Medicare." If you don't get it, ask. Pay particular attention to the part that says, "According to Federal law, your discharge date must be determined solely by your medical needs, and not by 'DRGs' or Medicare payments." If you are told to leave the hospital before you are ready, use the law and protest. It's a great help to take along a strong, forceful friend or relative to be your advocate. Here's what you can do:

Talk to your physician. Argue with the doctor, politely but firmly. Try to win him or her over as your advocate. Make it very clear that you are not well enough to go home. Show him or her the "Important Message from Medicare."

Ask to see the hospital's patients' representative. Many hospitals, especially those in urban areas, employ trained personnel called patients' representatives or patients' advocates to deal with patients' problems and complaints. Call hospital information, or ask your doctor or nurse to put you in touch with one.

"Patients' representatives can prompt physicians to reexamine a medical evaluation," says Navah Harlow, director of patients' representatives at New York's Beth Israel Hospital. "The DRG is not the all-decisive factor. Obviously, if there's a change in medical status, the situation will change."

Protest to the peer review organization (PRO). *This protest buys you a minimum of an additional two days in the hospital.* PROs are organizations of doctors set up by federal law to monitor cost containment efforts and quality of care under Medicare. (They are *not* located in the hospital.) Part of their job is to review complaints of patients who believe they are being sent home prematurely. Medicare has set up a formal procedure to complain to the PRO. Take advantage of it.

- Ask a hospital representative for a written Notice of Noncoverage. The notice says that Medicare is about to stop paying for your care and that you will be liable for the bill once Medicare stops paying. This is not an eviction notice; rather, it puts you on notice that you will be billed directly if you insist on staying.
- Appeal the Notice of Noncoverage. The notice will tell you how. Merely by lodging your protest, you will have gained two free days in the hospital to recuperate.
- Time your appeal on the basis of whether your doctor agrees or disagrees with the hospital's decision to release you. If your doctor and the hospital agree that you should be discharged, appeal by *noon of the next working day* (Monday through

Friday, excluding holidays) after you receive the Notice of Noncoverage. The PRO has one working day to rule on your appeal. You can't be charged until the following day. If your doctor and the hospital disagree, make an immediate appeal. The hospital cannot bill you until the third day after you receive the Notice of Noncoverage. Our advice is to leave after the second day, even if the PRO hasn't decided your case, to avoid being stuck with a bill for the third day.

Leaving the Hospital

What should you do if you are discharged from a hospital and you need further care? For example, home health, skilled nursing, or hospice care. Most hospitals have a discharge planner, often a social worker, who can help you arrange further treatment outside the hospital. "A lot of people don't know who to call," says Deborah Brialand Betts, national director of the Coalition for Long-Term Care, a Washington, D.C., advocacy group. "They equate social services with welfare. Yet we're talking about situations that six out of ten families encounter."

Coverage of Skilled Nursing Care

If you, like millions of other older people, need nursing home care only to help you walk, eat, or bathe, don't look to Medicare to pay for it. Medicare considers these custodial services and won't pay for them. (Medicaid, another government program, will if you are poor enough — see Chapter 12.)

Medicare pays for care only in Medicare-certified skilled nursing facilities. These tend to be high-tech sites where a specially trained staff works under doctors' orders. More and more, skilled nursing care seems to be available only to people who are hooked up to sophisticated equipment. Most nursing homes are not *"skilled nursing"* facilities.

To qualify for Medicare coverage of skilled nursing care, you must meet these criteria:

- You were in a hospital for at least three consecutive days and were transferred to a Medicare-certified skilled nursing facility within thirty days of discharge.
- You need skilled nursing or skilled rehabilitation services

daily. Your doctor must certify that you need, and are receiving, these services every day.

- The need must continue. Once you no longer need daily skilled nursing or rehabilitative care, Medicare stops paying the bill. Committees from the facility and the insurance company that bills Medicare monitor your need for skilled services.

If you qualify, Medicare covers up to 100 days of skilled nursing care in each benefit period, paying all costs for the first 20 days. You must pay $81.50 a day for days 21 through 100.

The nursing facility bills Medicare directly. If the facility believes a service is not covered, it must let you know in writing. About one out of five times, the nursing facility is wrong and Medicare will pay for the service. Diane Archer, executive director of the Medicare Beneficiaries Defense Fund in New York, says that you should have the nursing facility bill Medicare if there is any doubt about whether it is covered. You are not obligated to pay until Medicare denies payment.

Coverage of Home Health Care

Medicare pays the cost of skilled nursing care, rehabilitation therapy, and other health care delivered in your home under certain conditions. To qualify for Medicare payment of home health care, you must meet these criteria:

- You must be confined to your home. This means that you can leave home only infrequently or with the assistance of another person or a mechanical aid such as a wheelchair.
- You must be under the care of a doctor who sets up a treatment plan for you.
- Your care must be provided by a Medicare-certified home health care agency.
- You must need skilled nursing or skilled physical or speech therapy on a part-time or intermittent basis. How "part-time" or "intermittent" is defined in the context of Medicare is hard to understand and even harder to explain. The federal government's guidelines are all but incomprehensible, even to someone trained in the law. "As a rule of thumb, you must need

skilled services less than five days a week and as seldom as once in sixty days," says Diane Archer. In general, when the prognosis is uncertain and it is not clear how long the home care will last, Medicare pays for up to thirty-five hours a week of care that is provided either a few hours a day or a few days a week. Care can continue indefinitely as long as it is medically necessary. When the prognosis is clearer and the home care will end within a short period, Medicare can cover up to eight hours a day of home health care, including skilled services, seven days a week for up to twenty-one days, with the possibility of an extension.

Unlike eligibility for skilled nursing facility care, there is no requirement that you be hospitalized first in order to be eligible for Medicare's home health care benefits.

If you qualify, Medicare pays not only for skilled nursing care and rehabilitation therapy but also, if the doctor orders it, for unskilled home health aides to help with bathing, dressing, and the like. Medicare does not pay for round-the-clock nursing care or for such home care services as cleaning, cooking, and shopping.

The home health agency bills Medicare directly. You should not have to pay anything, with the possible exception of 20 percent of the cost of durable medical equipment such as a ventilator or an oxygen tent.

Home health agencies, believing they will not be reimbursed by Medicare, sometimes limit their care only to short periods or refuse to provide services unless the person is acutely ill. "Often they are wrong," says Ms. Archer. "Once you have met the government's criteria, you are eligible for Medicare." If it happens to you, she suggests you sign a form agreeing to pay the home health agency privately if Medicare turns down the claim, insist that the agency bill Medicare, and have your doctor prepare a letter describing the need for services. Even if the claim is denied initially, there is a 60 percent reversal rate on appeal.

Coverage of Hospice Care
Hospice care aims to relieve pain and provide comfort for the terminally ill. It is generally provided in a patient's home or the

home of a family member, although there are also inpatient hospices.

To be eligible you must meet the following conditions:

- A doctor certifies that the patient is terminally ill.
- The patient chooses to receive hospice benefits instead of the standard Part A and Part B benefits.
- Care is provided by a Medicare-certified agency.

If these conditions are satisfied, Medicare pays just about all the costs of hospice care, except for a small amount toward the cost of drugs and inpatient care. There is no limit to the length of hospice coverage.

Health Maintenance Organizations

Medicare gives seniors the option of joining a health maintenance organization (HMO) or a similar group, called a competitive medical plan, that has contracted with the government to serve Medicare beneficiaries. If you elect to join an HMO instead of the traditional fee-for-service Medicare system, you will receive all your health care through it without having to worry about deductibles, coinsurance payments, and benefit periods. Your Part B premium will go to the HMO, which is also allowed to charge you a monthly fee in lieu of deductibles and coinsurance. We discuss the pros and cons of HMOs in Chapter 3.

Paying the Bills: Part B of Medicare

What Is — and Is Not — Covered

Part B of Medicare covers part of your doctors' bills, lab tests, medical equipment and supplies, and other outpatient care. Insurance companies, such as Blue Cross and Aetna, are designated by Medicare as *carriers* to administer the Medicare program in specific areas. Although the Medicare law requires doctors to submit claims directly, you will be the one to correspond with these insurance carriers if a claim is denied or you receive less money than you are due. You may have to cope with mountains of paperwork and even end up fighting the bureaucracy.

In the past, Medicare paid the reasonable cost of medically necessary services. In 1992 the government began a new system of paying doctors (and other health professionals). It established a fee schedule that specifies the amount Medicare will pay for any diagnostic procedure or treatment. By federal law, a doctor cannot bill you for more than 20 percent above the amount set by the fee schedule; that figure will be lowered to 15 percent in 1993. Some states, like New York, have lower caps or forbid balance billing altogether.

Congress and the U.S. Department of Health and Human Services determine what services are covered and what are not, and the insurance carrier tries to interpret their wishes. The list of what is in and what is out may change somewhat from year to year. Pap smears and mammograms were not covered for a long time but now are. Among the services Medicare *does not* pay for are prescription drugs, routine dental, hearing, vision, and foot care — including dentures, eyeglasses (except for post–cataract surgery), and hearing aids — checkups, and most chiropractic visits and immunizations.

Medicare Part B *does* pay the reasonable cost of other medically necessary services, including:

- Drugs that a doctor or nurse must administer
- Outpatient hospital services, including emergency room
- Laboratory and diagnostic tests
- Prosthetic devices, braces, and artificial limbs
- Durable medical equipment such as wheelchairs or crutches
- Physical, occupational, or speech therapists' services
- Ambulances, under certain conditions
- Kidney dialysis machines, supplies, and services
- Blood for outpatient use, after the first three pints (which are not covered by Medicare)
- Home health care (for beneficiaries who do not have Part A)

If your doctor says that medical services are necessary, have him or her bill Medicare unless it is absolutely clear that such services aren't covered (for example, a hearing aid). If the claim is denied, file an appeal. You have a good chance of winning.

Medicare Part B does not pay the total amount of your doctors' bills. It covers 80 percent of the scheduled amount. You must pay the remaining 20 percent — the *coinsurance* — and your doctors' charges in excess of what Medicare allows. You also pay an annual *deductible*.

The Deductible

The concept of a deductible is a straightforward one. Each year, you must pay the first part of your medical bills, up to a specified amount, which is currently $100. Once you have met the deductible, you have fulfilled your obligation until the following year.

Coinsurance Payments

After satisfying the deductible, you are responsible for paying 20 percent of that part of your doctor's bill which Medicare allows. Let's say that your internist sends you a bill for $1,100. Medicare allows $1,000 for the treatment. Assuming that your deductible was already paid, Medicare would pay $800 (80 percent of $1,000), leaving you responsible for the coinsurance ($200) plus the remaining $100 of that bill.

Assignment

Under Medicare, some doctors accept what is called assignment, which means that the doctor agrees to accept the amount that Medicare allows as the entire amount of the bill. Medicare sends the doctor 80 percent of the approved charge; you must pay the remaining 20 percent.

If a doctor does not accept assignment, you must pay the coinsurance plus the portion of the bill that Medicare won't cover, up to 20 percent of Medicare's allowable charge. In the example we used above of the internist who charged $1,100 for work that Medicare said was worth $1,000, Medicare would pay $800 and you, the patient, would pay the doctor $300 (the $200 coinsurance plus the $100 more than Medicare allowed). If the doctor accepted assignment, the charge would be $1,000; you would have to pay only the $200 coinsurance. Table 3 shows what services Medicare covers under Part B and what must come out of your pocket (unless you have Medicare supplement insurance, which we discuss later in this chapter).

TABLE 3

Medicare Part B: Medical Insurance — Covered Services per Calendar Year

Services	Benefit	Medicare Pays*	You Pay
Medical expense Physicians' services, inpatient and outpatient medical and surgical services and supplies, physical and speech therapy, diagnostic tests, durable medical equipment, etc.	Medicare pays for medical services in or out of the hospital.	80% of approved amount (after $100 deductible)	$100 deductible plus 20% of approved amount (plus excess charges up to 20% of approved amount)
Clinical laboratory services	Blood tests, biopsies, urinalysis, etc.	Full cost of services	Nothing for services
Home health care	Medically necessary skilled care, home health aide services, medical supplies, etc.	Full cost of services; 80% of approved amount for durable medical equipment	Nothing for services; 20% of approved amount for durable medical equipment
Outpatient hospital treatment	Unlimited if medically necessary	80% of approved amount (after $100 deductible)	Subject to deductible plus 20% of approved amount
Blood	Blood	80% of approved amount (after $100 deductible and starting with 4th pint)	For first 3 pints plus 20% of approved amount for additional pints (after $100 deductible)

*The amounts are for 1992 and subject to change each year.

Source: National Association of Insurance Commissioners and Health Care Financing Administration

You can find a doctor who accepts assignment in the U.S. government listing titled *The Medicare Participating Physician/ Supplier Directory.* The insurance carrier handling Medicare claims in your area, the Social Security office, area agencies on aging, and many senior citizen centers have copies.

Many doctors do not like to accept assignment. They feel that Medicare pays them such ridiculously low amounts that it is hardly worthwhile to handle Medicare patients. However, *it is to your great advantage to find a doctor who accepts assignment.* It will definitely save you money and probably cut down on your paperwork. Don't be shy about asking.

Even doctors who do not accept assignment as a matter of course make exceptions in individual cases. A call from your personal physician can often turn the trick. Remember that many doctors, ranging from family physicians to surgeons and anesthesiologists to other medical specialists, may be involved in your care. Try to get all of them to accept assignment.

Fighting Back

> Thomas A. was billed $3,100 for the implantation of a pacemaker, for which he paid out of his own pocket. Medicare initially awarded him $34.30. On review, he received $1,078. At the second level of review, he received another $1,163.

The big secret about Medicare is that over 60 percent of the people who appeal win. If you are reimbursed for less than 80 percent of your doctor's bill or your claim is turned down, appeal. It's your right and you will not be penalized. Just do it within six months. All it costs you is a postage stamp. Here's how it works.

The reason your claim was rejected is noted on the Explanation of Medicare Benefits (EOMB). When you get the EOMB, this is what to do:

- If you've been paid less money than you think you are entitled to, write a short letter to the carrier asking that your claim be reviewed (you don't have to write anything more than "Please review"), attach it to a copy of the EOMB, and send it to the insurance carrier whose address is listed in the upper right-hand corner of the EOMB. The insurance carrier will assign a person different from the one who reviewed it originally.

- If the claim was turned down for a specific reason or the carrier needs more information, ask your doctor to answer the carrier's questions. Attach this information to a letter you write. State why your claim should be covered, supported by the attached documentation from your doctor. Often your claim may be denied for inexplicable reasons. For example, some insurance carriers' computers are programmed to deny claims for more than six doctors' visits for the same condition during the same calendar year. If your claim is denied for a seventh visit, write a note to the carrier explaining that the visit was medically necessary, backed up by a letter from your physician. Make sure you keep a copy of all correspondence with the insurance carrier.

If you still are not satisfied, Medicare provides three additional appeal levels.

- If the amount in dispute is $100 or more, you have a right to request a formal hearing with the insurance carrier. Until then, your claim was reviewed by a claims adjuster. Now you will go before a specially appointed person at the insurance carrier to explain why it should pay your claim or why you should get more money. At this stage, we advise you to consult an attorney or one of the Medicare advocacy groups listed on page 269.
- If you are still not satisfied and the amount in dispute is at least $500, you can progress to the next level — an appeal to an administrative law judge to whom you will present your case. This is a formal proceeding and your attorney may act for you.
- Finally, you can go to a federal district court if you are arguing about more than $1,000. Make sure that the amount you stand to win is enough to cover your legal fees.

Where to Turn for Help

A number of nonprofit organizations are available to help Medicare beneficiaries. If you are frustrated, bewildered, or angry, call a nearby group for advice.

Medicare Beneficiaries Defense
  Fund
130 West 42nd Street
New York, NY 10036
(212) 869-3850

Medicare Advocacy Project
315 W. Ninth Street
Los Angeles, CA 90015
(213) 614-0991

The Center for Health Care Law
519 C Street, NE
Washington, DC 20002
(202) 547-5262

Senior Citizens Legal Services
343 Church Street
Santa Cruz, CA 95060
(408) 426-8824

Medicare Advocacy Project
606 Minnesota Building
St. Paul, MN 55101
(612) 228-0771

Greater Boston Elderly Legal
  Services
102 Norway Street
Boston, MA 02115
(617) 536-0400

Legal Assistance to Medicare
  Patients
P.O. Box 258
Willimantic, CT 06226
(203) 423-2556

Center for Medicare Advocacy, Inc.
P.O. Box 171
South Windham, CT 06266
(203) 456-7790

Medicare Advocacy Project
P.O. Box 887
Springfield, VT 05156
(802) 885-5753

Advocates for Medicare Patients
  Project of Legal Services for the
  Elderly, Inc.
P.O. Box 2723
Augusta, ME 04338-2723
(207) 289-2287

In addition, legal service groups can often help decipher Medicare. Call the National Senior Citizens Law Project, (202) 887-5280 or (213) 482-3550, for the name of a group in your area.

Medicare Supplement (Medigap) Insurance

Several years ago, when Helen L., a seventy-seven-year-old Tampa, Florida, widow suffering from arthritis, answered the doorbell one afternoon, she was surprised to see a nice-looking, well-dressed young man who asked for her by name. He said he was from Medicare, or something like that (Mrs. L., who gets confused easily, wasn't too sure), and that he had to talk with her about her insurance. Thinking he was from the government, she invited the young man in. He was, in fact, an insurance agent on the trail of an easy sale. For the next three hours, the young man told her why her current Medicare supplement insurance was no good, why it could easily leave her destitute, and why she needed a new policy. What the young man said was very frightening. He left with a check for $1,500 for a Medigap policy that was essentially the same as the one Mrs. L. already owned.

To the agent, Mrs. L. was a "mooch," an easy mark. Other words commonly used by unscrupulous agents include "twisting" or "churning" — talking a client out of an existing policy and selling a substitute — and "stacking" — convincing the client to buy an additional policy. Although these practices are illegal, they are still being used. Many companies are honest, but others employ sleazy agents who are trained to prey on the vulnerabilities of the elderly.

Since there are so many holes in Medicare coverage, two out of three seniors buy some kind of Medicare supplement — Medigap — policy. These policies may pay for the deductible, coinsurance, charges in excess of Medicare's approved amount, and various services and supplies that Medicare does not cover.

In 1990, the U.S. Congress passed a law that addressed many of the tawdry practices that characterized the sale of Medigap policies. Oddly enough, the drive to reform Medigap did not come as a result of an outcry from consumer groups. "Congress passed Medigap reform because it was the right thing to do, not because of intensive lobbying by the elderly," says Gail Shearer, Consumers Union's health policy expert in Washington.

The Options
In the 1990 legislation, Congress ordered the National Association of Insurance Commissioners (NAIC) to come up with just ten

TABLE 4

Medicare Supplement Standards

Ten different policies, labeled A to J, are available under the standards. The core package is included with all options.

	A	B	C	D	E	F	G	H	I	J
Core*	◆	◆	◆	◆	◆	◆	◆	◆	◆	◆
Skilled nursing home	—	—	◆	◆	◆	◆	◆	◆	◆	◆
Hospital deductible	—	◆	◆	◆	◆	◆	◆	◆	◆	◆
Doctor deductible	—	—	◆	—	—	—	—	◆	—	◆
Excess doctor charges	—	—	—	—	—	80%	—	100%	—	100%
Foreign travel	—	◆	◆	◆	◆	◆	◆	◆	◆	◆
At-home recovery	—	—	—	◆	—	◆	—	—	◆	◆
Prescription drugs†	—	—	—	—	Basic	—	—	—	Basic	Ext.
Preventive screen	—	—	—	—	—	—	◆	—	—	◆

*The core package includes payment of the patient's 20% share of coverage for doctors' services; the patient's per day contribution to hospital bills for the 61st through 90th day; the patient's contribution for blood; and coverage for up to a year in the hospital if Medicare benefits are exhausted.
†The basic coverage pays half the cost of prescription drugs up to $1,250 a year after a $250 deductible is met; the extended coverage is the same, except that the upper limit is $3,000.
Source: National Association of Insurance Commissioners.

model policies and ordered the states to pass laws that make these *the only ones* that can be sold. The insurance commissioners complied in 1991, and the states have been adopting the NAIC guidelines as their own law since then. They eliminate the staggering number of options that confused consumers just a few years back. The ten model policies are summarized in Table 4.

Under the NAIC guidelines, which apply to all Medigap plans except employer-sponsored ones and those sold in Massachusetts, Minnesota, and Wisconsin, companies must offer the core plan that covers many of the basic gaps in Medicare. While you are in a hospital, it must cover the daily coinsurance for days 61 through

90, and the lifetime reserve days. Moreover, it must cover an additional 365 days when your Medicare hospital benefits are exhausted. For doctors' bills, the core plan must cover the 20 percent coinsurance; for blood transfusions, it must cover the cost of the first three pints of blood.

Beyond this core package, companies can offer up to nine other plans that pay for a variety of services not covered by Medicare, such as the deductible for hospital care and doctors' services; skilled nursing care coinsurance; prescription drugs; excess doctors' charges (those above what Medicare will pay), and foreign travel.

Rather than relying on federal and state regulations, exercise caution when buying a Medigap policy. "Buyer beware" should be the thought uppermost in your mind. To help you become a knowledgeable buyer and avoid being victimized by unsavory sales tactics, we offer the following tips.

CHECKLIST: BUYING A MEDIGAP POLICY

- **Never buy more than one Medigap policy.** It is against the law for insurance agents to sell you a duplicate Medigap policy. Despite this, some of them try. Under the law an agent must get a written statement of the policies you already own and you must state in writing that you plan to drop your current coverage. An agent found in violation faces a fine of up to $25,000 and five years in jail.

- **Don't change policies unless you really have to.** Most people don't realize that an insurance agent earns a huge commission on the sale of a new policy — up to 50 percent of the first year's premiums — and a much lower commission on continuations. As a result, agents have a great incentive to sell new policies, whether people need one or not. If you decide to switch, the insurance company must waive its normal waiting period for a pre-existing condition.

  You should be able to answer three questions before you switch policies: Why are you switching? How will the new policy improve your coverage? Will you save money, and if so, how much?

- **Request an Outline of Coverage and the NAIC/HCFA Buyer's Guide.** The Outline of Coverage is a summary description of what a policy covers and how much it costs. The National Association of Insurance Commissioners and the Health Care Financing Administration of the U.S. Department of Health and Human Services publish a *Guide to Health Insurance for People with Medicare.* Insurance agents are supposed to leave these with you. Don't buy from anybody who won't.
- **Don't be pressured into buying.** With yearly premiums ranging from $400 to well over $1,000, you need time to think it over. Remember that high-pressure tactics are the refuge of the desperate. Don't be taken in by statements like "I have to have an answer now" or "The offer runs out at midnight. I won't be able to get you these rates ever again." If the agent won't leave, threaten to call the police — and do it. Somebody who won't leave your home when told to is a trespasser, and trespassing is against the law.
- **Fill out the application yourself or have a friend do it.** If you don't, an unscrupulous agent may omit medical information from the application. It's illegal, but watch out for it anyway. In one case, Families U.S.A., a Washington, D.C., advocacy group concerned with long-term care, found that an agent failed to note that an eighty-two-year-old applicant was confined to a wheelchair. *Be sure to include all the information about your health requested by the company.* If you lie and are found out, the company may refuse to pay your claims. Show the door to any agent who suggests that you conveniently "forget" about any of your health problems. Honesty can save you money and future aggravation.
- **Find out the company's policy on pre-existing conditions.** Federal law prohibits an insurance company from asking about your health — and turning you down because of a pre-existing health condition — if you apply for a Medigap insurance policy within six months of becoming eligible for Medicare. "This means that upon turning sixty-five, people have a one-time shot at the best Medigap policy available at the lowest price," says Consumers Union's Gail Shearer.

Remember, too, that an insurance company cannot turn you down or require a waiting period because of a pre-existing condition if you are switching from another Medigap policy that you have had for six months or longer.

If you miss the six-month deadline and are buying a new policy, ask about the company's coverage of pre-existing conditions.

- **Pay your premiums by check, made out to the insurance company.** Never pay cash. And never make your check payable to the agent. More than one has skipped town with the money.

- **Don't be fooled by companies implying that they are associated with the government or by sales pitches by celebrities.** Neither Medicare nor any branch of the government sells or endorses private insurance policies. It's against the law to make such a claim. As for celebrities, remember that even your favorite movie star is an actor, not an insurance expert who knows your needs.

- **Take advantage of the "free look" provision.** You have thirty days to look over a Medigap policy. If you're not happy with it, the company must refund your premium. We recommend that you have a lawyer or a trustworthy friend who understands insurance jargon check the policy to make sure you are getting what you think you are. If you cancel a policy, send it and your letter to the insurance company — not the agent — by certified mail, return receipt requested.

- **Check the financial health of the insurance company.** With some insurance companies having gone the way of S&Ls, it's vital to check the financial health of a potential insurer. You can do this by telephoning companies whose business it is to rate insurers. The major ones are: A. M. Best, (900) 420-0400 (the charge is $2.50 per minute); Standard and Poor's, (212) 208-1527; Moody's Investors Service, (212) 553-0377, and Duff & Phelps, (312) 368-0377. A newcomer is Weiss Research, (800) 289-9222 (the charge is $15 per report). The same information is also available at some public libraries. Buy only from a company given a top rating by two of these firms.

• **Remember: Medigap policies do not cover nursing home care,** at least not the kind of custodial care most people mean when they think of nursing homes. To get insurance protection for custodial care, you must buy a separate long-term care insurance policy. We discuss this subject in Chapter 12.

Where to Turn for Help

Many states — California, Illinois, Iowa, Maryland, Massachusetts, Minnesota, New Jersey, New Mexico, Ohio, Washington, Wisconsin — have volunteer-run programs to help elderly people understand Medicare, Medigap, and Social Security. They provide considerable help to seniors. Call your state insurance department (listed in Chapter 3) to find out if it provides a counseling program and, if so, whom to call. Other sources of assistance are area and state agencies on aging (see the end of Chapter 12 for addresses and telephone numbers), senior centers, and community services groups.

12

LONG-TERM CARE

CONTENTS

Long-term Care Alternatives

More than 11 million Americans need some form of long-term care as the result of a chronic illness or condition. About 7 million are elderly; the remainder are younger people with mental or physical disabilities. They range from those who need help with simple household tasks to those who are totally dependent on others. The vast majority live in the community: at home, with a son or daughter, or in some form of senior citizen housing.

As people age, their health deteriorates and their need for care increases. Eighty-seven percent of people between sixty-five and sixty-nine are able to get along on their own; less than half of those eighty-five years and up can say the same. The job of caregiver often falls to children, particularly the daughters, of older people.

Like Lucille F., a boutique manager, who has lived with her ninety-three-year-old mother, Rose, in the same Tampa, Florida, house for the past twenty years. About seven years ago, a stroke landed Rose in the hospital. Shortly thereafter she had two corneal transplants and lost her vision in one eye. Her hearing deteriorated. "The doctor said to me, 'Get someone to care for her,'" says Lucille, who found a home health worker to look after her mother during the day.

Rose's retirement plan pays for most of her medical costs not covered by Medicare and the premiums on her Medicare supplement policy. "Could she have managed in a nursing home?" asks Lucille. "Perhaps, but she preferred to be at home. Besides, the good ones cost $4,000 a month. I guess she'd finally have gone on Medicaid."

Rose is now receiving home hospice care, which is funded by Medicare. "She's gradually getting weaker," says her daughter.

Does Lucille regret her decision to care for her mother all these years? "A lot of people tell me they don't know how I do it. But Mother is very easy to manage. She has all of her mind."

The Continuum of Long-term Care

"Although people automatically think of nursing homes when the subject of long-term care for the elderly comes up, only 5 percent of people sixty-five or older live in one," says Ruth Bennett, a Columbia University professor and expert on elder care. "There is a wide range of support services and living arrangements for older people to consider. Many were established and are funded under the Older Americans Act." The continuum of long-term care includes:

- **Senior centers.** Open to anyone sixty or older, they provide everything from Meals on Wheels and recreation to counseling on government benefits.
- **Adult day care.** Provides medical, recreational, and social services in a group setting to physically or mentally impaired seniors.
- **Respite care.** Designed to give family members who care for their aging relatives a break from their responsibilities, it provides short-term relief.
- **Home care.** Elderly people living at home often need additional help, including high-tech care given by nurses; assistance in walking, eating, and going to the bathroom given by nurse's aides; and homemaker services such as cooking, cleaning, and shopping. We discuss home health care later in the chapter.
- **Housing for the elderly.** For independent older people no longer willing or able to live at home, many housing options are available, such as retirement communities, seniors' apartments, board-and-care arrangements, and continuing care retirement communities, which we discuss below.
- **Enriched housing.** This is a way for seniors who are handicapped to continue living in the community rather than in an institution. Residents live in a supervised apartment setting where they get help with housekeeping, transportation to medical facilities, and other support services.

- **Adult foster homes.** These are private homes where seniors with partial disabilities are cared for.
- **Nursing homes.** We discuss these later in this chapter.
- **Hospice care.** Nursing care, emotional comfort, and relief from pain are provided for a terminally ill person. For people who do not want to spend their final days in a hospital hooked up to machines, it can offer a preferable way of facing death. We discuss hospice care later in this chapter.

How to Investigate the Options
Many resources are available to help elderly people and their families discover the available options. Some of the key ones are:

- Area agencies on aging and state agencies on aging. Addresses and phone numbers of the state agencies which can direct you to a nearby area agency, are given at the end of this chapter.
- National Council on the Aging, 409 Third Street, SW, Washington, DC 20024, (202) 479 1200
- American Association of Retired Persons, 601 E Street, NW, Washington, DC 20049, (202) 434-2277
- American Association of Homes for the Aging, 1129 20th Street, NW, Washington, DC 20036, (202) 783-2242

In addition, local nonprofit groups, such as the New York City Friends and Relatives of the Institutionalized Aged (FRIA), 11 John Street, New York, NY 10038, (212) 732-4455, provide information and help solve problems. Contact the area agency on aging for the names of nearby groups.

A new field, geriatric care management, devoted to helping seniors and their families sift through their options, has sprung up. For a hefty fee, a geriatric care manager visits an older person and does a report on the various alternatives; for an additional fee, he or she makes the necessary arrangements for housing or care and monitors them. This can ease the burden for those living hundreds of miles away from an aged parent. But beware. Geriatric care management is not regulated by local, state, or federal government. Check out agencies very carefully. Demand references and make sure any agreements are in writing. The National Association of Geriatric Care Managers, 655 North Alveron Way, Tuscon,

AZ 85711, (602) 881-8008, and Children of Aging Parents, 1609 Woodbourne Road, Levittown, PA 19057, (215) 345-5104, can give you the names of geriatric care management agencies.

Continuing Care Retirement Communities

You've probably seen the ads. A spry, gray-haired couple frolic in a bucolic setting. The ads explain tactfully that all their future health needs will be taken care of — although the couple look as if they will jog into the sunset forever.

For those who can afford it, continuing care retirement communities (CCRCs), also known as life care communities, are catching on. For a substantial bite out of your assets (sometimes $100,000 plus) and a monthly fee, a CCRC promises a model apartment in peaceful surroundings where your meals, activities, and health needs will be attended to. While you're healthy, you live in the residential community with other active seniors. Should you get sick, the CCRC transfers you to the community's nursing home or to a nearby hospital.

Unlike purchasing a house or condominium, paying your CCRC entry fee buys an occupancy license, which gives you the right to live in the community as long as you pay the monthly fees. In some communities, your initial payment entitles you to housing plus all the medical and nursing care you need. More frequently, the cost of medical and nursing care is extra. The range of payment and care options is almost infinite. Highly reputed communities maintain waiting lists of seven years or longer.

If it sounds too good to be true, perhaps it is. The continuing care retirement community industry has been plagued by a history of "intentional fraud and unintentional mismanagement," according to a guide to life care communities published by the National Consumers League. Twenty-nine states have passed laws regulating continuing care retirement communities, but the protection varies widely. In some states, the communities must keep a large reserve fund in escrow. In others, they must only disclose certain information, such as financial statements, leaving it to you, the potential resident, to fend for yourself.

In an effort at self-policing, the American Association of Homes for the Aging established the Continuing Care Accreditation Commission to give, or withhold, its seal of approval. Accreditation indicates that a community has met the commission's standards for financial stability, management, and resident care. Contact the commission at 1129 20th Street, NW, Washington, DC 20036, (202) 828-9439, for a list of accredited facilities.

There are a lot of smooth operators out there and a lot of heartbreaking tales of CCRCs going bankrupt or seniors not getting what they thought they had bargained for. In addition to finding out about a facility's activities and getting a feel for the place, make sure you can answer some basic questions about its financial and legal status. It is best to seek qualified help before agreeing to anything. Here's what to ask:

CHECKLIST: CONTINUING
CARE RETIREMENT COMMUNITIES

- Is the CCRC or its parent company financially sound?
- Is the cost of nursing home or hospital care covered? If not, what is the arrangement?
- Are nursing home or hospital beds guaranteed? What happens if none is available when you need it?
- What is the fee arrangement if you or your spouse is transferred to the nursing care facility?
- Are there limits to the monthly charges?
- What is the refund policy should you decide to leave?
- If you die shortly after joining, are your heirs entitled to all or part of the amount you invested in the community? If so, what are the time limits?
- Does the facility require residents to enroll in Medicare, buy Medigap insurance, or purchase long-term-care insurance?
- Under what circumstances can the facility terminate the contract?
- What happens in case of remarriage?
- What is the facility's policy toward respecting the wishes of residents about continuation or termination of life-support systems?

Home Health Care

Given a choice, most people would rather be cared for in the comfort of their home than in the institutional coldness of a hospital or the confines of a nursing home. Thanks to modern medical wizardry, the home has become an outpatient section of a hospital. Kidney patients can get dialysis at home; cancer patients can receive nourishment with home therapy; and people with respiratory problems can breathe easier using a home ventilator. And with hospitals pushing to release patients before they have fully recovered and insurance companies looking for ways to save a buck, home health care has become a growth industry used daily by 4 million Americans needing everything from high-tech oxygen therapy to help in bathing or cooking.

Home health care can be a physical and financial lifesaver. But consumers should know about some of the risks.

Payment
The first risk of home health care is financial. As we discussed in Chapter 11, Medicare, the federal government program for the elderly, does not pay for custodial home care of those with debilitating chronic illnesses such as Alzheimer's. The tragic consequence is that many infirm elderly and their children exhaust their resources to pay for the nearly constant home care they require.

If you need home health care and Medicare has turned you down, don't give up. "The fact that the patient is chronically ill is irrelevant," says Diane Archer, executive director of the Medicare Beneficiaries Defense Fund. "The only basis for not covering home health care is that there is no need for skilled nursing care." See whether the focus on dementia-related custodial care for which Medicare won't pay may overshadow a medical condition that Medicare does cover. Carefully examine your private insurance policy for coverage of at least some home health care. Finally, look into Medicaid, the health program for the poor. If you qualify for Medicaid, you may be eligible for the nonskilled nursing home care that some states provide.

Don't hesitate to call a local support group such as the Alzheimer's Association. A nearby chapter may be able to give you the names of lawyers to call, advice on the possibility of getting government coverage, and help finding caregivers. Call the headquarters, (800) 631-0379, to request the number of a chapter in your vicinity. The American Association of Retired Persons Legal Counsel for the Elderly program, (202) 833-6720, refers callers to lawyers in its network and, in some states, maintains a hotline to answer legal questions. The Medicare advocacy groups (see Chapter 11) are a good source for answers to your questions about Medicare coverage.

Guarding Against Fraud and Abuse
Think about it. An elderly, perhaps demented, bedridden man or woman is dependent for the basic activities of daily living — washing, eating, going to the bathroom — on an undertrained, underpaid stranger. Perhaps the old person once had or has a fat bank account or is cranky and hard to get along with. Perhaps the health worker is fed up with caring for this person while her own children sit home alone. Then think about the potential for abuse.

Nor are home health care agencies themselves immune from greed. Reports of practices such as charging for medical equipment of little or no use or padding bills appear all too frequently. If you think this happens only to the elderly, read on.

When John R. Figueroa, a forty-three-year-old former flight attendant with AIDS, was released from a hospital in December 1990, he continued home treatment for pneumonia. A nurse from a home health care agency came to his home two hours a day to administer pentamidine intravenously. "Then I got a routine statement from my insurance company listing $6,000 a week for home health care," says Mr. Figueroa. "It nearly sent me through the roof."

He asked for an itemized bill from the home health care agency, which first refused to provide it and did so only when Mr. Figueroa threatened to have the insurance company withhold payment. The itemized bill listed many drugs he was not using. "Every three or four days, they would drop off a box of supplies. Some of them I didn't need." More revealing, Mr. Figueroa discovered that the Hickman catheter cap connected to a tube in his chest, through which he received medication, sold for 79 cents at his local pharmacy in pricey Greenwich Village. The service charged him $8.39. The tape the service urged him to keep on hand cost $2.00 at the pharmacy, $7.00 through the service. He found he was being charged 200 to 500 percent more than the retail price at the drugstore down the street. "Before this I had no idea how I was billed," says Mr. Figueroa. "I have limited lifetime coverage, and I want to keep some for my old age."

Mr. Figueroa's response is a textbook example of what to do next. He wrote a letter of complaint to the home health care agency. When the company justified the tremendous markup as "overhead," he sent copies of his letter and the company's response to the state attorney general, the state and city consumer protection agencies, various AIDS and consumer advocacy groups, the press, and his congressional representatives. As a result, the New York City Department of Consumers Affairs took up his case.

While fraud and abuse may not be the norm, you should know that home health care agencies are obligated to meet only minimal state and federal standards. To protect yourself and those you care about, take steps to select a reputable agency. Your doctor or the discharge planner at your hospital may have suggestions, as may family and friends. Contact the local area or state agency on aging (addresses and phone numbers are listed at the end of this chapter), a social worker at a senior center, or one of the community groups that help elderly people. The National Association for Home Care, (202) 547-7424, and the National Council on Aging, (202) 479-1200, can give you general information on home health care and specific referrals.

Unless there is a good reason not to do so, we would recommend using an accredited home health agency. You can call the following organizations for the names of agencies they have accredited: Community Health Assessment Program, (800) 847-8480; National Home Caring Council, (202) 547-6586; Joint Commission on the Accreditation of Health Care Organizations, (312) 642-6061.

Even though home health care decisions are often made during a crisis, get some basic information about the agency and the people with whom you will be sharing your life by asking the questions in the checklist:

CHECKLIST: HOME HEALTH CARE AGENCIES

- **Is the agency licensed?** Almost all states require home health care agencies to be licensed, which means that they must meet state government qualifications, usually set by the state department of health. Licensure provides no guarantee that a home health agency will provide high-quality care. On the other hand, lack of a license should set off warning bells in your head. Find out why the agency does not have one.
- **Is the agency accredited?** To gain accreditation, a home health care agency must pass the standards for patient care, financial stability, and administrative competence of one of the three independent agencies listed previously.
- **Is the agency Medicare certified?** Some home health care services may be covered by Medicare (see Chapter 11). If they are, the services must be provided by a Medicare-certified organization. Again, while certification does not guarantee quality, it does mean that the agency has met federal government standards.
- **Is the agency bonded?** This is a legal requirement in many states. The company must carry insurance to cover claims made against it by its customers. If you have to sue a home health care agency and you win, there is more likely to be money to pay you.
- **What are the qualifications of the staff who will provide your home care?** Are the professional staff — nurses, therapists, and dietitians — licensed or certified? How much training have the nonprofessional staff, such as aides and homemakers, had and in what areas? Have references and backgrounds been checked?
- **How often will a supervisor visit you at home?** The home health worker's supervisor should visit your home periodically. Make sure that you have a chance to talk with the supervisor privately and confidentially during these visits.
- **Does the doctor who recommended the home health care agency have a financial interest in it?** Doctors sometimes have a financial stake in the home health care agency to

which they refer patients. Although federal law and American Medical Association policy discourage these referrals, there is not necessarily a conflict of interest. You should know about it, however, and take it into consideration.

• **How much will it cost?** You would think it would be easy to get this information. It isn't. Although a home health care agency can tell you how much you will have to pay for the time of a nurse or nurse's aide, you will have more trouble getting a reliable estimate of the cost of drugs, equipment, and supplies. The best you can realistically hope for is a ball-park figure.

Once home health care has begun, scrutinize your bills carefully. If the charges appear to be too high, request a detailed breakdown. Home health care agencies can make a killing on "overhead" tacked on to charges for equipment, medication, and medical supplies. Excessive charges can take needed money out of your pocket and, if the care is covered by insurance, exhaust your lifetime limit very quickly.

• **Is it covered by Medicare, Medicaid, or your health insurance?** Ask the agency to tell you specifically what parts are covered and what the limits are.

• **Whom do you talk to if there is a problem?** A home health care agency should have a number you can call twenty-four hours a day, seven days a week should a problem arise. Keep it posted.

Nursing Homes

Every day, one out of twenty people over the age of sixty-five wakes up in a nursing home. For those over eighty-five, the number rises to one out of five. A study published in the *New England Journal of Medicine* indicated that nearly half the people who are sixty-five will spend at least some time in a nursing home, and a quarter will spend more than a year.

Nursing homes often are seen as the end of the line, a place where people go to die. Although it certainly is not true of all nursing homes, Bruce Vladeck, president of the New York United Hospital Fund, described the typical nursing home as "a pretty awful place" where the residents are not only old but isolated.

Most people do not have the luxury of leisurely examining their options for a nursing home. They typically enter one directly from a hospital. Those who do have the time to look for a nursing home before needing it should think about what is really important to them. For many, it means proximity to a support network of family and friends, for others a sophisticated rehabilitation program. Whatever your needs, visit at least once before you choose. "The best time to visit is 10:00 or 10:30 in the morning," says Lynne Katzmann, president of Juniper Partners, which owns several nursing homes. "By that time, the residents should be up and dressed, activities should be under way, and the place should be pretty much cleaned." She suggests that you use common sense when evaluating a nursing home and ask yourself whether it is a place in which you could live comfortably. If it smells awful and is dirty, if the residents still aren't dressed or appear to be in a drugged stupor, get out.

Many books can advise you about how to find a nursing home and what to look for in choosing one. Check your local library. The American Health Care Association, 1201 L Street, NW, Washington, DC 20005, (202) 842-4444, which represents for profit nursing homes, and the American Association of Homes for the Aging, 1129 20th Street, NW, Washington, DC 20036, (202) 296-5960, which represents not-for-profit nursing homes, publish a variety of helpful pamphlets and brochures. Friends and Relatives of the Institutionalized Aged, 11 John Street, New York, NY 10038, (212) 732-4455, publishes a loose-leaf book, *Eldercare in the 90's*, filled with useful information on finding and paying for a nursing home. The long-term-care ombudsman's office in your state (see the end of this chapter for addresses and telephone numbers) also has information about nursing homes.

Know Your Rights
In 1987, Congress passed a law intended to eliminate the most serious abuses in nursing homes. Every nursing home that receives Medicare or Medicaid funds is supposed to comply with the Nursing Home Reform law. Under the law, the nursing home exists for

the residents, not the other way around. Rather than merely being spectators, nursing home residents, or their representatives, are to participate in their own care. By law, nursing homes must provide a high level of care, one that will "attain or maintain the highest practicable physical, mental, and psychological well-being of each resident." To meet this lofty goal, the law sets minimum standards that nursing homes must meet: for example, a licensed nurse must be on the premises at all times and a registered nurse must be there at least eight hours a day. Nurse's aides, the woefully underpaid and overworked backbone of nursing homes, must receive at least seventy-five hours of training within their first four months on the job.

The new law addresses some of the more prevalent abuses and outlaws most discrimination against residents who may become Medicaid patients. Since in most states a nursing home receives less for Medicaid residents than private ones, nursing homes try to limit such residents. As a result, Medicaid applicants often have to wait twice as long for a bed as private payers. Although the law does not ban this practice and require nursing homes to take residents on a first-come, first-served basis, it does prohibit some of the more common practices used to keep out Medicaid residents. It is against the law for a nursing home to demand that a resident agree not to apply for Medicaid for a specified period of time, to exact a "contribution" as the price of admission, or to require that a friend or family member guarantee payment.

The most important component of the law is a bill of rights for nursing home residents, including the following:

- The right to be free from abuse, corporal punishment, and involuntary seclusion
- The right to be free from physical restraints, tranquilizers, and mind-bending drugs except when a doctor orders them for medical or safety reasons
- The right to have immediate access to the ombudsman, the physician, and family members
- The right to participate in resident or family councils and to express grievances
- The right to use your own doctor
- The right to privacy, including receiving unopened mail

- The right to remain in the nursing home. Residents can be transferred or discharged only for medical reasons, to protect their own (and others') health and safety, and for nonpayment. Before an involuntary transfer, the nursing home must give thirty days' notice and information about how to appeal the decision.
- The right to an *individual* plan of care based on an assessment of a resident's needs. A resident and his or her representative has the right to participate in drawing up the plan and modifying it on the basis of periodic evaluations of the person's condition. Under the law, nursing homes must screen out mentally retarded and mentally ill people, except those with Alzheimer's disease, who can be better served elsewhere.

Asserting Residents' Rights

Although the Nursing Home Reform Act has been in effect since 1990, the federal government has been lax in enforcing it, and many state governments, which are responsible for monitoring compliance, have dragged their feet. The main reason is cost. Although the law is a wish list for a high-quality nursing home, the states, the federal government, and nursing home owners are fighting about who pays for the upgraded standards.

Nursing home residents need an advocate to assert their rights. Of course, residents can and should stand up for themselves, but as a member of a vulnerable captive population, an assertive person runs the risk of being labeled a troublemaker or being subject to retaliation. Far better that a family member or friend be seen as the protector. David Murray, director of the New York State ombudsman's office, says that nursing home staff tend to do a better job when they see a relative visiting regularly. He suggests that when you visit, you keep your eye out for signs of problems. In this, there is no substitute for common sense.

The first place to discuss problems is within the nursing home itself. Seek out the person responsible or a person with whom you have some rapport and discuss it with him or her. If, for example, you suspect that your mother is being drugged, ask the nurse what is going on or call the doctor (you have to call because doctors are not always on the premises). Bring an apparent problem with bed sores to the attention of the nurse's aides. If you get no satisfaction, bring the problem to the attention of those charged with supervision, on up to the administrator of the facility. Deirdre Rye, a health advocacy specialist for the American Association of Retired Persons, says that most problems can be solved by discussing them with the staff in a nonconfrontational manner.

The resident or family council, if one exists, is a good place to raise problems. By law, residents and their families have the right to form such councils, and nursing homes must make space available for them. They can be a good place to air problems and bring them to the attention of the administration. There is often strength in numbers.

Use the formal grievance procedure of the nursing home if necessary. All nursing homes must have one. If a problem cannot be resolved within the facility, take your complaint to somebody who can do something outside the home. The best place to start is with the long-term-care ombudsman. Under the Older Americans Act, every state is required to have an ombudsman who serves as an advocate for residents of nursing homes and whose job is to protect their interests. The ombudsman's office investigates complaints and tries to resolve problems. It will act on your behalf without revealing your name if you request anonymity. The addresses and phone numbers of these offices are listed at the end of this chapter.

The state department of health is another place to turn. It licenses nursing homes and their administrators and inspects nursing homes at least once a year. To complain, contact your state's department. Addresses and phone numbers are given at the end of Chapter 2.

Community groups sometimes act as advocates for elderly people in nursing homes. The ombudsman's office can steer you to a nearby group.

A number of national organizations can give you information about enforcing your rights or those of a family member in a nursing home. They include:

- National Citizen's Coalition for Nursing Home Reform, 1224 M Street, NW, Washington, DC 20005, (202) 393-2018
- National Senior Citizen's Law Center, 1815 H Street, NW, Washington, DC 20006, (202) 887-5280, or 1052 West 6th Street, Los Angeles, CA 90017, (213) 482-3550

Finally, if abuse or neglect is serious enough, you can bring a lawsuit. In 1990, the families of Margie Berryhill and Frederick Bolian, two deceased residents of a nursing home in McComb, Mississippi, won $250,000 each from the owner of the home, part of a chain called Beverly Enterprises. The families charged, and proved to the satisfaction of a jury, that the nursing home had allowed their relatives to wallow in their own excrement, verbally abused them, forced them to live in stinking rooms, and failed to bathe them.

Nursing Homes and Medicaid: Avoid Going Broke

To Mary M., a retired seventy-three-year-old administrator, the problem was creating a major stress in her life. Her husband of forty-seven years was confined to a wheelchair and was beginning to deteriorate mentally and physically. After much agony, Ms. M. saw that she might have to put him in a nursing home. Now came what she thought would be the easier part — paying for the care. She quickly discovered that the cost of nursing home care could easily lead to financial ruin. There was no way she could pay almost $3,000 a month, exclusive of doctor bills, lab services, and physical therapy. She came to me wanting to know whether she would be responsible for her husband's bills in a nursing home. How could she avoid going broke? Would the government cover the costs? Could she save some of their life savings so that their two children would be left with a decent inheritance? Would she have to get divorced?

Unfortunately, the answers to her questions were anything but easy. With proper planning, I told Ms. M., Medicaid would cover the cost of a nursing home, and she could still protect a large part of their life savings. Her concerns touched on a complex area of law concerning state and federal legislation on taxation, estate planning, and Medicaid. If you are in this situation, we advise you to consult an experienced lawyer before making any decisions.

Remember that *Medicare* does not cover custodial care in a nursing home. *Medicaid*, however, does. Medicaid is a health program for the poor funded by both the U.S. and state governments. National policy is set by Congress, but the program is administered by the states. Once a person becomes sufficiently impoverished, it picks up the costs of nursing home care. The bills of six out of ten people in nursing homes are paid by Medicaid.

In the past, with nursing home charges running up to $50,000 annually, many couples quickly ran through their life savings and sank into poverty. Changes in the Medicaid law that went into effect in 1989 give married couples some protection. They still have to "spend down," that is, exhaust their savings until they qualify for Medicaid, but the spouse who remains in their home — the "community spouse" — is not forced to lose everything. This is how it works.

Married Couples and Medicaid

For a spouse in a nursing home to qualify for Medicaid, assets — house, bank accounts, stocks — and income — retirement benefits, interest, dividends — at the time the spouse enters a nursing home must fall below a certain level. Set by the states, it is very low: a few thousand dollars or less. Remember, Medicaid is a program for poor people.

The law gives married couples a break. When calculating their assets, they can exclude the value of their home plus some other items, the most important of which are a car, wedding and engagement rings, and household goods. They can also exclude half their savings, up to a maximum level set by the states, ranging from $13,000 to $65,000 (it rises slightly every year). As a practical matter, this means that the community spouse can avoid nearly total impoverishment by keeping the home — often a couple's most important asset — some money, and the other items listed above. The rest, with the exception of a small living allowance, goes to pay for nursing home care.

For the purposes of Medicaid eligibility, it doesn't matter whose name the *assets* are in — Medicaid lumps them together. A bank account in the husband's name is considered joint property, as is a house in the wife's name. When calculating *income,* most states follow the "name on the check" rule. If a check is made out to the husband, it's considered his; if it's made out to the wife, it's considered hers. If both names are on the check, it's divided equally. So if the husband goes into a nursing home and dividends are sent in the wife's name, she gets to keep them; if the dividends are in the husband's name, they go to the nursing home.

Single People and Medicaid

The law is biased in favor of married couples. The situation is much worse for the 80 percent of Americans who are single or widowed when they enter a nursing home. Unless you take advantage of the legal ways to protect your assets, almost all of them will go to the nursing home. This includes your home in most states, unless you plan to return there. You may keep a small monthly allowance and get credit toward payments the nursing home makes for Medicare, other health insurance premiums, and medical expenditures not covered by Medicare or Medicaid. In half the states, a nursing home resident can get an allowance, for up to six months, to maintain a home in anticipation of returning there.

You Can't Just Give It Away

If you want your children, rather than a nursing home, to inherit whatever you've been able to save, why not simply give them almost everything, go on Medicaid, and let the government pay for your care? Alas, Congress thought of this first. It passed a provision to keep people — single and married — from disposing of their assets so that they could qualify for Medicaid.

Under the law, if you give away or sell your assets for less than their fair market value within thirty months of applying for Medicaid, the government will assume that you did so to qualify for the program and will deny your application for a period of time. Here's where it gets tricky. The length of time that an applicant is excluded from Medicaid depends on the value of the assets transferred and the cost of nursing home care. The government divides the value of the assets you transferred by the average monthly nursing home cost. The maximum time your Medicaid application can be denied is thirty months.

Let's say your dad gives you IBM stock worth $60,000. Three months later, he applies for Medicaid. Nursing home costs in the state average $4,000 a month. According to the formula, $60,000 ÷ $4,000/month = 15 months. Dad would be eligible for Medicaid in fifteen months.

How to Protect Your Life Savings

Despite the penalty for transfers made within thirty months of applying for Medicaid, there are legal ways to shield your assets so that they will go to loved ones rather than a nursing home. However, they involve intricate areas of state and federal law. Again, we recommend that you consult an attorney experienced in estate planning and Medicaid. Among the legal ways to protect your assets are:

- **Take advantage of the so-called permissible transfers, which are not penalized even if you make them the day before applying for Medicaid.** For example, parents can give their house to a son or daughter who cared for them there for at least two years prior to admission to a nursing home. An elderly person can give assets to his or her blind or disabled child. A married person can transfer title to a house to his or her spouse.
- **Increase the value of your home, the one big asset that is exempt.** Think about paying off your mortgage, adding the home improvements that you have talked about, or even buying a new home.
- **Transfer your home while retaining a life estate.** By doing this, you transfer ownership of the property to a son or daughter while retaining the right to live there during your lifetime. It guarantees that you can stay at home as long as you're able and protects some of the equity in the home.
- **Give someone you trust a durable power of attorney,** which we discuss in Chapter 13. Let's say you give one to your daughter and she transfers $500,000 of your money the day before you enter a nursing home and you then apply for Medicaid. Before you can become eligible, you must pay the nursing home for thirty months of care. The balance is protected, although there are gift and estate tax considerations.
- **Set up a Medicaid trust.** By so doing, you put your assets into a separate legal entity, called a trust, which is managed by the trustee you name — perhaps a son or daughter — for your benefit. "You must give up control of the assets you put in the trust," cautions Cleveland attorney Armond Budish. "Also, a Medicaid trust must be irrevocable. Once you have set it up, you can't undo it or change it."

- **Get a divorce.** Seriously, this is an alternative, although clearly a last-ditch one. Remember that although in most states a wife must pay the nursing home costs of her husband, an ex-wife has no such obligation.

Hospice Care

The purpose of hospice care is to help terminally ill patients live as comfortably as possible during their last days, weeks, or months. It makes no attempt to extend life beyond its natural end. Rather than life-prolonging medication or surgery, it offers management of pain, nursing care, and emotional support. Both the patient and family should understand this to avoid a conflict if there is a turn for the worse and a choice arises between hospitalization or simply providing comfort.

Hospice care may be provided in a person's home, a hospice facility, or a hospital. A doctor specializing in gerontology or the discharge planner at your hospital should be able to refer you to hospices. The National Hospice Organization, whose membership includes over twelve hundred hospice programs, has a toll-free hotline, (800) 658-8898. Its operators can give you the names of nearby hospices as well as answer questions about hospice care. Make sure that the hospice is Medicare certified if you expect Medicare to pay for it.

Long-term Care Insurance

With nursing homes costing upward of $30,000 per year, many seniors turn to long-term-care insurance to protect themselves against financial ruin. Sound like a good idea? Insurance companies think so. In 1983, only six companies sold such policies. Today the market is crowded, with at least 130 companies offering policies. For buyers, long-term care insurance as a cure for the high cost of care may be worse than the disease. "There's less regulation on long-term care insurance than any other insurance," says Keith Whalen, a consultant formerly with the Coalition for Long Term Care. The result, notes Mr. Whalen, is that abuse is widespread. As an all-too-typical example, he cites a California woman who bought such a policy for her aging mother. After her mother went into a nursing home, the company refused to pay. "She had clearly fulfilled the policy requirements," says Whalen. "She was in the home for two years before her daughter hired a lawyer. A year later, the mother died, but by that time, the family was bankrupt. It took four years for the insurance company to pay up."

Long-term care insurance is expensive, confusing, often misleading, and sometimes even fraudulent. It is not regulated by any government agency. This free-for-all has created a chaotic situation in which abuse is rampant, no basic benefit packages exist, and there is no standard for definitions and terms. A report by Families USA found long-term care policies to be so expensive that 85 percent of older Americans could not afford them. Another study, carried out by the United Seniors Health Cooperative, found that long-term care policies would not pay *any* benefits to 61 percent of the policyholders entering a nursing home. Many policies don't cover the one thing that the buyer wants — normal nursing home care.

Three kinds of abuses are most common. First, agents misrepresent the policy. Second, people have difficulty collecting benefits. Third, people have trouble getting their money back if they decide to cancel the policy. "Policyholders can build up a sizable equity after fifteen or twenty years," says Gail Shearer, Consumers Union's health policy expert. "But with rare exceptions, companies offer no benefits to consumers who let their policies lapse."

Particularly odious is a practice called post-claims underwriting, in which an insurance agent does not ask about or report an applicant's medical history. Later, when a claim is made, the insurance company refuses to pay on the ground that the person had an undisclosed pre-existing medical condition.

Take the case of Ms. L., a Georgetown, New York, woman who wanted to buy a nursing home insurance policy for her eighty-three-year-old aunt with arthritis and suspected Alzheimer's. According to a Families USA report, an insurance agent sold Ms. L. a policy after assuring her that it would cover her aunt even if she had Alzheimer's. Nine months later, Ms. L. checked her aunt into a nursing home. When the nursing home tried to collect payment, the insurance company denied the claim. It stated that information about the aunt's Alzheimer's had not been provided at the time of the application. Ms. L. had to pay $7,000 for her aunt's first two months of nursing home care plus a retainer of $1,000 for a lawyer — and her aunt had to apply for Medicaid.

About thirty-five states have passed laws addressing abuses in the sale of long-term care insurance. They base their laws on a model developed by the National Association of Insurance Commissioners. The problem is that states pick and choose which sections of the model law to enact. Only a handful of states prohibit the practice of post-claims underwriting, for example.

Since you are pretty much on your own, exercise great caution. Before you buy a nursing home insurance policy, make sure you can answer the following questions:

CHECKLIST: BUYING LONG-TERM CARE INSURANCE

- **Does the policy cover custodial care?** Many companies make a big deal about their coverage of skilled or intermediate nursing care. That's nice, but not a big deal. Make sure that the policy covers *custodial* care in a nursing home.
- **Does the policy cover Alzheimer's disease?** More than 50 percent of nursing home patients are victims of Alzheimer's, yet insurance companies sometimes try to avoid paying for it. Make sure that coverage for Alzheimer's is specifically included in the policy.
- **Is home health care covered?** Although people usually buy long-term care policies to protect themselves against the catastrophe of paying for a nursing home, some policies cover home health care as well. But there's a catch. "Home health care coverage is meaningless in the way a lot of policies define it — limiting it, for example, to highly skilled nursing or therapy," says Ms. Shearer. "Look for a policy that covers home health aides or, better yet, homemaker services."
- **Must you be in a hospital or a skilled nursing facility before going to a nursing home?** Beware of long-term care policies that require a prior stay in a hospital or skilled nursing facility. People with Alzheimer's and other chronic ill-

nesses tend to enter a nursing establishment directly from home. If your policy requires prior hospitalization or skilled nursing facility treatment and you go directly to a nursing home, you will not be covered.

- **When do you become eligible for benefits?** Some policies require that care be "medically necessary for sickness or injury." This can be very restrictive for people who are not sick or injured but need custodial care, particularly if an insurance company interprets it narrowly. Policies that begin coverage when a doctor orders the care or when the policyholder can no longer carry out two or three "activities of daily living," such as walking, eating, or going to the toilet, are less restrictive.
- **Are you insurable?** Some companies will not insure people who are already ill. Or they exclude coverage related to mental illness, alcohol or chemical dependency, heart disease and cancer, diabetes, and other conditions. Check the "Exclusions" section very carefully. Many companies will not sell a policy to people over seventy-five or eighty.
- **How long do you have to wait before pre-existing conditions are covered?** You will be asked to tell the insurance company about your health problems in the past, perhaps as long as three years ago. These are called pre-existing conditions. When it learns that you had a health problem, the company may refuse to insure you altogether; it may offer to cover you for a higher premium, or it may make you wait before coverage starts. Try to get a policy with a waiting period of six months or less. Do not hide an illness or health problem from the insurance company, even if you think the condition might keep you from getting insurance.
- **Is the insurance company financially sound?** Since you are buying *long-term* protection, it is important to know that the company will be there when you need it in ten to fifteen years. You can check out the financial health of a potential insurer by telephoning companies whose business it is to rate insurers. The major ones are: A. M. Best, (900) 420-0400 (the charge is $2.50 per minute); Standard and Poor's, (212) 208-1527; Moody's Investors Service, (212) 553-0377,

and Duff & Phelps, (312) 368-0377. A newcomer is Weiss Research, (800) 289-9222 (the charge is $15 per report). The same information is also available at some public libraries. Buy only from a company given a top rating by two of these firms. A word of warning: Even the rating companies cannot predict well into the future. There is no completely certain way of predicting a company's future financial health.

- **How much does the policy pay to a nursing home?** Almost all nursing home insurance policies pay a fixed daily amount, which may be $40 or $100. It almost certainly will not cover the full cost of the nursing home. Subtract the daily benefit from the daily cost to calculate how much you will have to pay.

- **Is there a yearly adjustment for inflation?** A benefit of $80 or $100 a day may seem satisfactory today if the average nursing home in your area now charges $110. Tomorrow it might be a pittance if the same care costs $200. Most companies allow you to buy a rider, or include a provision in the base policy, that increases benefits every year, usually by 5 percent. It may add 25 to 60 percent to your premiums, but is likely to be worth it. Without it, your coverage may prove illusory.

- **How long before benefits begin?** Nursing home policies do not start paying the moment you enter the door. There is a waiting period — sometimes called a deductible or elimination period — before the policy begins to pay. The shorter the waiting period, the higher the premium. In some policies, the deductible is set as a dollar amount that you must pay before the insurance kicks in.

- **How long does nursing home coverage last?** The best policy, one that pays for an unlimited number of days in a nursing home, is likely to be very costly. Since older people average 3.8 years in a nursing home, you want a policy that covers at least four years.

- **How much are the premiums?** Nursing home insurance isn't cheap. The older you are when you apply and the better your benefits, the more expensive your premiums. The average yearly premium a sixty-five-year-old has to pay for a so-so policy is $1,250; a seventy-nine-year-old we know paid nearly $4,000 a year.

Remember, premiums can, and probably will, increase, sometimes astronomically. A 1991 congressional report cited the case of a ninety-five-year-old Illinois man who purchased a long-term care policy in 1981 for a premium of $1,000 a year. By 1985 it had shot up to over $5,000 a year and in 1987 it was raised to $8,000. He was forced to drop his coverage and now requires nursing home care. Cost? $20,000 a year.

Don't be taken in by low premiums. Some companies intentionally underprice them to attract customers and, as a result, risk going under.

- **Can the company cancel the policy?** Buy only a guaranteed renewable or noncancelable policy. This means that the company cannot drop you; it must continue a renewable policy as long as you pay the premiums. You have to realize, however, that the company can raise those premiums. A noncancelable policy, which is an endangered species, assures that your rates will never go up.
- **Must you continue to pay premiums while you are in a nursing home?** Most policies allow you to stop paying premiums after you have been in a nursing home for a specified period, usually ninety days. This feature is called a waiver of premium.
- **Can you get your money back if you cancel or your coverage lapses?** With most companies, if you cancel or let the policy lapse, you lose all the money you have paid in premiums. Some companies offer to refund part of your money or provide some portion of your benefits if your policy lapses or you cancel. The National Association of Insurance Commissioners forecasts that such "nonforfeiture" benefits will become increasingly common in nursing home insurance policies.
- **Is there a thirty-day free look?** Almost every company offers to refund your money if you change your mind within thirty days. Be sure your company offers you this option.

Most of the tips we provided for buying Medigap policies (see Chapter 11) also apply to long-term care insurance:

- Request an Outline of Coverage.
- Don't be pressured into buying.
- Fill out the application yourself or have a knowledgeable friend or relative help you do it. Never pay cash.
- Pay your premiums by check made out to the insurance company.
- Don't be fooled by agents who imply that their policies are endorsed by the government.
- Be wary of celebrities touting a specific policy.

Is It Right for You?

Perhaps the hardest question of all is whether long-term care insurance is worth it for you. It's an expensive proposition for something you may never need. On the other hand, owning a policy can give you peace of mind.

In our opinion, it makes sense to buy only a long-term-care insurance policy that offers generous coverage. Why spend your hard-earned money on a policy that merely keeps you off Medicaid for a short period? This limits your options to the high-end policies. It also assumes that you have the means to pay the premiums year after year. If you have the money, the decision becomes a personal one, based on such factors as the following:

- *Your tolerance for risk.* The comfort of knowing that their later years are taken care of is worth a lot to some people. To others it is less important. How much is peace of mind worth?
- *The alternative uses of your money.* Money spent for insurance premiums is not available for other investments. Interest, dividends, and rental income can be used to pay for a nursing home if you need one, and is money in your pocket if you don't.
- *The desire to avoid Medicaid.* For many people, this is a matter of pride, apart from any finances involved. Also, Medicaid patients may have a harder time getting into nursing

homes than private-pay patients and may not receive the same quality of care.

It is said that you have to be healthy and wealthy to buy a long-term care insurance policy. Whether you are wise depends on you.

Where to Turn for Help
The volunteer counseling services offered by many states may help you decipher long-term-care insurance. Contact your state insurance department (see Chapter 3 for numbers) to learn what assistance is available for confused seniors. Community organizations sometimes advise on long-term-care insurance. Check your local senior center or area agency on aging.

Several national organizations can provide written material and may be able to refer you to a nearby source of assistance. They include:

American Association of Retired
  Persons
601 E Street, NW
Washington, DC 20049
(202) 434-2277

Health Insurance Association of
  America
1025 Connecticut Avenue, NW
Washington, DC 20036
(202) 223-7780

Families USA
1334 G Street, NW
Washington, DC 20005
(202) 628-3030

United Seniors Health Cooperative
1331 H Street, NW
Washington, DC 20005
(202) 393-6222

National Association of Insurance
  Commissioners
120 West 12th Street
Kansas City, MO 64105
(816) 842-3600

National Council on the Aging
409 Third Street, NW
Washington, DC 20024
(202) 479-1200

Consumer Reports, 101 Truman Avenue, Yonkers, NY 10703, (914) 378-2000, publishes occasional articles comparing various long-term care insurance plans.

We urge you to have a lawyer or an unbiased, knowledgeable person look over a policy. It is an extra expense, but compared to what you stand to lose if you're not protected, it's worth it.

When Older People Can No Longer Make Decisions

Annette B., a Minneapolis teacher, tells the story of her late mother's gradual disintegration. "About the time my mother turned eighty-eight, her condition started to get worse. Mom, who ran a farm for many years and raised five children, became forgetful and would repeat the same things over and over. Sometimes she wouldn't recognize me. She began to wander in the streets at all hours, day or night. We moved her to an apartment nearby, but that turned out to be a disaster. She left the gas on and almost asphyxiated herself and her neighbor. And she didn't clean, so the place began to smell. (We finally arranged for someone to come in twice a week.) We suggested she get a roommate, but she would hear none of it. She became suspicious of other people. Paranoid, really.

"Some friends said we had better do something about her financial affairs, since she obviously was no longer capable of handling them. I applied to be her legal guardian. It involved a hearing before a judge. I testified about her condition. My lawyer presented affidavits showing she was no longer competent to manage her affairs. Her doctor testified that she was suffering from Alzheimer's disease and that it was getting worse. The court-appointed guardian concluded it was in Mom's best interest to appoint a guardian. The judge agreed and named me. The whole process was easier than I had expected.

"We finally placed Mom in a nursing home. The cost of her care went up, and I had to sell her farm. Before I could do this, I had to go to court to get the judge's approval. As Mom got older, her health deteriorated. She became blind, incontinent, and unable to recognize anybody. She fell a lot and was tied to a chair for long periods. She would sit for hours on end staring vacantly into space. My four brothers and sisters and I signed a form authorizing the nursing home to withhold lifesaving care but requiring it to take measures that would make her as comfortable as possible. One night Mom died in her sleep. She was ninety-nine years old."

Sadly, this is not an unusual story. As people live to increasingly older ages, they sometimes outlive their ability to make financial and medical decisions. Illness, accident, Alzheimer's, can all rob a person of the mental faculties needed to make decisions. If you are worried about this happening to you, or are the concerned child of an aging parent, you can take a number of steps.

Protecting Money and Property

Execute a durable power of attorney. This legal document authorizes another person to act as your agent in carrying out your business and personal matters. You decide whom you trust enough and how much authority you want the person to have. You can give your agent as much or as little authority as you want — for example, power over all your property or, say, certain bank accounts. Because it is "durable," the power of attorney continues in the event that you become incapacitated.

Remember that the agent you appoint has as much power over your property as you do and can act in your stead. Make sure you have full confidence in the person you name. Remember, too, that your power of attorney can be revoked in writing at any time.

Many people are reluctant, while they are alive and well, to give another, even a beloved son or daughter, the power, for instance, to withdraw money from a bank or sell stock. If you fall into this camp, think about a newer mechanism called a "springing" power of attorney, which is allowed in a few states. It springs into life if you become incapacitated or a specified contingency occurs.

Set up a revocable living trust. With this option, you place some or all of your assets in a trust so that the property belongs to the trust, which is a separate legal entity, not to you as an individual. The property in the trust is managed by the trustees, whom you name. You can name yourself or anybody else.

There are many ways to set up a living trust. A common one is to appoint yourself as trustee and your children as cotrustees. The trust document can specify that your children become the sole trustees if you become incapacitated. A living trust should be made revocable upon the written instruction of the person who establishes it.

Here is how it works in practice. Miriam Y., an elderly widow living in Los Angeles, owned a house and a portfolio of stocks and bonds. She wanted the comfort of knowing that these would pass to her two daughters upon her death and that the children would be responsible for them should she become incapacitated. Ms. Y set up a living trust in which she placed all her assets. She named herself and her daughters as cotrustees and specified that, while she was competent, she alone had power to make decisions about the trust property. If she became incapacitated, as determined by two physicians, the daughters would become the trustees. Upon her death, the assets in the trust would pass to the daughters, who were named as beneficiaries.

Establishing a living trust is a legal procedure used in many states as a way of avoiding probate. You need a lawyer knowledgeable in estate planning to draw one up.

Guardianship. Although more and more older people are using durable powers of attorney and living trusts to transfer decision making about their property if they become incapacitated, it frequently happens that an older person is unable to make decisions because of mental deterioration and has not named anyone to do so. In that case, it is not unusual for one or more of the children to ask to be named as a guardian. This involves a formal petition to a court in which the children ask the judge to find that their parent is no longer able to manage his or her financial affairs and to appoint them as guardians. Any "interested party" — usually interpreted to mean a family member or close friend — has the right to file a guardianship petition in most states.

The determination whether a person is incapacitated, or incompetent, as it is termed in some states, is made by a judge at a legal proceeding called a hearing. The judge listens to testimony or reads affidavits from the family, doctors, therapists, and others whose perspective is of help. He or she interviews the elderly person, if possible. Usually the judge appoints a person, called a guardian *ad litem*, to provide an independent report.

The judge bases the decision about the parent's capacity on criteria set out in the state's law. If the parent is found incapable of managing his or her affairs, the judge names a guardian, or conservator in some states. The judge may give the guardian broad powers to make financial and medical decisions or limit the power to specific matters like finances. The guardianship appointment usually lasts indefinitely, although a court can establish it for a limited period or terminate it if the trust is abused.

Decisions on Medical Treatment

In some states, a guardian or an agent named in a durable power of attorney can make decisions to authorize or withhold medical care. In other states, the agent's authority is limited to financial decisions. Whatever the law in your state, it makes sense to separate your wishes on medical treatment decisions from those on financial matters. As we discuss in Chapter 13, almost all states have a law authorizing you to appoint a person — either a health care "proxy" or an agent named under a durable power of attorney — to make medical decisions if you are incapacitated or to write a living will. All patients entering hospitals or nursing homes that receive federal funds must, by law, be advised of their right under state law to specify in advance how medical care decisions should be made and who should make them.

STATE AGENCIES ON AGING

Note: State units on aging provide information and assistance, house long-term-care ombudsmen, and can direct you to a nearby area agency on aging. If the address or phone number listed below has changed, you can get the new one by contacting the National Association of State Units on Aging, 2033 K Street, NW, Washington, DC 20006, (202) 785-0707, or the National Association of Area Agencies on Aging, 1112 Sixteenth Street, Washington, DC 20036, (202) 296-8130.

Alabama
Commission on Aging
770 Washington Avenue
Montgomery, AL 36130
(205) 242-5743
toll free in state:
(800) 243-5463

Alaska
Older Alaskans Commission
P.O. Box C
Juneau, AK 99811-0209
(907) 465-3250

Arizona
Aging and Adult Administration
1400 West Washington
Phoenix, AZ 85007
(602) 542-4446

Arkansas
Office of Aging and Adult Services
Department of Human Services
P.O. Box 1437
Little Rock, AR 72203
(501) 682-2441

California
California Department of Aging
1600 K Street
Sacramento, CA 95814
(916) 322-5290

Colorado
Aging and Adult Services Division
Department of Social Services
1575 Sherman Street
Denver, CO 80203-1714
(303) 866-3851

Connecticut
Department on Aging
175 Main Street
Hartford, CT 06106
(203) 566-3238
toll free in state:
(800) 443-9946

Delaware
Department of Health and Social
   Services
Division of Aging
1901 N. DuPont Highway
New Castle, DE 19720
(302) 421-6791
toll free in state:
(800) 223-9074

District of Columbia
D.C. Office on Aging
1424 K Street, NW
Washington, DC 20005
(202) 724-5626

Florida
Aging and Adult Services
1317 Winewood Boulevard
Tallahassee, FL 32301
(904) 488-8922

Georgia
Office of Aging
878 Peachtree Street, NE
Atlanta, GA 30309
(404) 894-5333

Hawaii
Executive Office on Aging
Office of the Governor
335 Merchant Street
Honolulu, HI 96813
(808) 586-0100

Idaho
Idaho Office on Aging
Statehouse
Boise, ID 83720
(208) 334-3833

Illinois
Department on Aging
421 East Capitol Avenue
Springfield, IL 62701
(217) 785-2870
toll free nationwide:
(800) 252-8966

Indiana
Aging Division
Department of Human Services
P.O. Box 7083
Indianapolis, IN 46207-7083
(317) 232-7020
toll free in state:
(800) 622-4972

Iowa
Department of Elder Affairs
914 Grand Avenue
Des Moines, IA 50319
(515) 281-5187
toll free in state:
(800) 532-3213

Kansas
Department on Aging
Docking State Office Building
915 Southwest Harrison Street
Topeka, KS 66612-1500
(913) 296-4986
toll free in state:
(800) 432-3535

Kentucky
Division for Aging Services
275 East Main Street
Frankfort, KY 40621
(502) 564-6930
toll free in state:
(800) 372-2991

Louisiana
Office of Elderly Affairs
P.O. Box 80374
Baton Rouge, LA 70806
(504) 925-1700

Maine
Bureau of Elder and Adult Services
Statehouse, Station 11
Augusta, ME 04333-0011
(207) 626-5335

Maryland
Office on Aging
301 West Preston Street
Baltimore, MD 21201
(301) 225-1100
toll free in state:
(800) 243-3425

Massachusetts
Executive Office of Elder Affairs
38 Chauncy Street
Boston, MA 02111
(617) 727-7750

Michigan
Office of Services to the Aging
P.O. Box 30026
Lansing, MI 48909
(517) 373-8230

Minnesota
Minnesota Board on Aging
444 Lafayette Road
St. Paul, MN 55155-3843
(612) 296-2770
toll free in state:
(800) 652-9747

Mississippi
Division of Aging and Adult
    Services
421 West Pascagoula Street
Jackson, MS 39203-3524
(601) 949-2070
toll free in state:
(800) 222-7622

Missouri
Division of Aging
Department of Social Services
P.O. Box 1337
Jefferson City, MO 65102-1337
(314) 751-3082
toll free in state:
(800) 392-0210

Montana
The Governor's Office on Aging
State Capitol Building
Capitol Station
Helena, MT 59620
(406) 444-3111
toll free in state:
(800) 332-2272

Nebraska
Nebraska Department on Aging
301 Centennial Mall South
P.O. Box 95044
Lincoln, NE 68509
(402) 471-2306

Nevada
Division of Aging Services
Department of Human Resources
340 North 11th Street
Las Vegas, NV 89101
(702) 486-3545

New Hampshire
Division of Elderly and Adult
  Services
6 Hazen Drive
Concord, NH 03301-6501
(603) 271-4680
toll free in state:
(800) 351-1888

New Jersey
Division on Aging
Department of Community Affairs
South Broad and Front Streets
CN 807
Trenton, NJ 08625-0807
(609) 292-4833
toll free in state:
(800) 792-8820

New Mexico
State Agency on Aging
224 E. Palace Avenue
Santa Fe, NM 87501
(505) 827-7640
toll free in state:
(800) 432-2080

New York
New York State Office for the Aging
Agency Building 2
Albany, NY 12223
(518) 474-4425
toll free in state:
(800) 342-9871

North Carolina
Division of Aging
Department of Human Resources
693 Palmer Drive
Raleigh, NC 27603
(919) 733-3983
toll free in state:
(800) 662-7030

North Dakota
Aging Services
Department of Human Services
600 East Boulevard
Bismarck, ND 58505
(701) 224-2577
toll free in state:
(800) 472-2622

Ohio
Ohio Department of Aging
50 West Broad Street
Columbus, OH 43266-0501
(614) 466-5500

Oklahoma
Aging Services Division
Department of Human Services
P.O. Box 25352
Oklahoma City, OK 73125
(405) 521-2327

Oregon
Senior and Disabled Services
  Division
Department of Human Resources
313 Public Service Building
Salem, OR 97310
(503) 378-4728
toll free in state:
(800) 232-3020

Pennsylvania
Department of Aging
231 State Street
Harrisburg, PA 17101-1195
(717) 783-1550

Rhode Island
Department of Elderly Affairs
160 Pine Street
Providence, RI 02903-3708
(401) 277-2858
toll free in state:
(800) 322-2880

South Carolina
Commission on Aging
400 Arbor Lake Drive
Columbia, SC 29223
(803) 735-0210

South Dakota
Office of Adult Services and Aging
700 North Illinois Street
Pierre, SD 57501
(605) 773-3656

Tennessee
Commission on Aging
706 Church Street
Nashville, TN 37243-0860
(615) 741-2056

Texas
Texas Department on Aging
P.O. Box 12786
Capitol Station
Austin, TX 78741
(512) 444-2727
toll free in state:
(800) 252-9240

Utah
Division of Aging and Adult
    Services
Department of Social Service
P.O. Box 45500
Salt Lake City, UT 84145
(801) 538-3910

Vermont
Department of Aging and
    Disabilities

103 South Main Street
Waterbury, VT 05676
(802) 241-2400

Virginia
Department for the Aging
700 East Franklin Street
Richmond, VA 23219-2327
(804) 225-2271
toll free in state:
(800) 552-4464

Washington
Aging and Adult Services
    Administration
Department of Social and Health
    Services
OB-44A
Olympia, WA 98504
(206) 586-3768
toll free in state:
(800) 422-3263

West Virginia
Commission on Aging
State Capitol
Charleston, WV 25305
(304) 348-3317
toll free in state:
(800) 642-3671

Wisconsin
Bureau of Aging
Division of Community Services
217 South Hamilton Street
Madison, WI 53707
(608) 266-2536

Wyoming
Commission on Aging
Hathaway Building
Cheyenne, WY 82002-0710
(307) 777-7986
toll free in state:
(800) 442-2766

NURSING HOME OMBUDSMEN

Note: If an address or phone number listed below has changed, you can get the new one by contacting the National Association of State Units on Aging, 2033 K Street, NW, Washington, DC 20006, (202) 785-0707.

Alabama
Commission on Aging
770 Washington Avenue
Montgomery, AL 36160
(205) 261-5743

Alaska
Office of the Older Alaskans
    Ombudsmen
3601 C Street
Anchorage, AK 99503-5209
(907) 279-2232
(also accepts collect calls from older
    persons)

Arizona
Aging and Adult Administration
P.O. Box 6123-950A
1400 West Washington Street
Phoenix, AZ 85007
(602) 542-4446

Arkansas
Division of Aging and Adult
    Services
1417 Donaghey Plaza South
P.O. Box 1437
7th and Maine Streets
Little Rock, AR 72203-1437
(501) 682-2441

California
Department on Aging
1600 K Street
Sacramento, CA 95814
(916) 323-6681
toll free in state:
(800) 231-4024

Colorado
The Legal Center
455 Sherman Street
Denver, CO 80203
(303) 722-0300
toll free in state:
(800) 332-6356

Connecticut
Department on Aging
175 Main Street
Hartford, CT 06106
(203) 566-7770
toll free in state:
(800) 233-9074

Delaware
Division on Aging
1113 Church Avenue
Milford, DE 19963
(302) 422-1386
toll free in state:
(800) 223-9074

District of Columbia
Legal Counsel for the Elderly
601 E Street, NW
Washington, DC 20049
(202) 662-4933

Florida
State LTC Ombudsman Council
Office of the Governor
154 Holland Building
Tallahassee, FL 32399-0001
(904) 488-6190

Georgia
Office of Aging
Department of Human Resources
878 Peachtree Street, NE
Atlanta, GA 30389
(404) 894-5336

Hawaii
Executive Office on Aging
335 Merchant Street
Honolulu, HI 96813
(808) 548-2593

Idaho
Office on Aging
State House
Boise, ID 83720
(208) 334-3833

Illinois
Department on Aging
421 East Capitol Avenue
Springfield, IL 62701
(217) 785-3140
toll free in state:
(800) 252-8966

Indiana
Aging In-Home Services Division
Department of Human Services
251 N. Illinois
P.O. Box 7083
Indianapolis, IN 46207-7083
(317) 232-7020
toll free in state:
(800) 622-4484

Iowa
Department of Elder Affairs
916 Grand Avenue
Des Moines, IA 50319
(515) 281-5187
toll free in state:
(800) 532-3213

Kansas
Department on Aging
Docking State Office Building
915 Southwest Harrison Street
Topeka, KS 66612-1500
(913) 296-4986
toll free in state:
(800) 432-3535

Kentucky
Division for Aging Services
Cabinet for Social Services
275 East Main Street
Frankfort, KY 40621
(502) 564-6930
toll free in state:
(800) 372-2991

Louisiana
Governor's Office of Elder Affairs
4550 N. Boulevard
P.O. Box 80374
Baton Rouge, LA 70898-3074
(504) 925-1700

Maine
Commission on Aging
State House, Station 127
Augusta, ME 04333
(207) 289-3658
toll free in state:
(800) 452-1912

Maryland
Office on Aging
301 West Preston
Baltimore, MD 21201
(301) 225-1083
toll free in state:
(800) 243-3425

Massachusetts
Executive Office of Elder Affairs
38 Chauncy Street
Boston, MA 02111
(617) 727-7750
toll free in state:
(800) 872-0166

Michigan
Citizens for Better Care
1627 E. Kalamazoo
Lansing, MI 48912
(517) 482-1297
toll free in state:
(800) 292-7852

Minnesota
Board on Aging
Office of Ombudsman for Older
  Minnesotans
444 Lafayette Road
St. Paul, MN 55155-3843
(612) 296-0382
toll free in state:
(800) 652-9747

Mississippi
Council on Aging
421 West Pascagoula Street
Jackson, MS 39203-3524
(601) 949-2070
toll free in state:
(800) 222-7622

Missouri
Division of Aging
P.O. Box 1337
Jefferson City, MO 65102
(314) 751-3082
toll free in state:
(800) 392-0210

Montana
Seniors' Office of Legal and
  Ombudsman Services
P.O. Box 232
Capitol Station
Helena, MT 59620
(406) 444-4676
toll free in state:
(800) 332-2272

Nebraska
Department on Aging
301 Centennial Mall South
P.O. Box 95044
Lincoln, NE 86509-5044
(402) 471-2306, 2307

Nevada
Division for Aging Services
Department of Human Resources
505 East King Street
Carson City, NV 89710
(702) 885-4210

New Hampshire
Division of Elderly and Adult
  Services
6 Hazen Drive
Concord, NH 03301-6508
(603) 271-4375
toll free in state:
(800) 442-5640

New Jersey
Office of the Ombudsman for the
  Institutionalized Elderly
28 West State Street, CN 808
Trenton, NJ 08625-0807
(609) 292-8016
toll free in state:
(800) 624-4262

New Mexico
State Agency on Aging
224 East Palace Avenue
Santa Fe, NM 87501
(505) 827-7640
toll free in state:
(800) 432-2080

New York
Office for the Aging
Agency Building 2
Albany, NY 12223
(518) 474-7329
toll free in state:
(800) 342-9871

North Carolina
Division of Aging
Department of Human Resources
693 Palmer Drive
Raleigh, NC 27603
(919) 733-8400
toll free in state:
(800) 662-7030

North Dakota
Aging Services Division
Department of Human Services
600 East Boulevard
Bismarck, ND 58505
(701) 224-2577
toll free in state:
(800) 472-2622

Ohio
Department of Aging
50 West Broad Street
Columbia, OH 43266-0501
(614) 466-1221
toll free in state:
(800) 282-1206

Oklahoma
Division of Aging Services
Department of Human Services
P.O. Box 25352
Oklahoma City, OK 73125
(405) 521-6734

Oregon
Office of LTC Ombudsman
2475 Lancaster Drive
Building B, #9
Salem, OR 97310
(503) 378-6533
toll free in state:
(800) 522-2602

Pennsylvania
Department of Aging
231 State Street
Harrisburg, PA 17101
(717) 783-7247

Rhode Island
Department of Elderly Affairs
160 Pine Street
Providence, RI 02903
(401) 277-6883
toll free in state:
(800) 322-2880

South Carolina
Office of the Governor
Division of Ombudsman and
    Citizen's Service
1205 Pendleton Street
Columbia, SC 29201
(803) 734-0457

South Dakota
Office of Adult Services and Aging
Department of Social Services
700 N. Illinois Street
Pierre, SD 57501-2291
(605) 773-3656

Tennessee
Commission on Aging
706 Church Street
Nashville, TN 37219-5573
(615) 741-2056

Texas
Department on Aging
P.O. Box 12786
Capitol Station
Austin, TX 78741-3702
(512) 444-2727
toll free in state:
(800) 252-9240

Utah
Division of Social Services
120 North — 200 West
P.O. Box 45500
Salt Lake City, UT 84145-0500
(801) 538-3920

Vermont
Office on Aging
103 South Main Street
Waterbury, VT 05676
(802) 241-2400
toll free in state:
(800) 642-5119

Virginia
Department for the Aging
700 East Franklin Street
Richmond, VA 23219-2327
(804) 225-2271
toll free in state:
(800) 552-3402

Washington
South King County Multi-Service
  Center
1200 South, 336 Street
Federal Way, WA 98003
(206) 838-6810
toll free in state:
(800) 422-1384

West Virginia
Commission on Aging
State Capitol Complex
Charleston, WV 25305
(304) 348-3317
toll free in state:
(800) 642-3671

Wisconsin
Board on Aging and Long Term Care
214 North Hamilton Street
Madison, WI 53703
(608) 266-8944

Wyoming
Wyoming State Bar Association
900 8th Street
Wheatland, WY 82201
(307) 322-5553

13

THE RIGHT TO DIE

CONTENTS

Forty-five-year-old diane went to Dr. Timothy Quill, complaining of fatigue and a rash. A blood test confirmed the worst: acute myelomonocytic leukemia. Survival rate: 25 percent. Diane had overcome alcoholism and vaginal cancer, had a thriving business, and lived a completely abstinent life with her husband and college-age son. Chemotherapy was scheduled to begin immediately. But then Diane told Dr. Quill, who had treated her for eight years, that she did not want any treatment. Rather, she wanted to remain in control and spend her remaining time with her husband and son. Home hospice care was arranged, with the door left open for her to change her mind. What Diane ultimately wanted profoundly affected Dr. Quill and sparked a national debate when he wrote about it in the *New England Journal of Medicine*:

> It was extraordinarily important to Diane to maintain control of herself and her own dignity during the time remaining to her. When this was no longer possible, she clearly wanted to die. When the time came, she wanted to take her life in the least painful way possible.
>
> A week later, she phoned me with a request for barbiturates for sleep. Since I knew that this was an essential ingredient in a suicide, I asked her to come to the office to talk things over. In our discussion, it was apparent that she was having trouble sleeping, but it was also evident that the security of having enough barbiturates available to commit suicide when and if the time came would leave her secure enough to live fully and concentrate on the present. I wrote the prescription with an uneasy feeling about the boundaries I was exploring — spiritual, legal, professional, and personal. Yet I also felt strongly that I was setting her free to get the most out of the time she had left, and to maintain dignity and control on her own terms until her death.
>
> After three tumultuous months, bone pain, weakness, fatigue, and fevers began to dominate her life. It was clear that the end was approaching. She called up her closest friends and asked them to come over to say goodbye. As we had agreed, she let me know as well. When we met, it was clear that she knew what she was doing.

Two days later, her husband called to say that Diane had died. She had said her final goodbyes to her husband and son that morning, and asked them to leave her alone for an hour. They found her on the couch, lying very still and covered by her favorite shawl. There was no sign of a struggle. She seemed to be at peace.

A grand jury refused to indict Dr. Quill, and the state medical society declined to discipline him. One of the few physicians to admit his role publicly, Dr. Quill broadened the controversy about a patient's right to die to include doctor-assisted suicide.

Less than a year earlier, in 1990, Janet Adkins, fifty-four, a schoolteacher who liked hang gliding, mountain climbing, and flute playing, contacted Dr. Jack Kevorkian, a retired pathologist she had seen on the *Donahue* show. Ms. Adkins had early Alzheimer's disease; Dr. Kevorkian had invented a suicide machine. Two days later, Ms. Adkins lay on a cot in his rusty 1968 Volkswagen van, which was parked in a Michigan campsite. Dr. Kevorkian set up the machine — three vials suspended over a metal box containing an electric motor — and connected an intravenous tube to Ms. Adkins's arm. She pressed the button. First, saline solution flowed into her veins, then thiopental, which made her unconscious, and finally potassium chloride, which stopped her heart. Since assisting a suicide is not illegal under Michigan law, prosecutors attempted to charge Dr. Kevorkian with murder. A judge dismissed the charges. When Dr. Kevorkian assisted two more women to kill themselves in 1991 with the aid of a new, improved suicide machine, his license was suspended and he was charged with murder.

Cases such as these have brought assisted suicide out in the open. Witness the success of *Final Exit*, a how-to book on suicide by Derek Humphry, head of the Oregon-based National Hemlock Society. And Initiative 119 in the state of Washington in 1991 on legalizing doctor-assisted suicide for the terminally ill. The initiative lost but received nearly 50 percent of the votes cast. Assisted suicide remains a legal and moral gray area, troubling doctors, lawyers, and ethicists alike. The American Medical Association takes the position that a doctor may give medication to relieve suffering but should not intentionally cause death. Yet in an article appearing in the *New England Journal of Medicine*, ten out of twelve of the physician-authors concluded, "It is not immoral for a physician to assist in the rational suicide of a terminally-ill person."

The Right to Refuse Medical Treatment

Modern medical technology has changed the very meaning of life and death. Chemotherapy buys time for cancer patients. Dialysis gives a reprieve to people with nonfunctioning kidneys. Bone marrow, liver, and heart transplants offer the hope of new life. Yet many who would have died naturally twenty years ago are now "kept alive" indefinitely by respirators and feeding tubes, existing in a twilight zone of the living dead.

Some are in a persistent vegetative state — they have no higher brain functions and are permanently unconscious. But because the brain stem still functions, they can respond to stimuli such as light or noise. Karen Quinlan, whose plight first brought attention to the right to die, was in such a state. She was a twenty-two-year-old New Jersey woman who stopped breathing one night in April 1975 and was left in a chronic and persistent vegetative state, kept alive by the respirator to which she was attached, with no reasonable hope of recovery. Her parents, with guidance from their parish priest, asked the hospital to remove the respirator. The hospital refused to do so without the approval of a court. After years of agony and untold personal, emotional, and financial cost, the New Jersey Supreme Court, in a landmark decision, said that Karen's parents could authorize removal of the respirator. She lived another nine years, tethered to a feeding tube.

Every year, 2 million people die, 80 percent in hospitals, hospices, or nursing homes — perhaps 70 percent of them after a decision to forgo life-sustaining treatment has been made. For most, the end comes gradually. Chronic illnesses, such as heart disease and cancer, account for more than two thirds of the nation's deaths. Some people want their doctors to do everything humanly possible for them and to make sure that lifesaving measures are not withdrawn. Many others do not want to end up attached to sophisticated equipment that can never cure, only keep them alive. On any given day, ten thousand patients exist in this twilight zone. The condition of Alzheimer's patients brings up other controversial issues. They, and their families, fear the onset of dementia. What if the patient forgets how to swallow? Should a feeding tube be inserted?

Although it's a closely guarded secret in the medical community, you should know that you have the right to refuse medical treatment — even treatment others consider "good for you" — that may prolong or save your life. The U.S. Supreme Court indicated in 1990 that the right to refuse life-prolonging treatment is guaranteed by the Constitution.

One tragic case that exemplified the need for such a ruling was that of Elizabeth Bouvia, a completely bedridden young woman stricken with cerebral palsy. At twenty-three, she was a paraplegic, unable to use a wheelchair, sit up, move any part of her body beyond a few fingers of her right hand or her facial muscles, and dependent on others to feed, wash, and help her with bodily functions. She was in constant pain. In 1983, she tried to starve herself to death in a Los Angeles hospital. When the hospital insisted on force-feeding her, a California court supported the hospital. Three years later, Elizabeth Bouvia lay in another Los Angeles hospital, being force-fed through a tube in her stomach. She sued to have the tube removed, and this time she won. The court stated that "a competent adult patient has the legal right to refuse medical treatment." It ordered the hospital to remove the feeding tube and give her medication to alleviate her pain.

For Elizabeth Bouvia, and many others who want to determine their own fate, refusing medical treatment isn't easy. Doctors are trained to save lives, not to end them. Some physicians believe, as a matter of medical ethics, that they must use every means available to prolong life. Mostly, however, physicians and hospitals are worried about lawsuits, a fear that has little basis in reality. "No doctor or hospital has ever been sued successfully for terminating treatment of a hopelessly ill patient in response to a request from the person or the family," says M. Rose Gasner, former general counsel of Choice in Dying.

Legal Documents

If you are completely certain that you do not want to be kept alive by machines or tubes, make your wishes known in advance. One way is to write a living will. Another is to appoint a close friend or relative to make medical decisions, should you become incapacitated, by signing a durable power of attorney or health care proxy. Because living wills may be interpreted by courts and your wishes frustrated, many attorneys consider a durable power of attorney or health care proxy to be preferable. The legal term for these documents is "advance directives."

Living Will

A living will is a formal legal document you sign, usually in the presence of two witnesses, when you are competent. Unlike a normal will, it takes effect while you are still alive but are unable to communicate your desires about treatment, for example, in a coma. Although the specific wording of a living will varies according to state law and your needs, generally it says that if you have a terminal illness from which there is no reasonable hope of recovery, you do not want your life to be prolonged by the use of life-support measures. In effect, a living will tells your doctors that you have thought about the end of life and prefer to die naturally rather than be subjected to technology that will let you exist but not recover.

No one symbolized the need for a living will more than Nancy Cruzan. On January 11, 1983, life as the twenty-five-year-old young woman knew it came to an end as she lay unconscious in her overturned Nash Rambler outside Carthage, Missouri. Her brain was deprived of oxygen for twenty minutes before paramedics could restart her heart. Rushed to a hospital, Ms. Cruzan lay unconscious for seven years, sustained by feeding tubes. Doctors agreed that she had no chance of recovering. Convinced that their daughter would not have wanted to exist that way, her parents sued to have the feeding tubes disconnected. By the time her case reached the Supreme Court, Nancy Cruzan had become a symbol. In its 1990 landmark decision, the Court found that she had a constitutional right to refuse life-prolonging medical treatment. If, while she was competent, she had clearly and convincingly said that she would have wanted life-support measures removed, her wishes would have had to be respected when she was unconscious. However, like most Americans, Ms. Cruzan had not left a living will or unequivocally expressed her desires. As a result, the Supreme Court refused to authorize removal of the tubes.

The publicity prompted three of Ms. Cruzan's friends to come forward. They testified that Nancy had told them she would never want to "live like a vegetable" on medical machines. Because their testimony gave the clear and convincing proof of Ms. Cruzan's desires, a Missouri court authorized removal of the feeding tubes. Nancy Cruzan died on December 26, 1990.

As you write a living will, think about what could happen to you and what you would want done in various circumstances. Here are some decisions to consider:

- Do you want to be kept alive by a respirator?
- Should food and water delivered through a tube be withheld?
- Do you want cardiopulmonary resuscitation (CPR) in case of a heart attack? CPR is not a gentle kiss of life. It is violent and highly intrusive; it can involve someone pounding your heart, applying electric shocks to it, shoving breathing tubes down your throat, and performing open heart massage. Many people do not want it, particularly if it will only extend a painful existence for a few more days or weeks. CPR is practically a reflex procedure in most hospitals, almost all of which have rules specifying when it should be used. New York State law requires doctors to ask their entering hospital patients whether they want a "do not resuscitate" order entered on their chart.
- Do you want chemotherapy? Kidney dialysis?
- Do you want major surgery? Minor surgery? Blood transfusions? Antibiotics?
- Do you want maximum pain relief even if it shortens your life?
- If you have dementia or advanced Alzheimer's and can no longer swallow, do you want to have a feeding tube inserted?

Remember that you have the option of saying that you want everything medically possible done to keep you alive and that you always have the right to change your mind.

Living wills present two problems. First, the laws of some states are restrictive. For example, California, which passed the first law authorizing living wills, limits their use to the terminally ill faced with imminent death, thus excluding people who are permanently unconscious.

Second, nobody has a crystal ball. Who can predict what is going to happen to them? In some states, if you fail to predict your specific condition toward the end of your life, your wishes may not be carried out. This happened to Mary O'Connor, a seventy-seven-year-old New Yorker who had suffered a series of strokes. Confined to a nursing home, Ms. O'Connor was paralyzed, severely demented, and no longer recognized her two daughters who visited her daily. Before her stroke, Ms. O'Connor had frequently expressed her view that artificial means should not be used to sustain life. In one conversation about Karen Quinlan, she said, that it was "monstrous to keep someone alive . . . by using machinery and things like that when they were not going to get better." Her two daughters refused to allow the nursing home to insert a feeding tube. The nursing home went to court. New York's highest court ordered the tubes inserted on the grounds that Ms. O'Connor had never talked specifically about dying from starvation and about artificial feeding.

Durable Power of Attorney and Health Care Proxy

To avoid the problem of anticipating every possibility, you can sign a durable power of attorney or health care proxy. These legal documents authorize another person to make medical — *including life-and-death* — decisions if you become incapacitated and are unable to communicate. A durable power of attorney can also authorize your agent to make financial decisions for you (see Chapter 12). The person you appoint will make decisions on the basis of your specific instructions or their knowledge of your personality, character, tastes, and desires. In case of unforeseen circumstances, your agent will have the flexibility to make the decisions you would have wanted made.

Most people appoint a spouse, a relative, or a close friend. Above all, appoint someone you trust and have confidence in, someone who is familiar with your feelings about terminal and other care, who supports them, and who would be likely to make the same decisions for you that you would make for yourself. Be sure to choose someone who will act for you and not shrink from making difficult and painful decisions.

Since your proxy or agent will be making life-and-death decisions on your behalf, it is important to discuss your feelings about medical treatment with him or her. Talk about your attitudes toward respirators, tube feeding, surgery, antibiotics, dialysis, chemotherapy, and pain relief.

Know Your State's Law

State laws on living wills, durable powers of attorney, and health proxies are a patchwork quilt. Nearly every state has a law recognizing living wills, but that is where the similarity ends. They differ about such basics as when a living will can be used and whether food and water can be withdrawn. For example, if you were in a persistent vegetative state and your living will specified that you did not want to be kept alive in that condition, it would not do you any good in Oklahoma, whose law recognizes living wills only for people with a few hours or days of life remaining. By contrast, it would be recognized in South Dakota, where the law allows wishes expressed in a living will to govern treatment decisions of people in a persistent vegetative state. If you were terminally ill in Montana, feeding tubes could be withdrawn. In Kentucky, they would have to remain.

Under the federal Patient Self-Determination Act, most hospitals and nursing homes must tell entering patients about their rights to refuse treatment under state law. They also must document whether a patient has a living will, power of attorney, or health care proxy.

Where to Turn for Help

Because state laws differ so dramatically and because advance directives — living wills, durable powers of attorney, and health care proxies — are formal legal documents, be sure that your wishes are expressed in a form that will be recognized in your state. Choice in Dying can advise you about the law in your state and send you, free of charge, appropriate forms to use when you write or call: 250 West 57th Street, New York, NY 10107, (212) 246-6973.

Give your doctor, clergyman, and close family members a copy of your living will, durable power of attorney, or health care proxy. Discuss your wishes with them, not only to inform them but also to help you clarify your own thoughts. Carry in your wallet or purse a card stating that you have an advance directive and indicating where it is kept.

What If There Is No Legal Document?

Families, Doctors, and Courts

If you haven't clearly expressed your wishes, someone will have to divine what they are. Doctors usually turn to close family members, who are presumed to know what the patient would have wanted and how his or her best interests would be served. For most of the 1.1 million who die every year after life support is terminated, family members decide in consultation with doctors, perhaps with the guidance of a hospital ethics committee. The vast majority of Americans believe this is proper. In a Harris poll, more than 80 percent of those asked said that family and doctors should decide about life-support measures when patients are unable to.

Sometimes cases end up in court, usually because a hospital or nursing home, fearing a lawsuit, refuses to terminate treatment, but sometimes because family members can't agree. These cases involve hard legal and ethical decisions that people must make when faced with disconnecting a respirator or withdrawing feeding tubes from a person who has lost the ability to communicate. Karen Quinlan and Nancy Cruzan were two permanently unconscious people whose families had to go to court.

Paul Brophy, a forty-six-year-old Easton, Massachusetts, firefighter and emergency medical technician who loved fishing, hunting, and gardening, was another. In March 1983, Mr. Brophy complained of a splitting headache and fainted. He was rushed to a hospital, where doctors found a ruptured blood vessel in his brain and performed emergency surgery. Since Mr. Brophy could not swallow, his wife of twenty-seven years authorized the hospital to insert a feeding tube.

Mr. Brophy, who never regained consciousness, lapsed into a persistent vegetative state. Although his higher brain functions were severely damaged, he still responded to stimuli, blinking, for example, if someone shone a flashlight in his eyes. Damage to his brain was so severe that neurologists declared he would never recover. Supported by their five adult children, Mr. Brophy's seven brothers and sisters, and their parish priest, Mrs. Brophy asked the hospital to remove the feeding tube.

The hospital refused and Mrs. Brophy went to court. The evidence was quite clear that Mr. Brophy would not want to be kept alive. He had once received a commendation for rescuing a man from a burning truck. The man died three months later of severe burns. Mr. Brophy threw the medal away. "I should have been five minutes later. It would have been all over for him," he told one of his brothers. "If I'm ever like that, just shoot me."

Despite this evidence, the judge refused to authorize removal of the tube. Mrs. Brophy appealed. The Supreme Judicial Court of Massachusetts found that Paul Brophy had a right to refuse life-prolonging medical treatment. Since he could not exercise his right, his wife could do it for him. The court ordered the hospital to transfer Mr. Brophy to another facility or to his home, where the tube could be removed. He died eight days later, on October 24, 1986.

Life-and-Death Decisions for Another

Suppose you are asked to decide about starting, stopping, or continuing life-prolonging treatment for a close relative in a hospital or nursing home. How do you go about making such momentous decisions? The following steps can provide guidance:

Make sure that the person is not competent to make the decision. A person is considered competent if he or she can understand the nature and consequences of an illness and its treatment. Obviously, someone in a coma cannot make medical decisions. However, a patient who is conscious and rational, must make them, no matter how upsetting it may be to you. The decision about competence is often resolved at bedside by a doctor or a team of doctors in consultation with close family members. Doctors sometimes believe that nobody in his or her right mind would want to die and consider a person who refuses lifesaving measures to be incompetent. This is not true.

Find out whether someone was named to make health care decisions. Has the patient signed a durable power of attorney or health proxy? If the answer is yes, the person named in the document is responsible for making life-and-death decisions.

Get as accurate a medical picture as possible. Ask the doctors questions like these:

- What happened?
- What is the person's condition? Is he or she in a coma? Unconscious? In a persistent vegetative state? Severely brain damaged or brain dead? In pain?
- What are the prospects for recovery? Will he or she regain consciousness? Be aware of the surroundings or able to recognize people? Communicate? Will he or she lead a life of pain? What activities will he or she be able to do?
- What are the treatment alternatives and the pros and cons of each? Are they temporary or permanent measures? What about using a respirator? Hooking up feeding tubes? Continuing chemotherapy or dialysis? Treating infections with antibiotics? Giving pain relief?

Perfect accuracy is not possible, as the unusual case of Carrie Coons illustrates. Ms. Coons, an eighty-six-year-old New Yorker, suffered a massive stroke, which led to severe bleeding in the brain. After she was diagnosed as being in a hopeless and irreversible persistent vegetative state, a judge authorized removal of the feeding tubes. Before this could be done, Ms. Coons unexpectedly regained consciousness. Her doctor explained what had happened to her and asked what she wanted done about the feeding tube. She replied, "That's a very difficult decision to make," and promptly fell back unconscious.

Discover the patient's wishes, if known. Did he or she have a living will? Had he or she discussed what should be done in this situation? Did the patient say anything in reaction to the death of others? Ask as many family members and friends as you can.

The case of Brother Joseph Fox illustrates the kind of statements that indicate a person's desires. Brother Fox was a member of the Society of Mary, a Catholic religious order. In 1979, at the age of eighty-three, he developed a hernia while lifting some flower pots in a garden. During an operation to repair the hernia, Brother Fox had a heart attack, suffered massive brain damage, and was placed on a respirator, which maintained him in a vegetative state. The doctors said there was no reasonable hope of recovery. His close friend and confessor, Brother Eichner, asked the hospital to remove the respirator. The hospital refused to do so without court authorization.

New York State's highest court authorized removal of the respirator based on statements Brother Fox had made in the past. Discussing Karen Quinlan, Brother Fox said that he would not want any of this "extraordinary business" done on him. He expressed agreement with the Catholic church position that permits removal of life-support equipment from a person with no reasonable prospect of recovery. Shortly before the operation, he repeated that he would not want his life prolonged artificially if his condition were hopeless. The court found these statements to be clear and convincing evidence that Brother Fox did not want to be maintained in a vegetative state by a respirator.

If the person's wishes are not clearly stated, determine what he or she would have wanted done in the circumstances. Legally, this is known as substituted judgment or surrogate decision making. Most states allow close family members to make medical decisions for a person based on their knowledge of what the patient would have wanted done. The goal is to determine, insofar as possible, the decision the patient would have made if able to choose.

This involves looking at the patient's character, religious beliefs, opinion about medical treatment, and overall lifestyle. Did he or she hate all doctors and medical treatment? Refuse to take medication in the past? (In one case, a patient's earlier refusal to accept a pacemaker persuaded a judge that he would have refused life-support systems.) Was he or she an active and independent person who would loathe being bathed and changed by others?

Determine what is in the person's best interests. If the person has left no instructions, some states permit a decision to be made on the basis of the patient's "best interests." It means that you must weigh the burdens and the benefits of the treatment. What would life be like if treatment were continued? Would it be one of pain and suffering? Helplessness? Dependence on others for feeding, cleaning, and toilet functions? Is the treatment so intrusive that privacy and human dignity would be destroyed? Would the quality of life be so low in comparison with what it had previously been that no reasonable person would want to live it? These are the kinds of questions you must ask.

One famous case involved a profoundly retarded sixty-seven-year-old Massachusetts man suffering from leukemia who had the mental ability of a two-year-old and had spent his entire life in an institution. A decision had to be reached whether to treat his cancer with chemotherapy. Without treatment, he would die a relatively painless death within weeks or months. With chemotherapy, he would undergo great pain whose purpose he would not understand; at best, chemotherapy would produce a remission of only a year. Massachusetts's highest court ruled that chemotherapy could lawfully be withheld.

Withdrawing Food and Water

Legally and medically, withdrawing food and water is no different from disconnecting a respirator or turning off a dialysis machine. Emotionally, it is a red flag. Feeding the hungry, as ethicist Daniel Callahan notes, is the most fundamental of all human relationships. Withholding food and water condemns a patient to what many people feel instinctively must be a painful death by starvation. Without food and water, a person can live only a short time. Removing a respirator usually leads to death shortly afterward, but not always. As previously noted, Karen Quinlan lived for nine years after being taken off one.

Although the members of the Supreme Court issued five separate opinions in the Cruzan case, there was one issue all could agree on: withdrawing feeding tubes is no different from withdrawing other medical treatment. As Justice Sandra Day O'Connor stated, feeding a patient through a nasogastric tube requires a physician to insert a long flexible tube through the patient's nose, throat, and esophagus and into the stomach. A gastrostomy or jejunostomy tube must be surgically implanted in the stomach or small intestine. These are all uncomfortable invasive procedures, instituted by doctors, with significant risks.

The Supreme Court's view coincides with prevailing medical opinion. In 1986, the American Medical Association adopted the position that "life-prolonging treatment includes medication and artificially or technologically supplied respiration, nutrition, or hydration." Two years later, the American Academy of Neurology adopted a similar definition and added that patients in a persistent vegetative state do not have the capacity to experience pain. In other words, depriving a permanently unconscious person of food and water cannot cause suffering. Despite the near unanimity of views, some states have laws prohibiting it. The constitutionality of these laws may be tested in the courts in coming years.

If You Disagree with the Hospital

Suppose your father lies comatose in a hospital. Knowing that he wouldn't want to be kept alive that way, you ask the doctors to disconnect the respirator. The doctors, having consulted the hospital administration, refuse. What should you do if faced with such a situation?

First, try to get the matter resolved in the hospital. Discuss it with the patient representative or hospital ethics committee, if there is one. Find out the reasons for the hospital's refusal. It may be that it's too early to tell about the patient's condition. Neurologists say, for example, that it takes one to three months to tell whether severe brain damage is likely to be permanent. Or the hospital may be waiting to get the opinion of other family members.

If the hospital persists in its refusal and you are convinced that you are carrying out the person's wishes or serving his or her best interests, call your area agency on aging (see Chapter 12) or Choice in Dying for advice. Hospice or home care, or transfer to another facility, may be another option. As a last resort, you can hire a lawyer and sue to compel the hospital to remove the life-support systems.

Whether you must pay for medical care forced on you against

your wishes by a hospital or nursing home is not yet clear. One New York judge ruled in the negative. On July 30, 1986, sixty-year-old Jean Elbaum was admitted to North Shore Hospital on Long Island after a blood vessel in her brain ruptured. She fell into a coma and was diagnosed as being in a persistent vegetative state with no hope of recovery. Although Ms. Elbaum had stated on several occasions that she would not want life-support systems if she were in such a hopeless state, the doctor pressured Murray Elbaum, her husband of thirty-six years, into consenting to insertion of a gastrointestinal feeding tube.

Ms. Elbaum was then transferred to Grace Plaza nursing home, where Mr. Elbaum repeatedly told the administrators that his wife would not want to be kept alive in her condition and requested that the feeding tube be removed. They refused. After demanding in writing that the tube be taken out, Mr. Elbaum stopped paying the bills. At that point, he went to court and got an order instructing the nursing home to transfer Ms. Elbaum to a facility that would remove the tube or, if none were available, to find a doctor who would do it there. Ms. Elbaum was moved to a hospice where the feeding tube was withdrawn. She died a week later. The nursing home then went to court to collect the more than $100,000 it claimed was owed for the care it had given Ms. Elbaum. The judge ruled that it was not entitled to be paid for unwanted medical treatment delivered over Mr. Elbaum's objections. The decision is being appealed.

Taking the Law into Your Own Hands

On August 2, 1988, six-month-old Samuel Linares swallowed a balloon, choked, and fell unconscious. Grabbing his son, Rudolfo Linares unsuccessfully tried mouth-to-mouth resuscitation, called 911, and then, clutching his son, ran a block to the nearest firehouse shouting, "Help me! Help me! My son is dying!" Firemen removed the balloon with a forceps, but by that time Samuel had stopped breathing. After the baby had spent twenty minutes without any vital signs, cardiopulmonary resuscitation succeeded in getting his heart beating again.

Eight months later, Samuel lay unconscious in Rush-Presbyterian–St. Luke's Medical Center in Chicago. An EEG showed minimal brain activity. Samuel was in a persistent vegetative state, and the doctors said there was no chance the baby would recover. The grief-stricken parents asked the hospital to disconnect the respirator. The hospital refused.

On April 25, 1989, Mr. Linares walked into the pediatric intensive care unit of the hospital and pulled out a .357 Magnum. "I am not going to hurt anyone," he said. "I just want to let my son die." He unplugged the respirator and held Samuel in his arms until the child stopped breathing. Then he slid the gun across the floor to the police. Mr. Linares was charged with first-degree murder. A grand jury refused to indict him. Ultimately he received a suspended sentence for illegal possession of a weapon.

Although desperate people resort to desperate measures, you cannot take the law into your own hands and pull the plug, even though you think your loved one's life will be mercifully ended. No matter how benevolent the motive, criminal law considers it murder. Roswell Gilbert spent five years in a Florida maximum security prison for what he contends was the mercy killing of his wife of fifty-one years. Seventy-two-year-old Emily Gilbert had Alzheimer's, and Mr. Gilbert, saying he couldn't bear to see her suffer, shot her twice and killed her. Convicted of first-degree murder in 1985, eighty-one-year-old Gilbert was pardoned by Governor Bob Martinez in 1990 on the basis of old age and ill health. The case so captured the attention of the public that it became the subject of a television movie starring Robert Young.

If You Want Aggressive Treatment

What if you must make a decision for your wife, who is comatose and unable to talk to you or anybody else about what she wants? What if the doctors tell you that her case is hopeless? What if you and your children decide you want every possible life-sustaining treatment continued?

It happened to Helga Wanglie, an eighty-seven-year-old former schoolteacher who lay unconscious and brain damaged for eight months, sustained by a respirator and feeding tube, in a Minneapolis hospital. Ms. Wanglie's tragic saga began on December 14, 1989, when she tripped on a scatter rug in the hall of her home and broke her right hip. After developing breathing problems, she was transferred to the Hennepin County Medical Center in Minneapolis, where she was put on a respirator. Several months later, she was transferred to a long-term-care facility, where she had a heart attack. By the time she was resuscitated, her brain had been deprived of oxygen. Brain damaged and respirator dependent, she was returned to the Hennepin County Medical Center.

Her doctors said she had no reasonable hope of regaining consciousness and requested authority to turn off the respirator. After meeting several times with the medical staff, Ms. Wanglie's husband of fifty-three years, retired Minneapolis lawyer Oliver Wanglie, and their children, Ruth, forty-eight, and David, forty-five, refused to agree to removal of the respirator. "It seems to me that they're trying to play God," Mr. Wanglie told the New York Times. "Who are they to determine who's to die and who's to live? I take the position that as long as her heart is beating, there's life there."

The Wanglie family also argued that Ms. Wanglie, the daughter of a Lutheran minister, wanted all life-sustaining treatment continued and that they were expressing her wishes. Finally, the hospital went to court. "It would be novel and ironic to conclude that this person has a right to remain on a ventilator in a country where there is no general right to health care," wrote Dr. Steven Miles, a member of an ethics committee assigned to this case. "It also does not strike me that the physician is imposing his quality-of-life standard on this patient in that he would provide treatment if this woman had any personal sensation of her quality of life."

The judge decided in favor of the family and gave Oliver Wanglie the right to make decisions for his wife. "He is in the best position to investigate and act upon Helga Wanglie's conscientious, religious, and moral beliefs," said Judge Patricia Belois. The respirator stayed on. After being in a persistent vegetative state for over a year, Helga Wanglie died on July 4, 1991.

Since the vast majority of disagreements involve patients or their families who want life-support systems terminated, cases such as Helga Wanglie's are rare. There may be some limits on how much futile treatment a patient or family can demand, but it is not yet clear what they are. The lesson of the Wanglie case is that if you want to have everything medically possible done to keep you alive, even if you become permanently unconscious, be sure to spell out your wishes in a living will or discussions with the person you appoint to make health care decisions for you.

14

WHEN YOU NEED A LAWYER

CONTENTS

LIKE FINDING a good doctor or a good plumber, finding a good lawyer appears to be one of life's eternal mysteries. Of course, there are those who seem blessed by a certain type of star that leads them to the right professional every time. And then there are the rest of us. Indeed, one of the questions I am always asked — by clients seeking a referral, by my students, and by audience members to whom I speak — is how to find a decent, competent lawyer who won't charge the moon.

This is not to suggest that you rush to an attorney at the slightest hint of a problem or immediately sue somebody who caused you minor discomfort. But many times you need a lawyer to help you assert your rights and protect your own and your family's interests. Take malpractice. According to a Harvard University study, if you go into a hospital for surgery, the chances are one in twenty-five that something will go wrong in the operation and one in a hundred that you will be injured by negligent treatment. If you were the victim of malpractice, would you know where to find a competent attorney?

Or take the emotional, financial, and physical dilemmas faced by the elderly. Added to the mess of Medicare and Medigap is the task of trying to figure out whether long-term-care insurance is a good idea, the fear of becoming seriously ill and being tethered to machines with no hope of recovery, and the fervent desire to ensure that life savings are passed on to children and heirs, not drained away on phenomenally costly and ultimately futile medical technology. If you are in this position, or have a parent who is, do you know where to go for sound legal advice?

What if you are getting sick from working in a harmful environment? Or instead of benefits from an insurance company or the government, all you are getting is a runaround? Or you face job discrimination because of a handicap? The list goes on and on. How do you go about finding a competent, reasonably priced lawyer? Beyond looking in the *Yellow Pages*, most people don't have a clue. Yet lawyers manage to unravel the mystery for themselves. They know where to look if *they* need a lawyer to represent them.

In this chapter we share some of these lawyers' secrets. We tell you how to find and talk to an attorney, what you should know about fees, and what takes place in a lawsuit. The process may be time-consuming, but following our advice should lead you to a skilled attorney who will work hard to protect your interests.

Finding Mr. or Ms. Right: The Three I's

If you placed an ad in a "Personals" section of a newspaper, it might read like this: "Wanted: highly skilled, well-trained, experienced lawyer, particularly knowledgeable in [the area of your problem]. Must be a lamb to the client and a lion to the opposition. Must be easily reachable, willing to keep client informed, and selfless in pursuit of client's interests. Affordable rates only."

It probably sounds too good to be true, but there are ways to find an attorney who fills at least part of the bill. (A classified ad is definitely *not* the way to go.) We've devised a system that should lead you to a capable lawyer who knows his or her stuff. Since attorneys are not known for their modesty, we call our system the three I's: *Investigate, Interview,* and *Identify.*

Investigate
Your first task is to put together a list of recommended attorneys. Then, do your homework. Here are some sources of referrals.

- **Family and friends.** A personal reference from somebody whose opinion you trust is the way to start. If your brother-in-law was happy with his lawyer, get the name, but find out why he hired the lawyer. An attorney who drafted a will competently may not be the best person to represent you in a workers' compensation case.
- **Lawyers.** Attorneys are usually well connected and have some idea about whether other lawyers are any good. If you know any lawyers, or have friends or business contacts who do, ask them for a referral.
- **Your state or local bar association.** Bar associations are the professional organizations of lawyers. Every state has one; so do many counties and large cities. They can be a good source of referrals if used properly.

Call the bar association and ask for the person who handles referrals. Tell that person about your problem and ask for the names of lawyers who can help you. The bar association should be able to give you the names of three lawyers who specialize in your area of need, say, personal injury or health insurance. Referral from a bar association is not a guarantee of excellence. Any attorney can claim expertise in a specific area and ask to be put on the referral list. As with doctor referral services, many successful attorneys do not place their names on such lists.

A better way is to ask for the names of lawyers who give continuing legal education courses in your problem area. "Bar associations sponsor these short, usually one-day, sessions in which specialists give lectures to other lawyers to bring them up to date on the latest developments in the field. For example, an 'elder law' specialist might give a lecture on protecting assets," says Robert L. Herbst, a New York City trial lawyer. If this is your problem, contact the attorney giving the course. You may want him or her to represent you or to recommend somebody else.

A third way is to get the name of the leaders and past leaders of the section that deals with your problem. Bar associations are divided into sections of specialists. If, for example, a soda bottle exploded in your hand and sent fragments of glass into your face, you would want to reach lawyers involved with the product liability section.

You can look up the state or local bar association in the phone directory. If you run into problems finding it, call the American Bar Association, (312) 988-5000.

- **Support and Advocacy Groups.** National and community groups concerned with your problem can be an excellent source of referrals to lawyers. The names of many of these groups are sprinkled throughout this book. For example, the American Association of Retired Persons could recommend a lawyer for an older person, Planned Parenthood a lawyer knowledgeable about abortion, and Committees on Occupational Safety and Health a legal expert in hazardous work environments.

- **Legal Defense Groups.** Not-for-profit legal services or legal defense funds can be a good source of referrals. Do not expect them to represent you. Short of money and staffed by dedicated, overworked lawyers, they have to pick the people they represent very carefully, most often those who are indigent or whose cases can establish important legal precedents. Among the groups are the American Civil Liberties Union, (212) 944-9800, and the National Health Law Program, (213) 204-6010. Other, more specialized groups such as the Lambda Legal Defense and Education Fund (for AIDS) or the Medicare Beneficiaries Defense Fund are mentioned throughout the book.

Interview

After you have compiled a list of lawyers you think can help you, the next step is the interview. When you call to set up the initial appointment, give the lawyer a brief summary of your situation and ask if he or she has handled this type of case and feels comfortable with it. Use this phone call to screen the lawyer by asking about his or her background, experience, and opinion of the case. The responses and kinds of questions the lawyer asks should give you an inkling of how you two would relate.

Some lawyers charge for the initial interview, whether or not you hire them. Find out in advance if there is a charge and how much it is. If it is prohibitive, go on to the next name on your list. Also ask whether you should bring any materials to the interview. Remember that each of you is interviewing the other at the initial meeting. You are trying to find out whether you feel comfortable with this person and whether he or she has the background, skill, time, and interest to do an excellent job for you at a price you can afford. On the other side of the desk, the attorney wants to determine your needs, your chances of winning if a lawsuit is involved, and whether you two are a good fit.

At your first meeting, tell the attorney why you're there. Be completely open and honest — and brief. Don't go off on tangents. No one wants to hear that you burned the chicken because Medicare turned down your claim. Or that you blew a key presentation because you found a packet of birth control pills in your daughter's underwear drawer. On the other hand, don't leave out facts because you think they will hurt you or gloss over details for fear the attorney won't take your case. "The worst thing you can do is lie to your lawyer," says Washington, D.C., attorney Stephen M. Nassau. Lawyers plan their strategy on the basis of what their clients tell them. If you lie, and your attorney is later surprised by the facts, you suffer. If you're tempted to refashion the truth, remember what Joe Friday used to say: "Just the facts, ma'am."

Many people are intimidated at the thought of interviewing a lawyer. Don't be. This is a person with whom you will be working closely, whom you must trust, and with whom you may share intimate secrets. It is important to find somebody who is not only qualified but with whom you feel comfortable. Keep in mind that *you* are the one purchasing the services and that lawyers need clients as much as clients need lawyers.

CHECKLIST: INTERVIEWING AN ATTORNEY

To help you get the most information on which you can base your choice of attorney, we have drawn up ten questions for you to ask an attorney during an initial interview.

- **Where did you get your law degree and how long have you been in practice?** This is good background information to have. You can check the lawyer's credentials in *Martindale-Hubbell*, a compendium of lawyers available in most libraries. Do not make the mistake of searching only for a lawyer who has gone to a prestigious law school like Harvard or Stanford. Many excellent lawyers graduate from local law schools that do not have an illustrious reputation.
- **What areas do you specialize in?** Clearly, you want somebody knowledgeable in the area of your problem. In smaller communities, lawyers handle all sorts of legal matters; in larger ones, they specialize. You don't want a tax specialist to prepare your medical malpractice case.
- **How many situations like mine have you handled?** This is a critical question. If the attorney never worked on a prob-

lem like yours, go elsewhere. You don't want to pay for on-the-job training.

- **What are the strengths and weaknesses of my case (if applicable)?** This tests the lawyer's analytical skills and lets you decide whether he or she really understands your situation.
- **What are the chances of my winning or getting a favorable settlement?** Beware of snow jobs. If the lawyer is very enthusiastic about your case, find out specifically why. On the other hand, if the response is negative, ask why the lawyer does not think you have a strong case.
- **What legal strategy do you have in mind?** The answer to this question reveals how the lawyer thinks and whether he or she can talk in terms you can understand. Determine whether the lawyer's views on settling or trying the case are compatible with yours.
- **How long will it take?** Don't be discouraged if the answer is in years, particularly if you are contemplating a lawsuit, which can drag on forever.
- **How will you keep me informed about what's happening?** You want a lawyer who is willing to share information with you. How often will the lawyer discuss the case with you? Will he or she send you copies of all relevant documents?
- **Will you handle the case personally?** In large firms, the senior lawyers farm out the scut work to lower-paid associates or make extensive use of specialists. It has the advantage of reducing costs and, perhaps, being more efficient. It may have the disadvantage of your lawyer's not being fully aware of all aspects of your case and, perhaps, not giving it the personal attention it deserves.
- **How much will it cost and how will you bill me?** We discuss lawyers' fees and expenses later in this chapter.

Identify

How will you know when you've identified Mr. or Ms. Right? After evaluating the lawyer's background, experience, and apparent skill, it comes down to the intangible: trust your instincts. The way the lawyer answers your questions, the respect with which he or she treats you, the ability with which he or she analyzes your case, can all give you a sense of whether the person is for you. Ask yourself whether this attorney is capable of representing your interests, willing to put in the time, and, finally, whether you feel comfortable with him or her.

"The key element is whether the attorney makes sense to you," says Robert Herbst. "Whatever else lawyers have to do, they must be able to present matters in understandable terms. If you can't figure out what a lawyer is talking about, find someone else."

Once you have made your decision, be sure to sign a retainer agreement. This contract between you and the lawyer specifies what he or she is going to do for you and how much it will cost or at least the basis for determining the cost. Most lawyers ask for a *retainer*, an advance payment, at this time. Don't hire a lawyer on the basis of an oral understanding. You don't want to go into shock when you get a huge bill you never anticipated for work you did not think you were authorizing.

All about Lawyers' Fees

Almost the only thing that makes people more nervous than talking to a lawyer is waiting for the lawyer's bill. Legal fees add up — quickly. You should know how you will be charged and what you can do to keep the fees within reasonable bounds. Lawyers bill their clients in three ways:

- **Hourly fees.** When lawyers draft contracts, handle business or family matters, or do the day-to-day work that occupies most of their time, they usually charge on an hourly basis. They tote up the number of hours spent on the case, multiply by their fee per hour, and bill the client. Hourly rates can vary from $50 to more than $400. In addition to determining the hourly rate, get an estimate of the number of hours the attorney expects to spend on the case. Request that you be told when the fees reach a specified level. Remember that lawyers also charge for phone conversations, so don't be overly chatty, unless you are willing to pay. "Find out whether an attorney charges a minimum amount of time, such as fifteen minutes, for each phone call or conversation, no matter how brief," advises Stephen Nassau.

- **Flat fees.** Some legal matters, such as drafting an uncomplicated will or reviewing a nursing home admission contract, can be done for an amount fixed in advance. Make sure to clarify whether the agreed-upon fee includes the attorney's expenses.

- **Contingency fees.** If you are bringing a lawsuit for an injury you have sustained, for example, through medical malpractice or a harmful product, the lawyer often takes the case on a contingency basis. This means that you do not have to pay a lawyer's fee if you lose. If you win, you give the lawyer a certain percentage, commonly one third, after expenses are deducted. To take a simple example, if you won a $1.1 million judgment and expenses were $100,000, the lawyer would first be reimbursed for out-of-pocket costs — $100,000 — and then take $333,000 from the remaining million dollars. You would walk away with $667,000. Some lawyers use a sliding scale, charging a smaller percentage if the case is settled out of court and a larger one if it has to be tried.

  In an effort to cut back on malpractice and product liability lawsuits, some states have limited the percentage a lawyer can take on contingency. If lawyers make less money, the theory goes, they will have less incentive to take marginal cases. California, for example, sets a sliding fee for contingency cases, starting with 40 percent of the first $50,000 recovered and going down to 15 percent of any award of over $600,000. In the federal system, lawyers representing clients in Social Security Disability cases are prohibited from charging more than 25 percent of any award their clients win for past injuries.

- **Expenses.** A word of caution. Win, lose, or draw, you are normally responsible for paying your lawyer's expenses, unless you have agreed on an all-inclusive flat fee or the state's ethical code for lawyers allows them to absorb the expenses and your lawyer agrees to do it. In addition to such charges as telephone calls, transportation, transcripts, and court filing fees, in a lawsuit you must pay for the time of expert witnesses, private investigators, and other people whose support is necessary for your case. These can quickly escalate into the thousands of dollars. A lawyer is allowed to advance you the money used to pay the expenses of a lawsuit, but you may ultimately have to cough it up.

Taking the Mystery out of Lawsuits

Carole W. was a vivacious, forty-four-year-old writer when she went to a noted New York orthopedist for recurrent pain in her big toe. He diagnosed her condition as *hallex rigidis*, an arthritic big toe, and recommended surgery. Looking at the impressive array of framed diplomas from top medical institutions on the richly paneled walls of his antique-filled office, and listening to his thoughtful explanation of her condition, Ms. W. agreed to the operation without even seeking a second opinion. After all, she was no novice to the medical profession and knew quality when it stared her in the face. Her father and brother-in-law were doctors. She liked what she heard and what she saw.

As soon as the anesthesia began to wear off after the operation, Ms. W. knew she was in trouble. Her toe was red and inflamed and the pain unbearable. She immediately called the doctor, who responded by telling her it was normal and sent her home. The toe became worse and worse. Whenever she put any weight on it, an excruciating bolt of pain shot through her. Yet every time she called the doctor, he replied calmly, "It's normal. It will get better." If it hadn't hurt so much, she would have kicked herself (and the doctor) for not getting another opinion before going through with the surgery. Finally, he suggested massage therapy, which proved completely ineffective. Because her toe was so painful, Ms. W. ended up spending long days in bed or sitting on a chair. Work was impossible. She continued to call the doctor, but after a while she stopped believing him and became angry at his lack of concern.

Then Ms. W. sought the opinion of another doctor, who said that the procedure was very unusual and outside the bounds of standard medical practice. He explained that too much cartilage had been removed during the (unnecessary) operation and the bones of the toe were rubbing together at the joint, causing the pain. He thought corrective surgery might be necessary but suggested that before taking that step, she try an orthopedic shoe to relieve the pressure. This to a woman who took vacations only to places where she could wear high heels to dinner.

That was when Ms. W. and her husband came to see me. They wanted to know if they had a malpractice case, whether I would represent them, and what would happen if they sued the doctor. I answered that, yes, they probably had a case; that I personally did not take medical malpractice cases but would recommend three lawyers whom I knew to be excellent; and that a malpractice case was a frustrating, unpleasant, time-consuming affair that was likely to leave them unhappy even if they won. Since lawsuits are such a nasty business, they should at least think about whether they really wanted to go through with it.

I also said that despite what they might have read, it's not so easy to find a lawyer to take a malpractice case. Since malpractice lawyers work on a contingency basis and get paid only if they win, a lawyer's first thought will be, "Is this case a winner?" The second is likely to be, "Even if it is, what's the payoff?" or, in this case, "How much is a toe worth?" I also reminded them that even though no lawyer's fees were involved unless they won or settled, they would probably be responsible for the expenses, likely to be in the thousands of dollars.

I then explained what they could expect if they decided to go ahead with their suit. Although every case is different, certain types of preparation and procedures are the same for every lawsuit. All involve a lot of time and money. Roughly, they can be divided into what goes on before, during, and after a trial — if there is one. A lot of cases are settled before the judge even puts on his robes.

Before the Trial

The Summons and the Complaint
To start the case, your lawyer drafts a summons and a complaint, which must be done within a certain period, often two or three years, after the injury occurred or was first noticed. The period, called the *statute of limitations*, differs from state to state. The *summons* informs the other party that you are bringing a lawsuit. The *complaint* is a legal document that briefly describes what happened to you, why you are suing, and the amount you are

asking in damages. The summons and complaint are delivered, usually by a process server or certified mail, to the defendant — the person bringing the lawsuit is the *plaintiff*; the person being sued is the *defendant*. The defendant has a period of time, usually twenty to thirty days, to prepare an *answer* in response to the charges. The answer often denies any and all wrongdoing, but it may also claim that you or someone else was responsible for the injury or offer some other defense.

In their case, I said that Ms. W. would probably charge the doctor with malpractice for negligently performing the operation and failing to warn Ms. W. of its potentially damaging consequences. The doctor would probably deny any negligence in performing the operation and furthermore claim that Ms. W. herself contributed to the injury by walking when she should have been resting the toe.

Pretrial Discovery

The complaint and answer trigger a detailed investigation into the case by the lawyers for both sides. During this process, called *discovery*, the defendant's lawyers try to find out exactly what your case is about and what its strengths and weaknesses are. Your lawyers attempt to learn exactly what happened and anything else they can about the case. Although most people, except lawyers, are not familiar with pretrial discovery, it is a critical element, perhaps *the* critical element, of a lawsuit. It is through this detailed, painstaking effort that the groundwork for the case is built.

Although the rules differ somewhat from state to state, in pretrial discovery witnesses are interviewed, records pored over, investigations carried out. You may be asked to respond under oath to a long list of very detailed questions, called *written interrogatories*. These are questions about your claim, how the injury occurred, any damages that you are asking, and other matters that may or may not be relevant (wide latitude is given in pretrial discovery). On your side, your lawyer may send a list of written questions to the defendant in an effort to discover exactly what happened, who was present during the incident — particularly important for a plaintiff alleging injuries that occurred under anesthesia — and the strengths and weaknesses of the defense. Each side may also ask the other for copies of relevant documents — lots of them, including medical records. You should know that once you bring a malpractice action, your medical records are no longer considered confidential. You will also be examined by the defendant's medical experts and, if you are claiming emotional damages, by psychiatrists as well.

The most important part of the discovery process is often the taking of *depositions*. A deposition is a formal legal proceeding in which the opposing lawyer questions a witness about the case. Depositions are usually taken from the plaintiff, the defendant, and key witnesses. Expect to be questioned. Giving testimony at a deposition is like being a witness at a trial, except that it takes place in a lawyer's office and the opposing lawyer can ask questions that would not be allowed in a courtroom. You testify under oath. A court stenographer is present to transcribe the questions and answers. If your testimony at the deposition differs from your testimony during the trial, the opposing lawyer may seize on the discrepancy to raise questions about your credibility. Your lawyer should advise you beforehand on what to expect.

Settlement

All during this time, settlement offers may fly back and forth and the judge may push both parties to settle. There are likely to be many pretrial settlement conferences. A case can be settled at any time up to the moment a jury delivers its verdict, or after, if the case is appealed. As the case approaches trial, the settlement offers tend to become more serious.

Because of the sheer volume of malpractice cases, many states have taken steps to eliminate probable losers and encourage settlement. Some require that claims be submitted to a mediation or arbitration panel. In my talk with Mr. and Ms. W., I told them that until recently New York State required the parties to present their cases before a medical malpractice panel. The panel, consisting of a judge, a doctor, and a lawyer, offered a written opinion about whether the plaintiff had a viable lawsuit, which could be introduced during the trial. Obviously, if an independent panel of experts doesn't think you have a case and the jury knows it, it's pretty damaging to your side. The panels in New York were dropped when it was discovered that they were not weeding out frivolous claims or leading the parties to settle but were simply delaying cases.

Going Through the Motions

Both before and during the trial, both sides will pepper the judge with *motions,* or formal legal requests for the judge to take some action. For example, I told Mr. and Ms. W. that if the doctor's side refused to provide the relevant medical records, their lawyer would submit a motion to compel the defendants to produce them. And that, frequently, one or both sides submit a *motion for summary judgment,* which says, in effect, that the other side has such a weak case that the judge should throw it out immediately.

The Trial

Finally, after months or even years of preparation, comes the trial. Since most people have watched enough *L.A. Law* or *Perry Mason* reruns on television, we will not delve into the anatomy of a trial in any detail. In brief, for a jury trial, the members of the jury are selected; the attorneys present their opening statements summarizing the facts that they will present; the plaintiff presents its side first, introducing evidence and calling witnesses, who can be cross-examined; next, the defense presents its side; then the plaintiff has a chance to rebut. After closing arguments by the opposing lawyers, the case goes to the judge or the jury.

What viewers of television courtroom drama may not know is that a judge can step in at any time and declare one side the winner. If the evidence is so favorable to one side that there are no substantial issues of fact to be decided, the judge can order summary judgment or direct a verdict in favor of one of the parties. A judge can even reverse the verdict of a jury if he or she believes that the decision was truly unreasonable.

You should know that there is a difference between civil and criminal lawsuits. Malpractice, product liability, and almost all the other lawsuits we discuss in this book are civil actions called *torts,* in which an injured plaintiff asks a court to award money damages or correct a harm that was done. The complaint is filed in a civil court in the name of the plaintiff, who must prove to the satisfaction of a jury that the defendant is probably guilty of the charge.

A criminal case, on the other hand, is brought by the government, as representative of the people. Most criminal cases involve serious property damage, such as arson, or bodily harm, such as homicide or assault — behavior prohibited by law that should be punished. Civil law remedies a wrong by compensating the victim; criminal law punishes the wrongdoer by imprisonment, fine, or both. Since a guilty defendant in a criminal case can land in jail, the jury must find the defendant guilty "beyond a reasonable doubt." A single vote for acquittal results in a hung jury, and the defendant either goes free or has to face a new trial.

In both criminal and civil trials, the defendant can waive the right to a jury and ask that the case be decided by the judge.

After the Trial
The loser has the option of filing an appeal if there was an error in a matter of law. The judge, for example, may have allowed a lawyer to ask a question that prejudiced the case or misinterpreted the law in instructing the jury. A lawyer who fails to object at the time an error is made can't use it as the basis of an appeal. That is why lawyers are always jumping up and shouting, "Objection."

Cases brought in the federal court system, which begin in a district court, can be appealed to one of the twelve courts of appeal. The next and last stop is the U.S. Supreme Court. Cases brought in state courts begin at the trial level, can be appealed to an intermediary appeals court in the larger states, then to the state's highest appeals court. An appeal can be expensive. The cost of copying the records alone can run into thousands of dollars.

Damages
Injured people can sue for two kinds of damages.

- **Compensatory damages,** which compensate for both tangible and intangible losses. *Special damages* are awarded for tangible losses and include items such as hospital expenses, doctors' bills, rehabilitation costs, lost earnings, and other expenses resulting from an injury. *General damages* compensate plaintiffs for pain and suffering and other emotional or psychological difficulties they incur because of the injury. These are harder to calculate and may, in the case of someone who has

sustained a permanent or particularly painful injury, run into hundreds of thousands or even millions of dollars.
- **Punitive damages,** which are intended to punish a defendant for particularly venal conduct. One judge found that punitive damages could be awarded when "malice, vindictiveness, ill-will, or wanton, willful, or reckless disregard of an injured person's rights" is shown. The award is supposed to teach the defendant a lesson and serve as an example to others.

As one example, a jury awarded Carrie Palmer $2.6 million in punitive damages from A. H. Robins Company, makers of the Dalkon Shield intrauterine device, which Ms. Palmer was using when she became pregnant. In her third month, a life-threatening infection raged through her body and she went into shock. To save her life, doctors did a total hysterectomy, removing her uterus, fallopian tubes, and ovaries. From that time on, Ms. Palmer suffered serious health problems. Like many other victims of this device, Ms. Palmer was able to prove to a jury that the Dalkon Shield caused her injuries and that although A. H. Robins knew the IUD was dangerous, the company continued to market it anyway.

Many of the gigantic awards for pain and suffering or punitive damages that make the headlines are frequently lowered on appeal. As part of a growing movement to limit liability for malpractice and harmful products and to reduce insurance premiums, at least twenty-five states have placed a cap on damages for pain and suffering and punitive damages, most commonly $250,000.

Collecting If You Win
Even if you win, don't expect to spend the money immediately. The check won't be in the mail until the legal proceedings are completely over, which can take years. An insurance company is likely to file an appeal, either contesting the verdict or objecting to the amount of the award.

After years of the appeals process, the court of appeals may reduce the size of the award. Or it may order a new trial. If this happens, your initial victory is wiped out and you have to start all over again. Or it may even reverse the verdict and dismiss the case, which means that it's over and you've lost. If none of this happens and the appeals court upholds the decision of the trial court, you are entitled to the award with interest from the date on which the trial court entered its judgment.

Lawsuits: A Long and Winding Road
The length of time and the uncertainty and aggravation of lawsuits motivate many injured people not to bring a lawsuit or to settle, even though they don't feel they have been justly compensated. After talking to several lawyers, Mr. and Ms. W. could not decide whether to pursue their case. Their indecision was not unusual. According to the Harvard University study mentioned earlier in this chapter, only 2 percent of medical malpractice victims decide to sue. If you are considering a lawsuit, the information in this chapter should give you a base on which to make your decision and the tools to find high-quality legal representation. If you do bring a lawsuit, our advice should ease your journey through the legal system.

Perhaps more important, our aim throughout this book has been to show you how to use the law to *avoid* lawsuits. Knowing what questions to ask and what the law does and does not allow can reduce your chances of ending up in court and arm you with the power to determine the course of your own health care.

CASES AND
SOURCES CITED

2. Your Rights as a Patient

the Committee on Small Business, House of Representatives, Apr. 29, 1991.

3. Health Insurance

PAGE

38   The precise number of uninsured people is not known. Harvard University's Center for National Health Program Studies placed the number at 34.7 million people, based on its analysis of U.S. Census data. David U. Himmelstein et al., *The Vanishing Health Care Safety Net: New Data on Uninsured Americans* (Cambridge, Mass.: Center for National Health Program Studies, 1991). The Employee Benefit Research Institute found that 35.7 million Americans under sixty-five have no private insurance coverage of any kind and are not eligible for public programs to finance health care. EBRI, "Sources of Health Insurance and Characteristics of the Uninsured, Analysis of the March 1991 Current Population Survey," *Special Report SR-14*, 1991. The U.S. Bipartisan Commission on Comprehensive Health Care (the Pepper Commission) placed it between 31 and 37 million. *Documentation of Findings*, 1990. According to these sources, two thirds of the uninsured are in families of steadily employed workers, most of whom hold full-time jobs. Nearly half of the uninsured are under twenty-four, and more than one out of every four are under eighteen years old.

38   Milt Freudenheim, "Employers Balk at High Cost of High-Tech Medicine," *New York Times*, Apr. 29, 1990.

38   Health care costs reached $738 billion in 1991 according to the U.S. Commerce Department. Philip Hilts, "U.S. Health Bill Expected to Rise by 11 Percent for '91," *New York Times*, Dec. 30, 1991. The cost of health care is comprehensively reviewed in the statement of Charles A. Bowsher, comptroller general of the United States, "U.S. Health Care Spending: Trends, Contributing Factors, and Proposals for Reform," before the Committee on Ways and Means, House of Representatives, Apr. 17, 1991 (GAO/T-HRD-91-16). A survey by the benefits consulting firm A. Foster Higgins estimated that employers paid, on the average, $3,600 a year per employee for health care in 1991. Milt Freudenheim, "Health Costs Up 12.1 Percent Last Year," *New York Times*, Jan. 28, 1992.

39   Jane Bryant Quinn, "A Buyer's Guide to Cheaper Rates," *Newsweek*, Apr. 23, 1990.

42   Alain Enthoven, "How Employers Boost Health Costs," *Wall Street Journal*, Jan. 24, 1992.

42   Jon Gabel et al., "Employer-Sponsored Health Care in America," *Health Affairs* 8 (2): 116–28 (Summer 1989); Rhonda L. Rundle, "Insurers Step Up Efforts to Reduce Use of Free-Choice Health Plans," *Wall Street Journal*, May 11, 1988.

PAGE

44 Group Health Association of America, *HMO Fact Sheet*, Dec. 1991.

45 Sylvia Law, *Blue Cross: What Went Wrong* (New Haven: Yale University Press, 1976).

45 Elizabeth M. Sloss et al., "Effects of a Health Maintenance Organization on Physiologic Health: Results from a Randomized Trial," *Annals of Internal Medicine* 106 (1): 130–38 (Jan. 1987).

51 National Insurance Consumers Organization, *Buyer's Guide to Insurance*, (1988).

58 Employee Benefit Research Institute, *Retiree Health Benefits: What Is the Promise?* (Washington, D.C.: EBRI, 1989).

4. On the Job

69 U.S. Bureau of Labor Statistics, *Survey of Occupational Injuries and Illnesses in 1990* (1991).

70 Ralph Nader, Introduction, in Joseph Page and Mary-Win O'Brien, *Bitter Wages* (New York: Gross, 1973).

71 Teresa M. Schnorr et al., "Video Display Terminals and the Risk of Spontaneous Abortion," *New England Journal of Medicine* 24 (11): 727–32 (1991).

80 People v. Film Recovery Systems, nos. 84C 5064 and 83C 11901 (Cir. Ct. of Cook County, Ill. June 14, 1985. The case and related cases are examined in Note, "Getting Away with Murder: Federal OSHA Preemption of State Criminal Prosecutions for Industrial Accidents," *Harvard Law Review* 101: 535–54 (1987).

80 Whirlpool Corp. v. Marshall, 445 U.S. 1 (1980).

83 Specialty Cabinet Co. v. Montoya, 734 P.2d 437 (Utah 1986).

84 Hansen v. Von Duprin, 507 N.E.2d 573 (Ind. 1987).

85 Young v. Mutual Savings Life Insurance, 541 So.2d 24 (Ala. Civ. App. 1989).

85 Scott v. Workers Compensation Board, 536 A.2d 492 (Pa. Common. 1988).

90 Arthur Larson, *Workman's Compensation Law*, vol. 2, sec. 13 (New York: Matthew Bender, 1952 with annual supplements).

90 Iverson v. Atlas Pacific Engineering, 191 Cal. Rptr. 696 (Cal. App. 1983).

90 Johns-Manville Products Corp. v. Superior Court of Contra Costa County, 612 P.2d 948 (Cal. 1980).

93 Health Insurance Association of America, *The Consumer's Guide to Disability Insurance* (1990).

103 Council on Scientific Affairs, American Medical Association, "Scientific Issues in Drug Testing," *Journal of the American Medical Association* 257 (22): 3110–14 (June 12, 1987).

104 Mark Rothstein, *Medical Screening and the Employee Health Cost Crisis*, 107 (Washington, D.C.: Bureau of National Affairs, 1989).

5. Leisure, Sports, and Torts

6. Dangerous Products and Hazardous Substances

PAGE

129 Advisory Committee on the FDA, *Final Report* (1991).

132 U.S. Department of Health and Human Services, "A Primer on Medicines," *FDA Consumer* (Nov. 1979).

133 U.S. Department of Health and Human Services, *HHS News* (Sept. 12, 1990).

134 American Academy of Family Physicians, *White Paper on Generic Drugs* (1989).

139 Interview with FDA Commissioner David Kessler, *New York Times*, Nov. 6, 1991.

140 Claude Bouchard, "Is Weight Fluctuation a Risk Factor?" *New England Journal of Medicine* 324 (26): 1887–88 (1991).

140 Ron Wyden, "Juvenile Dieting, Unsafe Over-the-Counter Diet Products, and Recent Enforcement Efforts by the Federal Trade Commission," Subcommittee on Regulation, Business Opportunities, and Energy of the Committee on Small Business, House of Representatives, Sept. 24, 1990.

141 Nancy Wellman, testimony before the Subcommittee on Regulation, Business Opportunities, and Energy of the Committee on Small Business, House of Representatives, March 26, 1990.

151 Public Citizen Health Research Group, *Health Letter* (April 1990).

153 Greenman v. Yuba Products, 377 P.2d 897 (Calif. 1963).

153 Grimshaw v. Ford Motor Co., 174 Cal. Rptr. 348 (Ct. App. 1981). The Grimshaw case is discussed in Francis T. Cullen et al., *Corporate Crime under Attack: The Ford Pinto Case and Beyond* (Cincinnati: Anderson, 1987).

154 Wright v. Carter Products, 244 F.2d 53 (2d Cir. 1957).

154 Kaempfe v. Lehn and Fink Products, 249 N.Y.S. 2d 840 (App. Div. 1964).

7. Contraception and Abortion

171 Griswold v. Connecticut, 381 U.S. 479 (1965).

173 The New York State Court of Appeals affirmed a lower court's opinion denying a woman who was born disabled the right to sue the manufacturer of DES that her grandmother had taken. Enright v. Eli Lilly & Co., 77 N.Y.2d 377 (1991).

174 Susan L. Perry and James L. Dawson, *Nightmare: Women and the Dalkon Shield* (New York: Macmillan, 1985).

175 Richard Koenig and Stephen Wermiel, "Supreme Court Refuses to Hear Challenges in A. H. Robbins Case," *Wall Street Journal*, Nov. 7, 1989; Alan Cooper, "Game Plan of Trust Emerges," *National Law Journal*, Aug. 5, 1991.

175 See, for example, Marder v. G. D. Searle, 630 F. Supp. 1087 (D. Md. 1986), *aff'd as* Wheelahan v. G. D. Searle, 814 F.2d 655 (4th Cir. 1987), and Beyette v. Ortho Pharmaceutical Corp., 823 F.2d 990 (6th Cir. 1987).

PAGE

176 MacDonald v. Ortho Pharmaceutical Corp., 475 N.E.2d 65 (Mass. 1985), *cert. den.* 106 Sup. Ct. 250 (1985).

176 Kociemba v. G. D. Searle, 680 F. Supp. 1293 (D.C. Minn. 1988); *motion for judgment n.o.v. denied,* 707 F. Supp. 1517 (D.C. Minn. 1989).

177 Wells v. Ortho Pharmaceutical Corp., 615 F. Supp. 262 (N.D. Ga. 1985), *aff'd.* 788 F.2d 741 (11th Cir. 1986), *cert. den.* 479 U.S. 950 (1987).

179 Lovelace Medical Center v. Mendez, 805 P.2d 603 (N.M. 1991); Butler v. Rolling Hill Hospital, 582 A.2d 1384 (Pa. Super. 1990).

180 Tully v. Tully, 146 Cal. Rptr. 266 (Ct. App. 1978).

180 Stump v. Sparkman, 435 U.S. 349 (1978).

181 Roe v. Wade, 410 U.S. 113 (1973).

181 Harris v. McRae, 448 U.S. 297 (1980).

182 Webster v. Reproductive Health Services, 492 U.S. 490 (1989).

182 Rust v. Sullivan, 111 Sup. Ct. 1759 (1991).

183 Tamar Lewin, "In Debate on Abortion, 2 Girls Make It Real," *New York Times,* Oct. 27, 1991.

184 Carey v. Population Services International, 431 U.S. 678 (1977).

184 Doe v. Irwin, 615 F.2d 1162 (6th Cir. 1980), *cert. den.* 449 U.S. 829 (1980).

184 Patricia Donovan, *Our Daughters Decisions* (New York: Alan Guttmacher Institute, 1992).

184 See, for example, Bellotti v. Baird, 443 U.S. 622 (1979); Hodgson v. Minnesota, 110 Sup. Ct. 2926 (1990); Ohio v. Akron Center for Reproductive Health, 110 Sup. Ct. 2972 (1990).

8. Infertility and New Reproductive Technologies

194 Davis v. Davis, 1990 Tenn. App. LEXIS 642 (Sept. 13, 1990).

195 U.S. Congress, Office of Technology Assessment, *Infertility: Medical and Social Choices* (1988).

195 Ronald Sullivan, "Sperm Mix-Up Lawsuit Is Settled," *New York Times,* Aug. 1, 1991.

196 Karin T. v. Michael T., 484 N.Y.S.2d 780 (Fam. Ct. 1985).

198 Matter of Baby M, 537 A.2d 1227 (N.J. 1988).

200 Johnson v. Calvert, no. 61-31-90 (Orange County Super. Ct. Oct. 22, 1990), *aff'd* Anna J. v. Mark C., 286 Cal. Rptr. 369 (Ct. App. 1991).

201 Gina Kolata, "When Grandmother Is the Mother, until Birth," *New York Times,* Aug. 5, 1991.

9. AIDS and the Law

207 U.S. Department of Health and Human Services, Centers for Disease Control, *Understanding AIDS: A Message from the Surgeon General* (1988).

PAGE

209 Ronald Bayer, "Public Health Policy and the AIDS Epidemic," *New England Journal of Medicine* 324 (21): 1500–09 (May 23, 1991).

210 Tarasoff v. Regents of the University of California, 551 P.2d 334 (Calif. 1976).

210 "Hudson's Lover Wins $7 Million More," *New York Times*, Feb. 18, 1989.

212 Randy Shiltz, *And the Band Played On* (New York: St. Martin's, 1987).

215 McGann v. H. & H. Music Co., 946 F.2d 401 (5th Cir. 1991).

217 Thomas P. McCormick, *The AIDS Benefits Handbook* (New Haven: Yale University Press, 1990).

218 Chalk v. U.S. District Court, 840 F.2d 701 (9th Cir. 1988). See also Victoria Slind-Flor, "At the Limits," *National Law Journal* 12 (51): 1 (Aug. 27, 1990).

220 Warren R. Janowitz, "Safety of the Blood Supply," *Journal of Legal Medicine* 9 (4): 611–22 (1988).

222 Estate of William Behringer v. Medical Center at Princeton, 592 A.2d 1251 (N.J. Super. 1991).

224 National Association of State Boards of Education, *Someone at School Has AIDS* (1989).

224 Thomas v. Atascadero Unified School District, 662 F. Supp. 376 (C.D. Cal. 1987).

225 District 27 Community School Board v. Board of Education, 502 N.Y.S.2d 325 (Sup. Ct. 1986).

10. Parents and Children

234 Siemieniec v. Lutheran General Hospital, 512 N.E.2d 691 (Ill. 1987).

234 Turpin v. Sortini, 643 P.2d 954 (Calif. 1981).

236 Dawn Johnsen, "From Driving to Drugs: Governmental Regulation of Pregnant Women's Lives after *Webster*," *University of Pennsylvania Law Review* 138: 179–215 (Nov. 1989).

236 John Robertson, "Procreative Liberty and the Control of Conception, Pregnancy, and Childbirth," *Virginia Law Review* 69: 405–64 (Apr. 1983).

237 National Association for Perinatal Addiction Research and Education survey, reported in *Christian Science Monitor*, Feb. 15, 1989.

237 Ira Chasnoff, "Drug Exposure in Pregnancy: Incidence and Effects," *Adoptalk* (North American Council on Adoptable Children, Fall 1991).

237 People v. Stewart, no. M508197 (San Diego, Calif., Mun. Ct. Feb. 23, 1987).

238 People v. Hardy, 469 N.W.2d 50 (Mich. App. 1991).

238 Wendy Chavkin, "Drug Addiction and Pregnancy," *American Journal of Public Health* 80 (4): 483–87 (Apr. 1990).

PAGE

239   In re A.C., 573 A.2d 1235 (D.C. App. 1990).

239   American College of Obstetricians and Gynecologists, Committee Opinion from the Committee on Ethics, *Patient Choice: Maternal-Fetal Conflict* (1990).

241   International Union v. Johnson Controls, 111 Sup. Ct. 1196 (1991).

243   In re Infant Doe, No. GU 8204-004A (Ind. Cir. Ct., Apr. 12, 1982), *cert. den.* 464 U.S. 961 (1983).

243   Bowen v. American Hospital Association, 476 U.S. 610 (1986).

243   Arthur Southwick, *The Law of Hospital and Health Care Administration* (Ann Arbor: Health Administration Press, 1988).

244   Raymond S. Duff and A. G. M. Campbell, "Moral and Ethical Dilemmas in the Special-Care Nursery," *New England Journal of Medicine* 289 (17): 890–94 (Oct. 25, 1973).

246   See, for example, "Boston Jury Convicts 2 Christian Scientists in Death of Son," *New York Times*, July 5, 1990; and David Margolick, "In Child Deaths, a Test for Christian Science," *New York Times*, Aug. 6, 1990.

247   Prince v. Massachusetts, 321 U.S. 158 (1944).

247   In re Seiferth, 127 N.E.2d 820 (N.Y. 1955).

247   In re Sampson, 328 N.Y.S.2d 686 (Ct. App. 1972).

247   In re E.G., 549 N.E.2d 322 (Ill. 1989).

247   Jacobson v. Massachusetts, 197 U.S. 11 (1905).

248   Michael de Courcy Hinds, "Judge Orders Measles Shots in Philadelphia," *New York Times*, Mar. 6, 1991.

11. Medicare and Medicare Supplement Insurance

253   Joseph L. Matthews, *Social Security, Medicare and Pensions: The Sourcebook for Older Americans* (Berkeley, Calif.: Nolo, 1990); and Carl Oshiro et al., *Medicare/Medigap: The Essential Guide for Older Americans and Their Families* (Mt. Vernon, N.Y.: Consumers Union, 1990), attempt to make Medicare comprehensible to the public.

271   National Association of Insurance Commissioners, *Revisions to NAIC Medicare Supplement Insurance Minimum Standards Model Act and Regulation, 1991*; see also "The New Medigap Plans," *Consumer Reports* (Sept. 1991).

12. Long-term Care

280   National Consumers League, *A Consumer Guide to Life-Care Communities* (1990).

286   Peter Kemper and Christopher M. Murtaugh, "Lifetime Use of Nursing Home Care," *New England Journal of Medicine* 324 (9): 595–600 (Feb. 28, 1991).

PAGE

287 Bruce C. Vladeck, *Unloving Care: The Nursing Home Tragedy* (New York: Basic Books, 1980).

291 See Tamar Lewin, "Jury Finds Nursing Home Liable for Routine Neglect," *New York Times,* July 12, 1990.

294 Armond Budish, *Avoiding the Medicaid Trap* (New York: Holt, 1989).

296 Families USA Foundation, *The Unaffordability of Nursing Home Insurance* (1990).

296 United Seniors Health Cooperative, *Long-Term Care Insurance: How Well Is It Meeting Consumers' and Public Policy Concerns* (1988).

296 Families USA Foundation, *Long-Term Care Insurance: A Preliminary Investigation* (1990).

297 U.S. General Accounting Office, *Long-Term Care Insurance: Risks to Consumers Should Be Reduced* (GAO/HRD 92-14, 1991).

297 Subcommittee on Health and Long-Term Care of the Select Committee on Aging and the Subcommittee on Regulation, Business Opportunities, and Energy Subcommittee of the Committee on Small Business, House of Representatives, *Abuses in the Sale of Long-Term Care Insurance to the Elderly* (June 1991).

13. The Right to Die

317 Timothy E. Quill, "A Case of Individualized Decision Making," *New England Journal of Medicine* 324 (10): 691–94 (Mar. 7, 1991).

318 Tamar Lewin, "Doctor Cleared of Murdering Woman with Suicide Machine," *New York Times,* Dec. 14, 1990; and "Michigan Board Suspends License of Doctor Who Aided in Suicides," *New York Times,* Nov. 21, 1991.

318 Derek Humphry, *Final Exit* (Eugene, Oreg.: Hemlock Society, 1991).

319 Sidney H. Wanzer et al., "The Physician's Responsibility Toward Hopelessly Ill Patients," *New England Journal of Medicine* 320 (13): 844–49 (Mar. 30, 1989).

319 Matter of Quinlan, 355 A.2d 647 (N.J. 1976), *cert. den.* 429 U.S. 922 (1976).

319 Humphrey Taylor of Louis Harris and Associates, letter to *New England Journal of Medicine* 32 (6): 1891–92 (June 28, 1990).

320 Bouvia v. Superior Court (Glenchur), 225 Cal. Rptr. 297 (Ct. App. 1986).

321 Cruzan v. Director, Missouri Department of Health, 110 Sup. Ct. 2841 (1990).

323 In re O'Connor, 531 N.E.2d 607 (N.Y. 1988).

325 Brophy v. New England Sinai Hospital, 497 N.E.2d 626 (Mass. 1986).

PAGE

327 See Bonnie Steinbock, "Recovery from Persistent Vegetative State? The Case of Carrie Coons," *Hastings Center Report* (July/Aug. 1989).

328 Matter of Storar, 420 N.E.2d 64 (N.Y. 1981), *cert. den.* 454 U.S. 858 (1981).

329 Superintendent of Belchertown v. Saikowitz, 370 N.E.2d 417 (Mass. 1977).

329 Daniel Callahan, "On Feeding the Dying," *Hastings Center Report* (Oct. 1983).

330 American Medical Association, Current Opinions of the Council on Ethical and Judicial Affairs, *Withholding or Withdrawing Life-Prolonging Medical Treatment* (1986).

330 American Academy of Neurology, *Position of the American Academy of Neurology on Certain Aspects of the Care and Management of the Persistent Vegetative State Patient* (1988).

331 Elbaum v. Grace Plaza of Great Neck, 544 N.Y.S. 840 (App. Div. 1989).

331 See Gilbert M. Goldman et al., "What Actually Happened: An Informed Review of the Linares Incident," *Law, Medicine and Health Care* 17 (4): 298–307 (Winter 1989); and John D. Lantos et al., "The Linares Affair," *Law, Medicine and Health Care* 17 (4): 308–15 (Winter 1989).

332 Charlotte Sutton, "Gilbert Freed Today," *St. Petersburg Times*, Aug. 2, 1990.

333 Lisa Belkin, "As Family Protests, Hospital Seeks an End to Woman's Life Support," *New York Times*, Jan. 10, 1991; Steven H. Miles, "The Case of Helga Wanglie," *New England Journal of Medicine* 325 (7): 511–15 (Aug. 15, 1991).

14. When You Need a Lawyer

336 Troyen A. Brennan et al., "Incidents of Adverse Events and Negligence in Hospitalized Patients," *New England Journal of Medicine* 324 (6): 370–76 (Feb. 7, 1991).

350 Wangen v. Ford Motor Company, 294 N.W.2d 437 (Wis. 1980).

350 Palmer v. A. H. Robbins Co., 684 P.2d 187 (Colo. 1984).

351 A. Russell Localio et al., "Relation Between Malpractice Claims and Adverse Events due to Negligence," *New England Journal of Medicine* 325 (4): 245–51 (July 25, 1991).

INDEX